Praise for *Energy Psychology*

"Michael Mayer gives us the breadth and depth of energy psychology, how it can be part of all of our healing."

—James S. Gordon, MD, founder and director of The Center for Mind-Body Medicine, former chairman of the White House Commission on Complementary and Alternative Medicine Policy, and author of *Unstuck: Your Guide to the Seven-Stage Journey Out of Depression*

" ... a seminal book that creates a truly comprehensive energy psychology, dazzling in its breadth and depth, and having substantial research behind it to support the efficacy of its methods. Beyond the commonly used tapping methods that many associate with energy psychology, Dr. Mayer taps into a wider field of cross-cultural healing practices and creates an integral East-West psychology that can change each of us at the core. *Energy Psychology* is a thrilling blueprint for the integration of body, mind, and spirit. This book rewrites the origin myth of psychology and transforms the very ground of psychology by adding Eastern energy practices, storytelling, kabbalistic techniques, and imaginal processes to psychology's roots. It takes the radical perspective that all psychology is energy psychology; and when we expand our scope of vision this way we discover a fertile field for revitalizing our primordial Selves and reclaiming our self-healing abilities. Stemming from his thirty years of training in Tai Chi and Qigong, Dr. Mayer brings forth a unique amalgamation of practical, mind-body health practices that derive from his tireless dedication to the path that he walks."

—Larry Dossey, MD, author of *Reinventing Medicine: Beyond Mind-Body to a New Era of Healing*

"The past decade has seen a creative explosion in the integration of ancient healing practices with modern psychotherapy. Michael Mayer provides an ambitious and welcome map for psychotherapists and other healers wishing to embark upon the life-changing journey of adapting these traditions into their own practices."

—David Feinstein, PhD, author of *The Promise of Energy Psychology: Revolutionary Tools for Dramatic Personal Change*

"*Energy Psychology* is a valuable addition to the literature on psychological transformation and integral healing, bringing energy into the center of its scope. The procedures described in Michael Mayer's splendid book embrace both mind and body, both East and West, and both "physical" and "mental" problems. Most importantly, they coordinate external behavior change with internal healing processes. The result is a self-healing program whose goal is lasting change rather than superficial symptom removal. Contemporary practitioners and their patients often opt for the "quick fix," but this temporary palliative does not satisfy Dr. Mayer or those who will benefit from reading his book."

—Stanley Krippner, PhD, professor of psychology, Saybrook Graduate School, and author of *Haunted by Combat: Understanding PTSD in War Veterans Including Women, Reservists, and Those Coming Back from Iraq*

"Energy is the most self-renewing quality of any organism—if the organism is functioning properly.... The energy that joins body to mind is the continuous current that flows through all of Michael Mayer's healing efforts. He brings a practical capacity to utilize Eastern and Western disciplines into relationship with his powerfully intuitive trust of bodymind in a way that is a delight to learn from."

—John Beebe, MD, Jungian analyst, former president, Jung Institute of San Francisco, and author of *Integrity in Depth*

"The most comprehensive study of the therapy scene—and more—that exists. Dr Mayer has done a brilliant job integrating all aspects of all schools of thought as well as techniques of mind/body healing."

—Jane Goldberg, PhD, psychoanalyst and author of *The Dark Side of Love: The Positive Role of Negative Feelings*

"Michael Mayer's practical synthesis and deep knowledge of Qigong and Tai Chi movement forms has greatly impressed me during my years administering the Esalen Institute Movement Arts Program. Michael traces the roots of these practices back to their origins and presents a very usable as well as spiritual approach to these ancient and very valuable systems. He stands out among the many teachers I've met and practiced with and has provided me with insights available from no other teacher. With this book Michael Mayer breaks new ground in the realm of bodymind healing approaches, putting his unique synthesis of ancient healing practices and cutting edge psychology into a highly readable form. This deeply researched, unique, and practical manual will undoubtedly bring life-changing experiences to many readers."

—Rick Cannon, Esalen Institute Coordinator, Movement Arts Program

"In the nineteen seventies Dr. Michael Mayer began his study of Tai Chi Chuan and Qigong with me in Berkeley, California. With continuous diligence, devotion, and skill he grows and ages with me as faithful student and friend. It delights my eyes and warms my heart to witness the masterful way Dr. Mayer integrates the ancient wisdom of the East with the psychotherapy of the West."

—Fong Ha, internationally recognized grand master of Tai Chi Chuan and Yi Chuan Qigong

ENERGY PSYCHOLOGY

Self-Healing Practices for Bodymind Health

MICHAEL MAYER, PhD

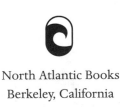

North Atlantic Books
Berkeley, California

Published by
North Atlantic Books
P.O. Box 12327
Berkeley, California 94712

Cover photo © iStockphoto / Damir Spanic
Cover design by Suzanne Albertson
Book design by Brad Greene

Printed in the United States of America

Energy Psychology: Self-Healing Practices for Bodymind Health is sponsored by the Society for the Study of Native Arts and Sciences, a nonprofit educational corporation whose goals are to develop an educational and cross-cultural perspective linking various scientific, social, and artistic fields; to nurture a holistic view of arts, sciences, humanities, and healing; and to publish and distribute literature on the relationship of mind, body, and nature.

North Atlantic Books' publications are available through most bookstores. For further information, visit our Web site at www.northatlanticbooks.com or call 800-733-3000.

Library of Congress Cataloging-in-Publication Data

Mayer, Michael, 1947–
Energy psychology: self-healing practices for bodymind health / Michael Mayer.
  p. cm.
Summary: "Merges Eastern practices with Western psychology to introduce self-healing tools"—Provided by publisher.
  ISBN 978-1-55643-724-3
  1. Energy psychology. I. Title.
  RC489.E53M39 2008
  616.89—dc22

2008025476

1 2 3 4 5 6 7 8 9 VERSA 14 13 12 11 10 09

This book is dedicated to healing the healer in each of us...
and to those who by necessity, calling, or love
have devoted their life energy to this path.

AUTHOR'S NOTE

The practices, ideas, and suggestions in this book are not intended as a substitute for medical attention. When considering applying these methods to various health-related issues, please consult with your medical doctor, psychotherapist, and/or other appropriate health professionals. Though benefit can be gained from reading about the integrated solutions to bodymind health issues in this book, caution should be exercised in undertaking the inward journeys suggested here. Such inner exploration is best done with a licensed mental-health professional. Please discuss these methods with your current health professionals to see whether, or how, they can be incorporated in your treatment. For more information on training in your area or finding a therapist trained or certified in these methods, please see www.bodymindhealing.com.

CONTENTS

SECTION I: Our Birthright: The Self-Healing Energy within Us . . . I

Chapter 5: Bodymind Healing Psychotherapy: The Psychotherapy of Shape-Shifting . . . 103

SECTION II: Case Illustrations for Common Mental and Physical Health Issues . . . 133

Chapter 6: Anxiety and Panic Disorders . . . 135

LIST OF ILLUSTRATIONS

ACKNOWLEDGMENTS

There is a creative source of energy in the universe that can be tapped if we can find the way to dowse for it. There have been many names for this wellspring. The Greeks called it the Fountain of the Muses and conceptualized it as created by Pegasus, the magical winged horse, after he was liberated from Medusa's head when it was severed by Perseus. As Pegasus leaped up into the sky, his hooves tapped a local mountain and out sprang the Fountain of the Muses. Rupert Sheldrake called this field of inspired creativity the *morphogenetic field;* Carl Jung called it the *collective unconscious.* Laszlo (2006)—drawing from Cheney's (1996) ideas about the Akashic records—called it the *A-field:* the all-pervasive information field that contains the imprint of the Self on the eternal, universal, electromagnetic atmosphere of primary substance (as cited in Krippner & Conti, 2006, p. 97). Many authors credit this field for the source of their inspiration. Francis Crick, the discoverer of DNA, said that he deduced the double-helix while using LSD, and Beethoven and Mozart and other musical geniuses gave credit to this mystical source of knowledge and creativity. Some call it God.

This is not a state relegated only to special people. Most of us have the experience of receiving messages from some unexplained source, some higher power "speaking" to us at some time during our day. Part of our work as human beings is to distinguish whether these messages are a call from this "higher Self" or a projection from a more limited aspect of ourselves. Rationalists would say this voice comes from our mind's synthesis of information and intuitive leaps. Those who have a spiritual stance toward life consider it to be more than that; perhaps, as Native Americans say, it is the voice of *Wakan-Tanka,* the Great Spirit or the Great Mystery. There are at least as many stances toward the ineffable as there are feet of human beings.

The fact that such creative surges often come when our conscious mind is least active (in the world of sleep) gave rise in psychology to theories of "the unconscious" and the understanding that rational thought is just one bandwidth of consciousness. Energetic bandwidths like REM sleep and delta wave sleep give access to other energetic bandwidths of consciousness that are equally important to our functioning and to our identities as human beings.

Regardless of what we call this creative source, for a period of one year, from the spring equinox of 2005 through the spring equinox of 2006, virtually every morning I woke up flooded with what felt like a compelling force leading me to what I was supposed to write that day. My job was to scribble down the notes first thing in the morning, as I woke from immersion in the hinter world of sleep, so I would not forget. And then, between my patient sessions and before workshop planning, I felt compelled to continue to write down what had come through me that morning. Though this period of creative flow built upon the edifice of my past writings, experiences, and thinking—which helped to gestate these perspectives—there was a felt sense of being a captive of something greater than what my rational mind could generate. So, first and foremost, I must acknowledge that this book stemmed from this creative source, though my twenty-seven years of private practice as a psychotherapist helped to open the door to the creative message of this book and gave it an appropriate container to hold its contents.

In the Preface, I acknowledge how my thirty years of training with Sifu (respected teacher) Fong Ha and other Qigong masters helped to form the container of my knowledge. I would like to thank again Master Fong Ha and the other masters whom he brought to train us, including Han Xingyuan, Cai Song-fang, and Sam Tam. As well, my Qigong knowledge and practice were enhanced by my work with Bryan O'Dea at the Acupressure Institute of Berkeley, California, and training in the animal forms of medical Qigong with Dr. Alex Feng. My training was also enhanced by a wide number of medical Qigong masters at various professional conferences. An avid addict of Qigong, I have also appreciated the knowledge gleaned in workshops from the teachings of Kumar Francis, Luke Chan, and Sat Chuen Hon. My friendship, sharing, and collegial relationship with Taoist scholar Ken Cohen was an important influence on my knowledge base in the arena of Qigong healing.

There were many influences of my early psychological training and on what would become Bodymind Healing Psychotherapy. At the forefront was Dr.

Eugene Gendlin, for whom I served as a Focusing training coordinator. John Beebe, MD, a Jungian analyst; Sam Keen, author extraordinaire; Bill McCreary, PhD, and Gordon Tappan, PhD, influenced me as they served on my doctoral committee. My early clinical supervisors, Larry Jaffe, PhD, and Ron Levinson, PhD, also deserve thanks. Many authors had a strong influence on my development, including James Hillman's archetypal psychology and Carl Jung's teachings about symbolic process. Various theorists of traditional psychotherapies—such as psychodynamic/neoanalytic, cognitive-behavioral, existential/humanistic, and transpersonal—and authors of the newly emerging energy psychology also had a major influence on my perspective. Additionally, authors in the area of behavioral medicine and medical hypnosis were important influences, and I would like to thank Ken Pelletier, PhD; Ernest Rossi, PhD; and Robert Sapolsky, PhD. Many of these authors are listed in the reference section in the back of this book. As a child who was taught to kiss a book if it fell on the ground (because of my family's belief that books are sacred), I am grateful to the authors whose books deserve to be kissed even when not on the ground.

Regarding the influences upon Bodymind Healing Psychotherapy from the wider age-old, cross-cultural traditions and esoteric sources that have helped to broaden my perspective to psychotherapy, I have appreciated the writings of Mircea Eliade and Joseph Campbell on cross-cultural mythology, Felicitas Goodman's teachings about postural initiation, Edward Edinger's approach to psychotherapy as alchemy, and C.A. Meier's insights about psychotherapy as an initiatory process. And my personal meetings with Dane Rudhyar and Manly Hall will always be with me.

It is customary to thank individuals in an Acknowledgment section, but other spheres of existence have been equally significant in helping authors write through the ages. Therefore, I would like to honor my temple, Chochmat Halev—meaning wisdom of the heart—for helping to restore my soul after long hours of writing. No less a temple is the special place in nature where I go to restore my soul. In this healing environment, which I call Bear Creek Mountain, I play my flute; practice Qigong; and watch the still egret, with one foot in the water and one foot on land, waiting for some morsel to emerge from the depths. I watch in awe the quick turns of the white terns, as their mastery of flying and diving into the depths could inspire the most blocked writer to shift into a new direction. And the deer, as it jumps over bramble bushes, could help even the most civilized among us to remember the power of primordial movements to overcome obstacles.

To acknowledge a major source of my instilled love for learning, I want to thank my parents, Abraham and Freda Mayer, who devoted a good portion of their lives to providing the fertile soil from which I could grow and receive the best education possible. My father would oftentimes jump up from the dinner table and go to the encyclopedia when a difficult question was asked; and as my mother served delicious food, my father came back serving morsels of wisdom, transmitting to me a love of research. Also, my mother's emotional intelligence was high-quality food for thought. Without my parents' loving efforts and sacrifices, the seeds from which this book was planted would have never met the ground.

I gratefully thank Dr. Len Saputo, with whom I cofounded the Health Medicine Institute, for his assistance in grounding my knowledge base in this medical setting. I also want to express my great appreciation to my other fellow multidisciplinary health professionals there, such as Colette Devore, acupuncturist; Steve Milligan, chiropractor; Bill Kneebone, chiropractor; Calista Hunter, MD; June Engle, MD; Linda Chrisman, bodyworker and trauma specialist; and Phillip Scott, Native American chief and ritualist. They helped me to see the power and potential of collaborative relationships in integrative medicine.

As well, to those other readers who gave me feedback on my book, I would like to thank Tarra Christoff; Mark Fromm, PhD; Gareth Hill, PhD; Jean Hayek; Sandy Rosenberg, PhD; Susan Schulman; Larry Stoler, PhD; and David Weinstein.

I want to thank North Atlantic Books, and its president Richard Grossinger, for having the belief in the marketability of this book and the desire to bring it to the public. I much appreciate Jessica Sevey, the editor and project manager of this book, for her adept juggling of various facets of the publication process and valuable editorial contributions. I'm grateful to Phyllis Baecker, a dedicated, conscientious copy editor, for her meticulous attention to details that helped to fine-tune this book. Thanks to Random House for distributing the seeds of this book to their wide distribution network.

Depth lies on the surface of things.
　　—Ludwig Wittgenstein

The Six-Year-Old Energy Psychologist in Each of Us

As a six-year-old child, I remember lying in bed trying to find the best posture to go to sleep. My favorite position was to sleep on my belly with my left leg outstretched and bent, with my left arm bent at the elbow with my fingers pointing up and my right arm pointing downward next to my straight right leg. I realized that the anxiety in my stomach from so much pressure from trying to excel at school was soothed by this posture of lying on my stomach, as my body pressed against my pillow, which lay on an angle from my right ear to my heart. As I slowly breathed and directed the breath alternately up and down the left and right sides of my body, there was some strange peaceful relaxed energy that was released from my left fingers pointing upward and my right fingers pointing downward that helped me release my tension and enter into the sought after world of dreams.

It was much later in my life that I learned that the experience of energy I felt as a six-year old is called *Qi* (also spelled *chi)* in Chinese, which is the focus for a practice of cultivating the energy of life for healing in the Chinese medical system of Qigong. I also found out that the awareness of energy moving up and down is called the *raising and lowering of the chi*. The use of intention to direct Qi is called *yi;* and in Qigong, it is said that "the yi leads the Qi."

I also noticed, as I was lying in my favorite sleep posture, that one hip felt more blocked than the other and that turning over and switching my position from my left leg out to my right leg being outstretched helped to bring balance to my body. Bringing balance to the body by switching postures from one side of the body to the other, I later discovered, is a fundamental part of the philosophy of medical Qigong and is called *balancing excess and deficiency.*

One of the oldest human activities according to the research of Dr. Felicitas Goodman, the anthropologist who coined the term *traditions of postural initiation,* was to assume various postures for hunting and survival purposes; and the shamans of a tribe would use postural stances as a method to enter into a trance state for the purpose of healing, divination, and metamorphosis (Gore, 1995, p. 14). However, we do not need to travel back to a premodern hunter-gatherer society, to go to a yoga class, or to practice sitting, standing, or moving meditation in order to experience traditions of postural initiation. Postures for expanding human consciousness are part of our everyday waking and sleeping lives. Every child discovers these postures naturally. What is your favorite sleep or waking posture and how is it a healing postural ritual that brings healing energy and balance into your life?

When I was sick in bed during my grammar school years, I remember not being able to sleep because I was so congested. I noticed that one nostril was more filled than the other. I instinctively rolled over to my side so that the congested side was higher; and in a few moments, the congested side flowed to the opposite nostril. As I turned from side to side, in those moments of clarity when there was no congestion, I was able to fall sleep. It was much later in my life that I realized this experience was an early entryway into one of the key healing pathways of the ancient art of Tai Chi Chuan,[1] which uses movements of filling and emptying to activate the healing powers of *yin* and *yang.*

Borne from my congestion was the inkling of another part of the path of Taoist healing that I would later discover. Finding the calm place after the out-breath whereby one enters into a zone of peace beyond the opposites of yin and yang that the early Taoists called *wuji* (the mother of yin and yang), the void from which creation and healing energy emerges. After many years of practicing Tai Chi, I was introduced to one of hidden purposes of Tai Chi practice: the movements of Tai Chi repeat the cosmogenic creation myth of moving from wuji to Tai Chi to become part of the creation in the world of opposites and from movement in the world of opposites (Tai Chi) to stillness (wuji). In our everyday lives we all repeat this cycle as we get caught in the world of opposites (of good and bad, right and wrong, stuck and unstuck) and need to find the relaxed center point of equilibrium to find peace. So, whether we are congested with a cold or with the psychological issues that encumber our free flow of Qi, we all are tested to look under the crosscurrents that pull us from side to side and find the sacred place of stillness deep within that is beyond the forces that disturb our equilibrium.

As an adolescent and not confident in myself, I saw that other more popular boys held their chests out more proudly than I did. I experimented with expanding my chest farther and felt a bit more confident. (It was a combination of experimenting with assuming this posture as if I was more confident and other inner work I did through the years that helped this stance to take hold gradually.) This was long before I discovered the ancient traditions of shape-shifting that would become one of my contributions to psychotherapy and Western bodymind healing methods. It is interesting to me how what we psychologists learn from our own lives often parallels the issues in our patients' lives. Along these lines in Chapter Fifteen, you will read of how one of my patients with severe impulse control problems, who pushed his chest out to exaggerate his machismo, benefited from energy psychology methods of postural initiation and finding a new "life stance."

When I was in high school, I had so much tension in my neck that I was at my wit's end to find a solution so that I could return to studying. I intuitively touched and pressed some points in my shoulders; and after a few (sometimes quite a few) breaths, the tension released. During my acupressure training many years later, I learned that the points I had touched as a teen were called *Gall Bladder 21* and that for thousands of years acupuncturists had discovered that these points were useful for releasing neck tension. I further found out, during my medical Qigong training, that the principle of touching points lower than a tense point high in the body to reduce tension is a key to Taoist healing, and is called *sinking the chi*.

So, not only the famous mythologist Mircea Eliade (1952) knew that the sacred is in the profane of everyday life, but each of us may experience in any moment a natural depth emerge onto the surface of our lives. It may be from a posture we assume while asleep or awake, a place we touch on our bodies, or from an illness we suffer.

Borne from all of our illnesses are the discoveries of healing pathways. These natural discoveries are part of every person's opening to the healing powers of his or her primordial Self. Whether we vary hot and cold water in the shower in the morning or let go of tension on our out-breath, these are the gifts of our human bodies and part of the treasure-house of energy that makes us human and lets us experience divine healing states. In spite of the importance of these healing pathways, we are not usually trained in cultivating these ways; we are taught about the fifty United States in geography classes but not the hundreds of useful state-specific, healing, energy states.

Imagine a tradition that spends as much time on educating these Self-healing energies as we do on reading, writing, arithmetic, television, and computers. The ancient Taoist tradition of Qigong is such a pathway, and how to cultivate the energy of life is the curriculum. As we combine that wisdom with our own natural introspection and our culture's psychological knowledge, we embark on the path of cultivating the vital energy of our primordial Selves.

My Professional Background: Tai Chi, Qigong, Psychotherapy, and Bodymind Healing

My early training in psychotherapy helped me to understand why there was such an imbalance between my mind and body, which manifested in my neck. I was ripe for the growing movement that sought an integrative approach to healing body, mind, and spirit. In the early 1970s, I went on a "quest to the West," where graduate programs existed that allowed people to study holistic ways of healing the psyche. At Saybrook Institute in San Francisco, I discovered a program that incorporated holistic psychology, which provided me the opportunity to study a wide variety of ancient healing traditions while obtaining my doctoral degree. In addition to traditional psychological methods, I was able to study symbolic process traditions of the so-called Western Mystery Traditions (Matthews & Matthews, 1986), including dreamwork, mythology, alchemy, and astrology. I wrote two books on these subjects entitled *The Mystery of Personal Identity* (1984) and *Trials of the Heart* (1993).

I knew that integrating the body was crucial for my own healing as well as to help in the healing of others. So I looked for a tradition of bodily healing to integrate with my mental/emotional healing path. I served as Dr. Eugene Gendlin's Focusing training coordinator of the San Francisco East Bay area for ten years. Focusing is a method of body-oriented psychotherapy that pays attention to the "felt sense" in the body in such a way that "felt meaning" of body blocks emerges and a "felt shift" of energy happens. This method helped to transform my way of being, as I hope it will do for you.

As I moved down the stream of my life, I cofounded the Transpersonal Psychology Department at John F. Kennedy University (JFKU) in Orinda, California—a place where East and West as well as body and mind were integrated into the training of therapists. I taught there for twelve years. Integrating different traditions became a trademark of my work as a therapist, and the method became Bodymind Healing Psychotherapy. At JFKU, I taught the first course to be offered at an accredited university on integrating astrology and psychotherapy. In 1979 *The Mystery of Personal Identity* (Mayer, 1984) won the World Astrology Prize from the Astrological Association of Great Britain for introducing a new phenomenological theoretical framework using astrology as a tool to explore one's life meaning rather than objectifying the correspondence between cosmos and personality.

A key concept of this three-semester, graduate psychology course was how to use astrology in counseling without ever mentioning the word *astrology*. Instead students learned in this class to use astrological metaphors to describe the energies of life—such as fire, earth, air, and water—and to reframe psychological issues, to transform pathological ways of viewing one's self and one's relationships, and to find new meaning in one's life by using this transpersonal tool. Following the theme of incorporating ancient sacred wisdom traditions to expand the healing tools of modern psychotherapy, I also taught symbolic process courses to psychotherapy interns at JFKU for five years. I wrote *Trials of the Heart: Healing the Wounds of Intimacy* (Mayer, 1993) to show how ancient myths can help couples deepen their perspective regarding the lessons that an intimate relationship provides. The Mythic Journey Process I developed was a tool for therapists to help their patients ground the expansive energies of archetypal myths by using their bodies' felt sense and Dr. Gendlin's Focusing method, while telling their life stories.

A major point in my healing came when I met Master Fong Ha, a lineage holder of one of the great rivers of bodymind healing knowledge based in ancient Chinese traditions and a greatly respected teacher of the art of Tai Chi Chuan (also spelled *T'ai Chi Ch'uan*). Master Ha represented a lineage that came through Dong Yingjie, a famous Yang stylist, and Yang Shouzhong, a lineage holder of the Yang family style of Tai Chi Chuan. In 1974 as I was looking around at many teachers of Tai Chi to help me "get into my body," I chose Master Ha not because of his credentials but because of the quality of his movements—embodying solidity and grace—and his personality, which was open and explorative. I felt a cross-discipline identification with him: I was seeking a psychotherapeutic style that was not rigidly attached to a single method as the answer to the quest for wholeness, and Sifu Ha was seeking the same in the area of the body. Through-out the three decades, I have studied with him, I have had an opportunity to grow with him as he has invited various masters from China to teach us. Three of these teachers who greatly influenced my development were standing med-itation masters: Han Xingyuan—a master of the *Yi Chuan* (the mind or inten-tionality behind the various systems of Chuan); Sam Tam—a master of Eagle Claw, Yi Chuan, and Tai Chi; and Cai Songfang—a master of Wuji Standing Meditation.

From my study in the circle of Master Ha, at his Integral Ch'uan Institute in Albany, California, I was able to find an age-old tradition of bodily energy heal-ing that helped to heal my imbalances. I went from there to the Acupressure Institute of Berkeley to further my study in oriental methods of healing and received a certificate in acupressure in 1990. For many years I kept the knowl-edge derived from my Tai Chi, Qigong, and acupressure training separate from my work as a therapist.

I was trained to believe that there were problems, detriments, and dangers involved in integrating Eastern modalities with Western psychology, and I inter-nalized and adhered to those beliefs. For example, psychology as a profession has a history of disapproving the integration of Eastern modalities and body prac-tices in part due to the belief that they are transcendental in nature. In this book, however, you will see how integrating *transcendent* and *transmuting* (meaning "rising above" and "working through" respectively) approaches is a key dialectic of an integrative paradigm of healing. Perhaps it was the memory of the importance of the healing, energetic and postural experiences of my childhood that gave me the courage to remember my purpose and find my way to a place of more expansive vision.

Combining the Eastern methods of Tai Chi, Qigong, and acupressure self-touch with other body-oriented traditions helped me to find the path that I was seeking to heal the bodymind split that was so much a part of my early life. Through the practices I learned over the years, I was able to find the way to heal the blocked energy in my neck and to find a bridge between traditions of the mind and body. Some of these traditions that influenced me, and later became fundamental parts of the approach to energy psychology that I was in the process of creating, included Western psychotherapy methods such as self-psychology, psychodynamic and object relations theory, cognitive-behavioral psychotherapy, symbolic process traditions, and Dr. Gendlin's Focusing method. Also, Tai Chi, Qigong, hypnosis, and acupressure self-touch became vital parts of the integrative approach called Bodymind Healing Psychotherapy.

I took the knowledge that I had been accumulating and taught the first program in the United States to master's level counseling students on the integration of Tai Chi, Qigong, and psychotherapy at John F. Kennedy University. This three-semester class ended with a counseling case seminar where students were able to apply their knowledge to cases in their internship program. Later the California Institute of Integral Studies invited me to teach the first two classes ever offered on the integration of Qigong and psychotherapy to doctoral students. Then I taught courses in Eastern perspectives on healing at San Francisco State University for three years, bringing this knowledge base to undergraduates— just as I would have liked to have happened for me in my early years.

While I was training therapists, I was also learning from my experience with my patients, to whom I am most grateful. My specialty became self-healing methods for physical and mental-health problems. My dharmic agenda was to reach a wider audience and to impact the way our culture looks at physical and mental health. My stream joined the larger stream of fellow travelers in mind-body medicine. At that point in our culture's evolution where corporate greed and multibillion-dollar pharmaceutical companies' agendas rule our approach to health, it is helpful to step out of the tide of commercialism and wonder what a more person-centered, holistic approach would be. What would be an approach that honors the wonders of modern medicine and gives due weight to the ancient reservoir of knowledge held by time-tested methods of age-old healing traditions? This type of approach, which is still evolving, is called *integrative medicine.*

My interest in this path led to my cofounding and practicing as a psychologist and Qigong teacher at the Health Medicine Institute (HMI) in Lafayette, California, where a multidisciplinary team of health practitioners practice integrative medicine.[2] Some of the illustrative cases that I put forth in this book come from my experience at HMI, others from my three decades as a psychotherapist.

I greatly appreciate that I have been able to share my methods at such venues as Alta Bates Summit Medical Center, Mt. Diablo Hospital Medical Center, Bryn Mawr College (Bryn Mawr, Pennsylvania), Institute of Imaginal Studies, Saybrook Institute, the National Institute for the Clinical Application of Behavioral Medicine, and Esalen Institute. I am grateful to be offering now two certification programs—one in Bodymind Healing Qigong and another for Bodymind Health Professionals.

Overview

Energy Psychology builds upon the two volume series of *The Tao of Bodymind Healing.* Volume I, *Secrets to Living Younger Longer: The Self-Healing Path of Qigong, Standing Meditation and Tai Chi* (Mayer, 2004b), is about Qigong and psychotherapy with the emphasis on Qigong; and Volume II, *Bodymind Healing Psychotherapy: Ancient Pathways to Modern Health* (Mayer, 2007), is about psychotherapy and Qigong with the emphasis on psychotherapy. *Bodymind Healing Psychotherapy* emphasized the incorporation of Qigong into both the psychotherapy and behavioral health arenas and showed how to bring Qigong into psychotherapy without a word about Qigong and without doing a Qigong movement.

Although Qigong originated in China, one of my favorite sayings is that Qigong is not just Chinese. All around the indigenous world, energy and intention as well as movement and metaphor have been used as sources of healing. Though the Chinese have perhaps done the best job of keeping intact the knowledge of specific methods of energy healing, in *Secrets to Living Younger Longer* (Mayer, 2004b), and now here, you will see how a broad array of traditions contribute to the root system of an integrative healing paradigm.

To help you heal your mind and body, I have created a comprehensive energy psychology, which is comprised of a variety of ancient pathways. These Western and Eastern traditions include (1) Chinese medicine approaches including Qigong and self-touch of acupressure points; (2) a full-spectrum approach to symbolic process methods that include psycho-mythological inner work using techniques such as the Mythic Journey Process and the River of Life Process, which integrates guided imagery with Microcosmic Orbit Breathing; (3) kabbalistic processes; and (4) methods drawn from ancient traditions of meditation and postural initiation. Bodymind Healing Psychotherapy's approach to energy psychology weaves these somatic and imaginal methods from ancient traditions together with modern psychological methods. Actually, as Carl Jung pointed out, symbols have the capacity to awaken healing energy, as all of us know when we hear an uplifting story.

The three books each touch on different facets of an integrated self-healing paradigm. Thus, those who are more interested in a focus on Qigong may want to read *Secrets to Living Younger Longer* (Mayer, 2004b), and they will also get information on the importance of the psychological dimension to make their Qigong practices more whole. Likewise, those who are more interested in psychotherapy may read just *Bodymind Healing Psychotherapy* (Mayer, 2007), and they will find some information on Qigong. Like a yin-yang symbol, each of these two books shows how a dot of each tradition is in the half circle of the other. In actuality, energy and psychotherapy cannot be separated into different volumes, nor into different facets of a whole crystal—each are integral parts of the whole gem of holistic healing.

In the chapters that follow, you will learn how I have integrated my experience as a psychologist and my Taoist practices into tools for self-healing in everyday

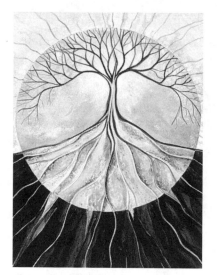

Figure 1. Finding Your Hidden Reservoir of Healing Energy

life. Though one of the major sources for energy psychology is from my psychotherapy methods, a comprehensive energy psychology requires breaking out of the confines of a psychotherapy office and finding the energy of life in our relationships with others and reflecting on our deepest issues.

For example, one cancer patient, with whom I used a guided visualization of a stream, told me that his chemotherapy and radiation left him so dry that he could not feel moisture. He said he felt so much like a dried-out tree next to a dried-out river that he could not even imagine a stream or a tree with moist leaves. I changed the metaphor; and by following his exhalation down into the roots of the dried-out tree, he was able to imagine and feel himself draw moisture and energy from an underground aquifer. A healing practice emerged for him that I later developed into an audiotape for other cancer patients and those suffering from various chronic diseases (Mayer, 2001a). You will later read how the guided visualization used by this cancer patient drew from The River of Life process, a key energy psychology method that I developed for my patients to practice outside of our sessions, and how this process combines a Taoist breathing technique with a guided visualization practice that can be of benefit in everyday life. We can use it to soothe us when we are having a hard time falling asleep, to calm us when we are anxious, to center us when we are verbally attacked by another, and to find a pathway to release mental and physical pain.

In the pages that follow, you will be initiated into the healing pathway that I have been on for over thirty years, which I have used with myself, in workshops, in training many hundreds of psychotherapy interns, and in my private practice as a therapist. It is a pathway that grew from a place where I sat as a child—a place where I listened to the sound of two rivers becoming one. Native Americans say that the places and experiences of our childhoods hold keys to our destinies. This was certainly true for me as I continued on my life path: exploring the Eastern part of the stream became various Taoist and Chinese medical practices for cultivating Qi and the Western stream became the study of Western bodymind healing traditions.

As each of us sits by the stream of our own life experience, as a child or as an adult, whether it is the postures we assume at a given moment, or in the breath we take, our awareness and the healing energy states we discover sanctifies the journey of our psyche down the stream of our lives. This is the journey of energy psychology.

You will see the path that evolved from that natural child's experiences to thirty years of my East/West exploration about how to balance the energies of the body and mind. You will learn how to tap on a primordial healing energy that is not limited to any culture—but is part of all our inner resources—whether you are a six-year-old child or a Chinese Qigong master. I consider it a great blessing to have you join me along this path to look beneath the surface of things and search deep within ourselves to activate our Self-healing resources. I hope that what you read helps you, as it has me, to serve in the healing of our Selves and others.

INTRODUCTION

It is probably true that, in general, the most fertile developments in the history of human thought are born at the intersection of two currents of ideas. These currents may originate in the midst of totally different cultural conditions, in diverse epochs and places. But from the time that they effectively meet and maintain a relationship sufficient for a real interaction to take place, one can hope for new and interesting developments to occur.

  —Werner Heisenberg

The Inner Revolution: Self-Healing Power to the People

The seeds of this book were planted in the turbulent era of the 1960s and 1970s, a time when chants of "Power to the People" rang out on the streets. During this revolutionary era of wanting to overthrow a government and worldview, which led to the Vietnam War, another revolution was taking place—a revolution of consciousness. This inner revolution was perhaps captured most succinctly by John Lennon who said, "You say you want a revolution . . . well, you better free your mind instead."

This revolution brought a wide variety of meditation methods from the East, such as yoga and sitting meditation, and indigenous traditions and LSD laboratories brought the use of plant medicines (psychedelics) and other methods to transform inner consciousness. A wave of this revolution swept me up and carried me from preparing to go to law school in Washington, D.C., to entering into a humanistic psychology program on the other side of the country in San Francisco. I was part of that subgroup of the revolution that followed John Lennon's belief that a most important part of changing the world is to begin with changing the inner landscape of our own minds.

During this era when Alan Watts wrote *Psychotherapy East and West* (1961), I learned about psychologist Eugene Gendlin in my doctoral psychology program. He was attempting to bring the knowledge of humanistic psychology to everyday folk so that we would have the tools to engage in the process of inward accessing and create deep meaningful change in our psychological patterns in an outwardly focused materialistic culture. His Focusing method came from his research with graduate students who listened to psychotherapy tapes and extracted the essence of what made therapy work in any system. These research assistants listened to Freudian, Jungian, and behavioral therapy sessions and asked clients: "What were the significant moments of change in your therapy, and what made them happen?" Then the work began to identify the essential processes that made these changes occur. From this, Dr. Gendlin derived his Focusing method.

Though Dr. Gendlin won the most distinguished psychologist of the year award from the American Psychological Association, his Focusing method is not very well known, similar to the way the temple of Psyche in ancient Greece remained a lesser-known, yet valuable, temple. This six step method, outlined later in this book, has been used by many people within and outside psychotherapy offices to empower people to have an essential tool to activate their inner process of change, and it has been used in a wide variety of healing contexts, such as the Simonton Cancer Center in Bridgeport, Texas. Focusing has become a center post of the integrative approach to energy psychology that I present in this book.

As one of his training coordinators, I oftentimes had conversations with Dr. Gendlin about bringing Taoist breathing practices into Focusing to help people clear an internal space to deal with their issues, and he was intrigued with the idea and supportive of my efforts. One of the most understated discoveries of Dr. Gendlin's work in the 1970s was a felt energetic shift that was at the center of the process of change once new meaning is discovered on a life issue.

Age-Old Roots of Current Energy Psychology

Though Dr. Gendlin's idea about the connection between energy and healing was revolutionary for the times, actually this idea was not new. The principle of healing with energy was a fundamental axiom of the Western and Eastern mystery traditions (see Chapter Three). But it would take many years before this concept of the importance of energy in healing would reemerge in psychotherapy with the advent of the field of energy psychology.

While the incorporation of energy into psychology was gestating through the following decades, I was practicing one of the oldest forms of energy self-healing methods. Tai Chi Chuan was a lifeline to relaxation and energy cultivation that occupied my hours when I was not seeing patients. Coming from a traditional family and trained in a psychology profession that looked askance at the incorporation of Eastern practices and energy healing into psychology, I kept my two worlds separate. Yet there was something about the revolutionary empowering ideas of bringing healing technologies to the public, regardless of boundaries between East and West or psychology and ancient traditions that helped me to take a conceptual leap and to become the first person to integrate Qigong and psychotherapy.

I called the psychoenergetic approach that I developed Bodymind Healing Psychotherapy (BMHP), and I self-published a professionally oriented book, which gratefully received endorsements from many leaders in mind-body medicine. This book is a transposition of the healing methods of that book into terms that will make those methods more available for everyday use to a broader range of people. Though using these methods with a trained therapist is certainly ideal, the purpose of this book is to make these methods accessible to the public for the healing that is so necessary as we deal with the uncertainties and stresses of life in today's "interesting times." As our *bodyminds* take on these issues, a pathway is opened for psychospiritual growth, soul making, and finding the source of healing as we embark on the journey using the methods outlined in this book.

Definition of Terms

Bodymind Healing

I use the term *bodymind* to capture the need for modern psychology to resolve the mind-body split of Cartesian dualism. This idea is receiving increased notice in the field; not just for academic and philosophic purposes, but because it relates a fundamental truth. Mind, body, and spirit may seem separate; but if we stop and reflect on them, all three levels exist as one inseparable whole in our everyday experience. For example, when we feel angry, our face often turns red, thoughts of aggression may fill our minds, and we may become out of harmony with our higher cognitive capacities—unable to differentiate between rage and constructive critique or between blame and constructive expression of anger. Similarly, we may lose connection with our higher intention and spiritual purpose—to approach the offending person with a higher intention, to clear things, and to have things be different in the future.

The first use of the term *bodymind* in Western thought, that I am aware of, came from Ken Dychtwald in his book *Bodymind*, written in 1977. Many people now use the term *mind-body* to describe this integration; but I prefer putting the body first in our overly mental culture, in which cognitive therapy is perhaps the best-known form of therapy and the most recognized treatment of choice for many psychological conditions. Joining the two words *body* and *mind* into one word *bodymind* expresses the core philosophic belief of Eastern thought: body, mind, and spirit are one inseparable whole. *Bodymind healing* is a term that emphasizes the need to activate all aspects of ourselves to achieve optimal mental, emotional, and spiritual health.

In the chapters that follow, you will read how integrating the body into psychotherapy has been shown by clinical research to be crucial to the process of healing and has advantages over psychotherapy's talk therapy. The body has formed a key building block of modern psychology in spite of the fact that many still associate psychology with the study of the mind. This book adds to the tradition of somatically oriented psychology by drawing from cross-cultural ancient sacred wisdom traditions and methods of postural initiation, including Qigong. You will learn how it took a few decades of brain research, cross-cultural anthropological investigations, and clinical experience from psychotherapists to improve John Lennon's statement and say more accurately, "If you want a real revolution, you need to free your *bodymind* instead."

Self-Healing

The term *Self-healing* has a depth of meaning behind it. The term *Self* with a capital *S* was initially coined by Carl Gustav Jung to mean a Self broader than the ego—a Self that incorporates the archetypes of the collective unconscious. Thus, the path of individuation, according to Dr. Jung, is to form an ego-Self axis, whereby the personal ego is connected with the transpersonal elements of the psyche. Later in Dr. Jung's work, he spoke of the importance of the *psychoid* (body-centered) elements of the psyche in the individuation process.

When the term *Self*, as in *Self-healing*, is used in this book, it is meant to convey not only the psychoid dimension of the Self but also the incorporation of the healing elements of the surrounding universe. The healing powers of the Self can indeed blossom when the archetypal possibilities of embodied life are brought to fruition. This follows the viewpoint that in order for the Self to be whole, the mind-body-universe split needs to be resolved, which can be accomplished through incorporating bodymind healing practices from the East, such as the ones outlined in this book.

What Creates Psychological Change?

All psychological theories have their hypotheses regarding what creates change, and so does Bodymind Healing Psychotherapy (BMHP). In general, psychodynamic therapists emphasize the insight gained from going back to our families of origin, cognitive-behavioral psychotherapists emphasize changes in beliefs and behavior, humanistic/existential psychotherapists emphasize choice, Jungians emphasize the role of symbolic process, and Dr. Eugene Gendlin emphasizes the energy shift that is experienced in the body and new meaning that emerges at key moments of change in psychotherapy. BMHP draws from all of these traditions and uses a mandala of psychotherapies. In addition to this integrative perspective, BMHP draws from certain traditions stemming from the ground of ancient sacred wisdom traditions. From these traditions there are three interrelated concepts woven together throughout this book: (1) transforming your life stance, (2) shape-shifting, and (3) repairing and cultivating your primordial Self.

Just as Dr. Gendlin attempted to extract the essence of what made therapy work to empower the process of change for people, I discovered these three interrelated concepts from my thirty years of practice of psychotherapy, Qigong, and ancient sacred wisdom traditions that seemed to capture the essence of what created energetic change for people.

Transforming Your Life Stance

Change needs to be embodied change, thus the use of the concept *transforming your life stance*. This is one of the quintessential elements of Bodymind Healing Psychotherapy (BMHP). Influenced by the traditions of Standing Meditation Qigong and postural initiation (Mayer, 2004b) as well as the recent advances showing the importance of the body in the role of psychological healing (van der Kolk, 1994, 2002), BMHP places the literal/physical and symbolic elements of transforming one's life stance at the hub of the wheel of its theory of change. Another way to speak of changing our life stance is to use the practices and metaphors of *shape-shifting*.

Shape-shifting

One of the earliest roots of psychotherapy involved traditions of shape-shifting that used transfiguring metaphors and practices to enhance the process of psychological transformation, loosen up fixated life patterns, and help to change a person's life stance. Virtually all age-old cultures have myths of the shape-shifting of human beings into forms that have an ability to heal and transform their souls. The two volumes of *The Tao of Bodymind Healing* (Mayer, 2004b, 2007) unfolded this perspective and took readers on a journey to the age-old traditions of our trans-temporal compatriots. There, I drew on the teachings of cross-cultural mythologies and shamanism, the first holistic healing center of the Western World (the temple of Aesclepius), the Kabbalah, as well as the traditions of postural initiation in Native America, Greece, India, and China. In

Bodymind Healing Psychotherapy (BMHP), I specifically applied this age-old knowledge of shape-shifting to help those in modern psychotherapy to increase vitality, add depth, promote healing, and discover the multifaceted form of our true selves.

In the following chapters, you will see how the somatic and imaginal methods outlined in those earlier books can be used by the general public for Self-healing in the deepest sense of the word.

Repairing and Cultivating Your Vital, Primordial Self

In colloquial usage we, as modern people, sense that when we talk about our selves we are usually speaking of the culturally embedded modern selves that we are, with our personal histories. We perhaps owe it to the Jungians to recognize that there exists a deeper self, a Self of the collective unconscious—and when one gets in touch with that Self, a deep layer of healing may emerge.

Literary critics adopted the term *primordial* from Jung's theory of the collective unconscious composed of archetypal symbols. *Encyclopedia Britannica Online* says that a primordial image is a character, or pattern of circumstances that recurs throughout literature and thought consistently enough to be considered universal. Such primordial images and archetypal symbols include the snake, whale, eagle, and vulture. An archetypal theme is the passage from innocence to experience; archetypal characters include the blood brother, rebel, and wise grandparent. Dr. Jung defined an *archetype* as an "energy potential." But long before Jung used the term *primordial,* in the Western mystery tradition, both Christian gnosticism (Matthews & Matthews, 1986) and the Jewish Kabbalah (Hoffman, 1981) described the importance of activating the energies of the "primordial human," called *Adam Kadmon*. In gnosticism, activating Adam Kadmon was an important part of "realizing the macrocosmic signatures within man the microcosm" (Matthews & Matthews, 1986, p. 146.) The Kabbalah states that "in the form of Adam Kadmon (the primordial human) the powers of the divine Sefirot also flow within each of us" (as cited in Hoffman, 1981, p. 55). The Sefirot are the Jewish archetypes of creation and symbolize the ten archetypal spheres of the tree of life, such as the paired opposites of strength and compassion.

However, you do not need to look at the cultivation of the primordial Self as something esoteric. In psychotherapists' everyday practices, the activation of the primordial Self is a common marker of psychological growth. For example, recently I worked with a woman who had a very demeaning husband. She had been trained in her Middle Eastern family always to defer to men. After three sessions of working on this issue and practicing how to appropriately express her feelings to her husband, she came into our fourth session with happy tears. She reported that she finally spoke up to her husband about how she wanted a change to take place in their relationship regarding his demeaning communication. She found the Self she was before acculturation—a Self who felt free to express her primordial need to be respected as a person, regardless of what her culture taught about the subservient role of women. Surprisingly to her, he received her comments well and agreed to work on this.

In the East the concept of the primordial Self can be seen in the Buddhist idea of "finding the face of yourself before you were born"; that is, before the conditioning of life covered over your essential nature. In Taoism cultivating the primordial energies of the universe was viewed as an essential part of developing the whole person. In China Taoist adepts spoke of a primordial Qi (*yuanqi*) that becomes separated into two essential souls and makes up the living person: the *hun,* or spirit soul of celestial origin, and the *po,* or material soul that belongs to earth. At times various animal forms of movements were suggested to develop the initiate's primordial chi, and it was said that for those following these movements "the hundred diseases will not arise."

The importance of incorporating animal movements in developing the primordial Self was captured well by Laurens van der Post after he spent time with the Kalahari Bushman. He said, "We cannot recreate the original wilderness man . . . But we can recover him because he exists in us. He is the foundation in spirit or psyche on which we build, and we are not complete until we have recovered him."

The implications for bringing imaginal and body-based ancient sacred wisdom traditions into psychotherapy and behavioral health care were outlined in the two volumes of my last series (Mayer, 2004b, 2007). Here, I take these breathtaking methods and bring them more into public view for self-empowering our everyday lives. I learned in my early training from studying the research of

Herbert Benson (1983), a Harvard doctor, that breathing was important in evoking the relaxation response; later I discovered from many psychoneuroimmunological researchers—including Rossi (1986), Achterberg (1985), as well as Ader and Felton (1991)—that not only does the relaxation response feel good, but also it has been scientifically shown to activate various aspects of the psychoneuroimmunological system, the parasympathetic nervous system, the brain, and electromagnetic elements of the body for healing. Little did I know that my path would lead to a thirty-year training curriculum in Qigong and Tai Chi—two significant, time-tested relaxation traditions from the East, as well as other age-old traditions of cultivating and recovering the primordial Self.[1] And as you will learn, the connection between specific types of breathing and specific energetic and healing states is a specialty of Tai Chi and Qigong.

When I use the term *vital, primordial Self*, a double meaning is intended. First, it is important to be with our primordial Selves at key moments in our lives. Secondly, the term *vital* is used to connote aliveness and a fullness of energy. This is an essential concept in psychology, not only for depressed patients but also for anyone who wishes to live a life filled with meaning and purpose.

We all hope that psychotherapy will help us access our vital reservoir of energy at those times when we are blocked because of an old psychological complex or a difficult life situation. Whether those blocks are from fear of rejection or inhibitions in being true to ourselves, summoning forth our coping skills requires us to draw from a place deeper than our entrenched, reactive patterns. How to do this is "the grail quest" of everyday life, the quest to bring liquid flow back to a depleted land. Therefore, it is interesting that psychology has yet to draw from these age-old traditions that specialize in the cultivation of vital energy and that have been a part of our ancestral, cross-cultural lineage as human beings for thousands of years.

Qigong: Ancient Cross-Cultural Path to Modern Health

One of the oldest energy-enhancing healing traditions is Qigong. Using posture, movement, breath, sound, touch, and awareness, Qigong has been practiced for many thousands of years as a way to cultivate the energy of life. Tai Chi is the best-known system of Qigong.

Qigong: Not Just Living Longer but Living a More Vital Life

People say that what we're all seeking is a meaning for life. I don't think that's what we're really seeking. I think that what we're seeking is an experience of being alive, so that our life experiences on the purely physical place will have resonances within our own innermost being and reality, so that we actually feel the rapture of being alive.

—Joseph Campbell

In *Secrets to Living Younger Longer* (2004b), I discussed the research showing how Qigong was associated with longer life. For example, I learned from a thirty-year study that a group of hypertensive patients in China who practiced Qigong lived longer compared to a control group who had fewer deaths from heart attacks and strokes (Kuang, Wang, Xu, & Qian, 1991). A wide number of well-researched studies have also shown that Qigong and Tai Chi enhance longevity by reducing many stress related disorders, lowering blood pressure, preventing deaths from falls amongst the elderly, enhancing immune system functioning, aiding in the treatment of arthritis, limbering joints, and so forth.

Herbert Benson, the Harvard Doctor who coined the term *relaxation response,* and those researchers who have built on his research showed that activating the parasympathetic nervous system's relaxation response is helpful in reducing the effects of free radicals, enhancing immunity, reducing stress, and promoting healing. In Chapter One you will read how the trance state that is created in Tai Chi and Qigong is a specific way of activating the relaxation response that has many advantages as compared to other methods of relaxation.

Many health products, vitamins, and exercise systems claim to extend the number of years of our lives. But the real key to the treasure of life is not just extending our lives but how we maintain our vitality in our everyday lives.

The initiate who is trained in the inner teachings of Qigong assumes the posture of a dragon as energy is whipped around the belt meridian, moves like a snake creeping low as a secret door to the sea of vitality is opened in the belly, or he or she raises two hands like a white crane spreading wings to uplift the spirit of the heart. But what is unique in the approach that follows is the addition of the power of Western bodymind healing methods to Qigong. What oftentimes robs us of energy are those everyday psychological issues that block the rivers of our chi, such as fear of speaking up due to fear of rejection, anxiety about not succeeding, and depression from our inner critics' voice putting us down. So the fountain of youth, my friends—as we all deeply know—is not to be found solely in a pill, the latest diet, or even in exercise; but in a holistic approach to life that helps us work through the issues that encumber our life energy and activate our soulful way of being in the world.

In the approach that follows, you will become armed with Self-healing methods from a combination of Qigong and Western psychology to cultivate Self-healing tools to deal with common ailments, transmute long-standing psychological patterns, and add soul to your way of working through these issues, using a Mythic Journey Process to defeat the inner demons that block your inner rivers of Qi from flowing naturally. From the energy psychology methods that follow you will be able to not just live longer, but to live a more vital life..

In *Secrets to Living Younger Longer*, Qigong was shown to be not just a Chinese tradition of healing (Mayer, 2004b). Using and respecting the healing power of the energy of life is a fundamental part of virtually every indigenous culture on earth. In addition I discussed the anthropological evidence for the existence of these traditions of "postural initiation" in China, India, Greece, Israel, and Native America. I also showed how in virtually all religions of the world, the concept of "the energy of life" forms a fundamental aspect of our relationship to God —whether it is in the Taoist idea of *Qi*, the Hindu idea of *prana,* or the Kabbalistic idea of *chiyyut*. I discussed the research showing how the Buddha was trained in traditions of energy cultivation, and I showed how pictures of the Dancing Shiva reveal this tradition of moving with divine energy.

In *Bodymind Healing Psychotherapy,* I proposed that it was time to incorporate more fully the healing knowledge of these traditions into modern psychotherapy (Mayer, 2007). In this book on energy psychology, I will show how there are two healing streams running through the land of Self-healing traditions through the ages. One is a transcendent tradition exemplified by certain Eastern approaches, which teach us how to enter into an altered state that helps us to merge into a larger sea of consciousness and energy where our individual life problems dissolve. This state is called *wuji* in Taoism, *satori* in Zen Buddhism, and *ain soph* in the Kabballah. There is another tradition that involves transmuting psychological issues. This tradition was perhaps best exemplified by the alchemical tradition and used metaphors of transforming lead into gold to speak of how to transform our psychological substances.

In the approach to energy psychology that follows, you will see how this false dichotomy is dissolved through the "transcending/transmuting dialectic" and how incorporating the benefits of both traditions gives you a double-edged sword to help you conquer your demons and heal your whole, vital, primordial Self in the way you approach everyday life.

Integrating Qigong and Psychology

The integration of Qigong and psychology did not come easily for me. Like many other Western-trained psychologists, I had been trained to keep the realms of psychotherapy and spiritual traditions separate. By keeping the two worlds completely separate, it was as if I were a "split personality"—a psychologist by day and an avid Tai Chi and Qigong practitioner in my off-work hours. But perhaps it was the memory of that strange energy from my childhood that came out of my fingers, and relaxed my tension as I assumed various postures, that helped me to have the courage to believe that there was some worthwhile healing power in walking on this path.

A Turning-Point Patient: Carpal Tunnel Syndrome

All therapists have their turning-point patients. For me, one of these patients—named Boris here—was a medical student working on a research project that required a lot of writing. In our depth psychotherapy sessions, he was often distracted by his diagnosed condition of carpal tunnel syndrome. At that time in my evolution, I was very careful about dual relationships, having been trained in the potential dangers of mixing other disciplines with psychotherapy. So I thought, why not just refer Boris out? What happens if using these health methods stops him from getting appropriate medical treatment? What happens if the complementary treatment does not work and it produces a transference issue that interferes with the therapeutic relationship?

While Boris was working mainly on issues with his father—who was a medical doctor—and the childhood physical abuse that occurred in their relationship—Boris came into our session week after week with his arm in a sling and a splint due to his diagnosed condition of carpal tunnel syndrome. The physical therapist he was working with said to keep his arm still, and she worked with him each week to strengthen his wrist through various exercises. One day my compassion overruled my considerations about being unduly cautious. I mentioned to Boris that I had something to tell him about my life that normally I would keep to myself, but it could be relevant to him healing his wrist. He expressed appreciation for my caring; and we agreed we would continue our long- standing practice of clearing any negative feelings, if they arose for him through this process. I then told him that I practiced Qigong and that some research (Garlinkle et al., 1998) showed that it was better to use relaxing, energizing movement to promote healing rather than to use splints and not move. I suggested that we might try this Qigong method, which combined stillness and movement, to explore together like scientists researching to see if these methods helped him. He agreed.

First I asked Boris to do the breathing method that, from our work together, had become one of his favorite ways of relaxing, called Microcosmic Orbit Breathing. Boris and I had never before discussed its roots in Qigong and Taoism. On this day we repeated this breathing method to activate a trancelike state. Then I asked him as he inhaled to imagine that he was in water up to his shoulders and that his hands were floating up, wrists leading the way. From this position on a long, unforced exhalation, I directed him to press the heels of the hands down slightly all the way to the level of the belly.[2] He repeated this quite a few times; and by the end of the session, his pain reduced from a self-reported 8 on the subjective units of distress scale (SUDS are measured on a 10-point scale, 10 being the most stress) to a level of 2 SUDS. Instead of practicing the movement while standing, Boris practiced it from a sitting position.

I was glad I had suggested to Boris to clear with me any negative feelings, because during the next session he said he was angry that the Qigong had worked in the session and had lasted a few days but then the pain had come back. Then he added, "My father was right about this Eastern stuff not working."

This was a good lesson for me: it told me that I needed to explain new methods more carefully. I told Boris that the underlying philosophy of Eastern methods of healing was not based on a "one-time fix" model; that even with Western drugs, one has to continue a medication regimen; and that there are usually side effects with Western medications. We discussed how his body was signaling him that he needed to get up and take more breaks. We discussed how Qigong was "a practice" that needed to be engaged in regularly, not a one-time curative event. So, Boris went home that week and did the Raising and Lowering the Qi movement. He came into our next session without his brace for the first time in months and never needed it again. He said that the pain would come back when he was working too long but that he was learning to use his pain as a signal to relax and practice his Tai Chi. Boris indicated he was grateful that I had stretched the therapeutic boundaries to introduce him to what he now described as "this cool new behavioral health method."

In addition to the healing that occurred, our process deepened our relationship and helped Boris begin to individuate from his father. Boris saw the limitations of his father's myopic view that Western medicine was the answer to all health concerns. The process helped to validate further Boris's choice to take some of the new courses offered in his medical school on alternative therapies, and it gave him strength in the future to stand up to his father when their opinions differed.

You will read about more of my turning-point patients later, and you will learn how to walk the pathways they discovered. For example, in Chapter Six you will read about a graphic artist with a panic disorder. From her inner work, you will learn some methods for relaxing and transforming your anxious states when you suffer from the overwhelming stresses of everyday life. In Chapters Six to Fourteen, you will read about how I began integrating my work with Qigong and other ancient sacred wisdom traditions with a wide array of patients with a variety of issues. The case examples in this book are being used for illustrative purposes. Sometimes these cases are composites, names are always altered, and details are changed to dis-identify patients, protect their identities, and to illustrate how ancient sacred wisdom traditions, in general, and Qigong, in particular, can aid patients' healing in psychotherapy. Thanks to the inner pathways they forged, you will see how the methods used in my psychotherapy office can be expanded into your everyday lives.

Energy Psychology Distinguished from Energy Psychotherapy

The sphere of energy psychology is wider than energy psychotherapy. In my approach to energy psychology, I have included such ancient traditions of postural initiation as Tai Chi Chuan and Qigong and practicing these traditions in a spiritual and "soulful" way (defined in Chapter Five).[3] Also energy psychology includes various symbolic process traditions—like dreamwork, guided imagery, various forms of storytelling, and the Mythic Journey Process—because these traditions are some of the deepest ways to infuse the path that we walk in life with energy. Various forms of energy psychotherapy are included in the sphere of energy Energy psychology, such as Thought Field Therapy and the Emotional Freedom Technique (Gallo, 2002).

Energy psychotherapy uses energy psychology methods, such as tapping and other meridian-based therapies. The particular form of energy psychotherapy I developed, *Bodymind Healing Psychotherapy*, as discussed in Chapters Five and Six, integrates various forms of traditional psychotherapy with certain ancient sacred wisdom traditions that have energy psychology methods at their core.

SECTION I

Our Birthright:
The Self-Healing Energy within Us

The energy of the human body is the foundation of our health. When our energy is at its peak, our immune system is at full strength. When our energy declines we become vulnerable.

All healing depends on energy. This energy can come to us in many ways, but ultimately it is our own reserves of energy that provide the inner strength, which keeps us healthy and enables us to overcome illness.

Energy is the foundation of life. Without energy we die. All the cells in our bodies depend on energy for their existence. It is energy, which keeps them constantly at work, reproducing and renewed.

If we learn how to increase our energy to higher levels, we can use it to support others and ourselves when we are hurt or unwell.

—Yi Chuan Master Lam Kam Chuen
The Way of Healing: Chi Kung

CHAPTER ONE

The Self-Healing Power
of the Bodymind

*At the beginning of time, the gods had just finished their divine work
of creating the first humans. One of the gods spoke up and said,
"Where should we hide the secret of their Self-healing?"*

The earth goddess said, "Let's hide it the center of the biggest mountain."
*"That's no good," replied another. "One day they'll have bulldozers
and find it too easily."*

*"What about hiding it in the depths of the deepest sea?" replied the
god of the sea.*
*The wise reply came, "They'll have submarines someday and will find
it without any inner work."*

*A third god suggested, "What about hiding it in the Great Pyramid in
a safe up a narrow shaft?"*
"Not really any better," replied another.
*"Some day they'll have mechanized little vehicles that can just go up
the shaft and open the safe."*

Then Thoth, the trickster god, spoke up with a wry smile,
*"Why don't we just hide the secret of Self-healing inside of their very
Selves?*
They'll never think of looking there."

And so it was decided.

—Michael Mayer
Retold and Adapted from the *Shamanic Oral Archives*

The Self-Healing Powers Hidden within Us

If computers can have self-repairing programs installed at the beginning of their making, are human beings' biocomputers any less evolved? Did not "our maker" install such self-healing abilities? Certainly, it is true that when we have a debilitating medical issue there is often merit to seeing a specialist. But it has been estimated that fifty percent of all primary care consultations and physical disorders are attributable to *somatization*—the phenomenon when a patient presents with a physical symptom that cannot be entirely explained by a physical disorder (Brown, Robertson, Kosa, & Alpert, 1971; Roberts, 1994).

But we do not need to read professional journals to find the evidence for how we somatize life's issues. Everyday stressors give us a chance to study the effects of stress in our own bodies, as we become students in an internal somatic education program, or face the consequences of truancy in the school of life. A female office worker develops an undiagnosable rash from the daily pressure of dealing with a demanding boss. An adolescent complains of stomachaches from too much homework and a grueling schedule of after-school activities to keep up with the other kids and prove he is college worthy. A housewife complains of headaches that strangely seem to occur when her husband is uncooperative in doing household chores.

In our everyday life experience, each ache or symptom in our body is a call to learn to read our body's language. Is our body saying that we have a serious problem that is there to teach us to let go of our self-healing arrogance and rely on the advice of a medical professional who can help us deal with an early warning sign of cancer or liver disease? Or are we giving away our power to the medical propaganda machine that benefits from convincing us that every symptom is a call to go the temple of Western medicine for relief? At those times when our own inner temple has the resources to heal us, it is empowering to activate those inner healing abilities and avoid the side effects of modern drugs. If these methods fail, then we may choose to move up the hierarchy of responses.

Among the most significant Self-healing "mechanisms" in the human organism is the energy that runs us. This should not be news to any of us, because we all know that the energy of the human body is the foundation of human health.

When our energy is high, our immune system is strong; and when our energy is low, we become vulnerable to disease. It has been known through the ages that healing depends on energy; that energy is the foundation of life; and that without energy, we die. In our everyday lives, we seek to increase our energy by the way we eat, the way we exercise, and the lifestyles we choose. In fact, much of our everyday lives involve a process of making choices about activating or relaxing our energy.

Low energy is the not-so-hidden epidemic of our times. It seems that Starbucks and other coffeehouses are appearing in our neighborhoods faster than restaurants. As a culture, we are starved for energy and gravitate toward almost anything that promises to give it to us. According to a Gallup Poll, forty percent of all Americans report a significant daytime tiredness. Low energy is the most frequent complaint pharmacists and physicians hear from their patients. Many surveys also indicate that fatigue and lack of energy is the most common complaint and symptom reported to physicians. For example, thirty-seven percent of 500 patients in a Boston health-center survey reported feeling tired. Shopping carts in corner store pharmacies are filling up with popular energy boosters. In a single year, Whole Foods reports that natural energy supplement sales have risen by fifteen percent. Our energy level is an indicator of our overall health. Those who are energetic are generally healthy, whereas those who are tired all the time are usually ill or about to be ill. A Yale University assessment of more than 300 nurses found that energy levels had the highest correlation with general health status. Energy was also found to be the best predictor of both physical and psychological health over time (Grauds & Childers, 2005).

The Real Scoop on Energy-Enhancing Substances

There is no shortage of externally based cures for low energy promoted in advertisements coming from our mass media. In a culture where sales of pharmaceuticals[1] and products are promoted far more often than are our self-healing abilities, we hear of energy drinks that have four times the amount of caffeine as compared to normal sugary sweet drinks (http://www.mercola.com/blog/2006/mar/30/the_caffeine_overdose_in_energy_drinks), and synthesized vitamin formulas that promise quick results. Even comedian Jerry Seinfeld wondered during one of his sketches whether the guys in advertisements on TV who are drinking those energy-boosting diet sodas, which purportedly create a life filled with enthusiastic smiles and jumping around on volleyball courts with those beautiful girls, are drinking the same soda that he is.

So it seems that Thoth in the mythical story at the beginning of this chapter is right: human beings seldom look inside for the Self-healing mechanisms that will restore their energy. Certainly, this is not an either-or proposition. As a strong advocate of integrative medicine, and having worked in an integrated medical clinic, I encourage my patients to draw from the realm of all aspects of the mandala of healing. For example, certainly nutritionally sound food, healing herbs, and nutritional supplements are part of this healing equation. However, when we are depressed about our lives, use self-denigrating messages toward ourselves, have debilitating anxiety about unachieved life goals, or have blocked communication with a loved one, is a pharmaceutical medication or a nutritious meal really going to create a felt shift in our energy in any substantial, long-term way? After a good differential diagnosis, we need to determine what it is at the root of sapping our energy at a given moment and apply the appropriate remedy.

In our materialistic culture, we are not inclined to focus on how the "secret Self-healing medicaments of the gods" are hidden within us. Yet, such songwriters as Donovan in the 1960s proclaimed the value of the ancient wisdom lineage of looking within when he said, "there is an ocean of vast proportion, and she flows within ourselves. . . . To take dips daily, we dive in gaily, he knows who goes within himself." Though traditional culture may call this inward-looking orientation self-indulgent "navel gazing," in fact, the orientation to "navel gazing" has actually led, throughout the ages, to profound healing states that go beyond contemporary ideological put-downs. Coincidentally, the navel center was one of the places that Taoist practitioners identified thousands of years ago as a vital center for energy cultivation and called it the *Tan Tien*. They said the Tan Tien is where an experiential ocean of energy, the Sea of Elixir, is located. According to Wilhelm's research in *The Secret of the Golden Flower* (1931; 1963), ancient Taoist texts indicate that their methods of taking dips in the Sea of Elixir brings health, longevity, and energy. Believing in its healing power, the modern psychologist Carl Jung wrote an introduction to Wilhelm's book, in which Jung described a type of breathing—called *microcosmic orbit breath*—that helps to activate the Tan Tien. You will learn how to do this type of breathing in Chapter Four.

Studying the vital healing force of the sea of life's energy in many of its manifestations is the subject of the newly emerging scientific study of energy, which now permeates many fields of modern research. How to sail in this sea to maximize our vitality and health is the voyage of energy psychology and energy medicine.

Energy Medicine

There is a profound evolutionary shift that is taking place in the world that can be seen in the growing recognition of the fundamental role that energy plays in healing (Benor, 1992). The grandfather of this revolution of energy healing in the West is Dr. Robert Becker. In the early 1980s, he was one of the first scientists to measure the "current of injury" associated with healing wounds and bone fractures. In his early research on the healing and regeneration of salamanders, Becker (1985) showed that the control system that started, regulated, and stopped healing was electrical (pp. 235–236).

Becker's work built upon the work of other scientists, such as Harold Burr, a Yale School of Medicine neuroanatomist who measured the electrical field around an unfertilized salamander and put forth research that physical illness is preceded by changes in an organism's electromagnetic field (Burr & Northrup, 1935). Scientist Owen Frazee reported in 1909 that passing electrical currents through water containing young salamanders speeded up the regeneration of amputated limbs (as cited in Becker, 1985, p. 82). Since that time, there have been numerous well-researched studies showing the efficacy of various forms of energy in healing.[2] Some have described this paradigm shift as a revolution, signaling a move from a Newtonian to an Einsteinian medicine model. From Einstein's insights about how energy is a key to opening the mysteries of the universe, and the physical sciences developing that idea further, we are now on the edge of harnessing those mysteries in the arena of medicine and healing. As paraphrased from Gerber (1996, p. 43):

> Newtonian thinkers see the human body as a series of intricate chemical systems powering a structure of nerve, muscle, flesh, and bones. The physical body is viewed as a supreme mechanism, intricate physical clockwork down to the very cellular structure. Einsteinian Medicine sees human beings as networks of complex energy fields that interface with physical/cellular systems. There is a hierarchy of subtle energetic systems that coordinate electrophysiological, hormonal, and cellular structure of the physical body. It is from these subtle levels that health and illness originate. These unique energy systems are powerfully affected by emotions, spiritual balance, nutrition, and environment. They influence cellular patterns of growth.[3]

This energy-related revolution is affecting a wide variety of disciplines, including physics, biology (Pert, 1997; Lipton, 2005), and medicine, and should no longer be considered fringe science—it is now thought to be mainstream. Western knowledge of energy in the human organism has come a long way from believing that nerves are the only part of the body that contain electricity. We now know that the body emits a broad spectrum of electromagnetic and acoustic radiation that has been measured by magnetic resonance imaging (MRI), electroencephalogram (EEG), electrocardiogram (EKG), electromylogram (EMG), thermography, and ultrasound. These instruments are used to monitor and diagnose diseases.

Behind the everyday use of instruments to measure energies lies a once-in-an-era change in the very foundation of science. It was Dr. Lipton (2005), cell biologist and author of *The Biology of Belief*, who wrote that the pyramid of science is changing. With this shift at the bottom of the pyramid showing physics changing from a Newtonian mechanistic view to one of quantum mechanics, energy and energy fields have come to the forefront of importance. Lipton says that once the bottom of the pyramid of science in physics shifts, all of the levels—chemistry, biology, and psychology—need to shift as well.

Although Western medicine uses instruments, such as the EEG, to read energy fields, it has not taken the next step in understanding the role energy plays in other ways, according to Dr. Lipton. He shows how animals, from single cells to humans, convert environmental stimuli into physiological and behavioral responses. Dr. Lipton says that scientific research has revealed that "every facet of biological regulation is profoundly impacted by the 'invisible forces' of the electromagnetic spectrum ... electromagnetic radiation regulates DNA, RNA and protein synthesis, alters protein shape and function, and controls gene regulation, cell division, cell differentiation, morphogenesis [the process by which cells assemble into organs and tissues], hormone secretion, nerve growth and function. ..." Dr. Lipton laments that "though these research studies have been published in some of the most respected mainstream biomedical journals, their revolutionary findings have not been incorporated into our medical school curriculum" (Lipton 2005, as cited by Feinstein & Eden, 2006b). Most important for this book, Dr. Lipton speaks about the implications of this for the field of psychology and shows how the newly identified cellular mechanisms include master switches through which our thoughts, attitudes, and beliefs create the conditions of our body and of our place in the world.

Energy medicine is increasingly becoming a part of the new theoretical underpinnings of "a medicine for the twenty-first century." Candace Pert, PhD, author of *Molecules of Emotion: The Science behind Mind-Body Medicine* (1997) and research professor at Georgetown University School of Medicine, calls this revolution "New Paradigm Medicine." She says, "While not well understood, subtle energies can be operationally defined as energies that cannot be measured using existing instrumentation but which, like gravity, are known for their effects. Energy is also hypothesized as being somehow involved in the elusive link between chemistry and consciousness" (Pert as cited in Feinstein, 2004a). Other frontier scientists report that they are able to measure "the biofield" with sensitive magnetometers, such as the SQUID (Rubik, 2002). The biofield is comprised of an extremely weak but measurable electromagnetic field with its own waveform, intensity, polarity, and modulation patterns that surrounds all living systems. And for those of us who believe that only big things can create big changes, it should be noted that Becker found that tiny currents, on the order of a billionth of an ampere, were more effective than larger currents in stimulating tissue regeneration (Becker, Spadao, & Marino, 1977).

Modern science has demonstrated that electromagnetic fields of the body are generated during various biological processes, including rapid cell division; during natural growth processes, such as growth of bone cells; as well as following fracture, intense nervous activity associated with mental processes, and various pathological conditions, such as abnormal cell growth with diseases like cancer. The distinction between conservative medical practitioners and the new proponents of energy medicine is summed up well by one of the early researchers in the field, Dr. Glen Rein (1992), who wrote:

> It is now well known that the human body emits a broad spectrum of electromagnetic and acoustic radiation. Traditional medicine looks at these as by-products of biochemical reactions in the body. They are not considered by most biomedical researchers to be involved with the basic functioning (or healing) of the body. The basic tenet of energy medicine is that these fields are not only involved with functioning of physical/chemical body but regulate these processes. (p. 7)

Dr. Rein is not alone in his views. A variety of scientists are now documenting how organizing fields of energy may be responsible for directing genes and biochemical processes like a conductor directs an unimaginably big orchestra (McTaggart, 2003, p. 45); and these organizing fields direct biochemical processes as decisively as a magnetic fields aligns metal filings (Liboff, 2004). This paradigm shift has major implications for an expanded approach to medicine. Does this field hold the key to the Grail Castle that that will restore our depleted inner land?

Energy medicine is used in the treatment of disease. It is now commonplace to hear of athletes using transcutaneous electrical nerve stimulation units (TENS) to deal with the effects of pain. Nurses in many hospitals use energy-healing methods (approved by the North American Nursing Diagnosis Association), such as therapeutic touch and its cousin—healing touch—to treat their patients. Research is also accumulating to show the efficacy of touch in reducing anxiety among institutionalized patients (Gagne & Toye, 1994), in alleviating depression in breast cancer patients (Nurse Healers-Professional Associates, 2000; Moreland, 1998), in enhancing immune system response (Quinn & Stelkaudal, 1993), and in accelerating wound healing (Wirth, 1991).

At leading-edge hospitals, energy medicine is being explored in a variety of ways. For example, at New York's Columbia Presbyterian Hospital, cardiac surgeon Dr. Memmot Oz has had Julie Motz, an energy healer, use energy-emission methods with her hands prior to, during, and following surgery for heart replacement surgery. It has been reported that there are less cardiac rejections when such energy-medicine procedures take place.[4]

Interestingly, Harold Saxton Burr, the neuroanatomist at Yale University, back in the 1930s showed that disease shows up in the patient's energy system before manifesting as symptoms, and he believed that restoring balance to a person's energy system could treat physical diseases. This early research has been followed up by recent research reported in the *Journal of Biology and Chemistry* that the uteruses of women with uterine cancer had a negative charge and that those without cancer had a positive charge. The negative charge in many tumors is assisting in the diagnosis and treatment of breast cancer.[5]

Treatments that influence the brain's electrical activity are being used to overcome a range of psychiatric and other medical disorders. The magnetic stimulation of specific areas of the brain has been shown in double-blinded, placebo-controlled research to help with major depression that did not respond to other therapies (Fitzgerald, 2003), and with bipolar disorder (Rohan, 2004). The surgical implantation of deep-brain stimulators that deliver targeted electrical stimulation in the brain have helped thousands of patients with Parkinson's disease to better control their symptoms; and these brain pacemakers are also used with some success to stimulate the vagus nerve in treating severe depression, compulsive disorders, and other neurological conditions (Archart-Treichel, 2003).

Differentiating between the energy that is electricity and the energy that is constellated in various human emanation and self-cultivation traditions is part of the work of the field of energy medicine. There is much research in each of these areas that is worthy of efforts to replicate further and substantiate initial results. For example, Dr. Bjorn Nordenstrom (1983) has experimented with electricity's effect on tumors and reports a cure or prevention rate in ten out of twenty patients.[6]

Chinese medicine in the form of acupuncture is now a well-accepted part of Western complementary health care and is a licensed health profession in many states. Scientific evidence is mounting to support the long-held empirical claims of acupuncturists. Among the mental-health conditions that the World Health Organization lists as being responsive to acupuncture are anxiety, depression, stress reactions, and insomnia. An acupuncture needle inserted into a specific point on the toe can be seen in a functional MRI as affecting blood activity in the brain—though no nerve, vascular, or other physical connections are known to exist there (Cho et al., 1998). Another study using an MRI demonstrated that stimulating specific points on the skin not only changed brain activity but also deactivated areas of the brain that are involved with the experience of fear and pain (Hui, 2000). Other components of the Chinese medical tradition, such as Tai Chi and Qigong, are also gaining acceptance. The *Journal of the American Medical Association* published a study showing that Tai Chi prevented more falls among the elderly than nine other forms of Western exercise (Province et al., 1995). Qigong is taught at California Pacific Medical Center in San Francisco and other leading-edge medical institutions. There are Qigong studies showing beneficial results on hypertension (Kuang et al., 1991) and many medical disorders (Sancier, 1996b). Determining which type of energy medicine should be used for different conditions, and at what times, is a next step for researchers.

The Six Pillars of Energy Medicine

An overview of the emerging field can be found in Feinstein & Eden's (2006b) article *Six Pillars of Energy Medicine*, which puts forth the following strengths of energy, compared with the traditional medical model. This article supports these propositions with scientific research:

Pillar 1: Energy medicine can influence certain fundamental biological processes in ways that conventional medicine cannot.

Pillar 2: Energy medicine embraces modern physics in ways that conventional medicine has not, resulting in greater methodological precision and flexibility.

Pillar 3: Energy interventions are faster, more efficient, and far safer than chemical interventions in biological regulation.

Pillar 4: Energy interventions are available that can be readily, economically, and noninvasively applied.

Pillar 5: Patients can utilize energy-medicine techniques on an at-home, self-help basis.

Pillar 6: Energy medicine focuses on the total person.

Qigong: An Age-Old Path for Cultivating the Energy of Life

For a moment reflect on a "breakthrough" intervention now being supported by decades of research from the National Institutes of Health. This breakthrough has been acknowledged by the American Medical Association and the United States Surgeon General. It has the documented effect of reducing virtually all forms of illness. It helps patients prevent or recover from high blood pressure, diabetes, osteoporosis, breast cancer, arthritis and chronic pain. It improves mental function, sleep, weight loss and muscle mass, and extends life expectancy. Miracle drug? New product of advanced genetic engineering? . . . None of the above. It is . . . exercise. Exercise is more important for health than most of the more exotic forms of CAM, and a great many forms of conventional medicine.

—K. R. Pelletier
(Pelletier, 2000, p. 34)

Given this understanding of the importance of exercise from Dr. Pelletier, it is interesting that Tai Chi and Qigong are not even more widely known in the West than they are because they represent some of the most time-tested methods of beneficial exercise.

When many people feel low energy, one of the things we often think of is getting some exercise: going for a long jog or going to the gym for a hard workout. In tune with our cultural conditioning, we think of pumping ourselves up to give us energy as we do our cars at the gas station. And the more we put in, the bigger and better is our tank . . . right? Wrong. Actually, recent research stemming from the Harvard Health Professionals Study shows that long runs decrease the size of our hearts and create more problems than short bursts of intense activity and then rest.[7] This is why, according to author Al Sears, MD, long-distance runners have a higher risk of sudden cardiac death than other athletes. This modern scientific discovery was well known by ancient Taoists who said that the secret to longevity was not overdoing, but instead using effort-less effort (*wu wei*), balancing effort (*yang*) and stillness (*yin*), and finding still-ness in movement and movement in stillness.

In a holistic approach to exercise, the healing dimensions of Tai Chi and Qigong can be balanced with the cardiovascular-enhancing attributes of bursts of aerobic exercise; and there are many unique gifts that Tai Chi and Qigong have to give to an integrated approach to "exercise":

- Tai Chi and Qigong are low impact so that instead of producing many of the injuries associated with running—including joint problems and injuries from running on hard pavement—these age-old practices provide benefits without negative side effects.

- Tai Chi and Qigong activate a type of energy called *sung*, or *fongsung*, defined as "relaxed awakeness." Just as Eskimos have many names for snow because they are long-term experts in snow, the Chinese Taoists coined many descriptive terms for energy because of their expertise in energy cultivation. We in the modern Western world have no word for combining energy and relaxation. But the Taoists speak of *fongsung*, which is like a totally relaxed cat that is ready to pounce. This has important real-life applications because as the practitioner trains in holding of stances like a cat, this is a way to practice activating the relaxation response in the midst of attack. To see how Tai Chi and Qigong practices can aid in the healing of post-traumatic stress, refer to Chapter Eight. The idea of combining energy and relaxation is a health message to us over eons of time to transmit a secret pathway to health and longevity.

- Tai Chi and Qigong emphasize mind and intention in particular sophisti-cated ways. For example, using the mind to direct energy to different parts of the body, to balance yin and yang (excesses and deficiencies), to use an attitude of no-force to create a greater force, to imagine a dangerous physical attack to activate the healing resources in the body, and to create a neurophysiology of harmony. As we imagine shape-shifting into various elements, such as a tree, ball, or caterpillar reeling silk, we can develop specific energetic states for different purposes.

- Tai Chi and Qigong derive from ancient traditions of postural initiation where exercise is not split off from other aspects of holistic healing in the deepest sense of the word. These ancient "exercise traditions" have physical exercise intertwined with an awareness that is oriented to self-healing, spiritual unfoldment, self-defense, and changing our life stances.

Tai Chi and Qigong: Age-Old Methods of Mind-Body Medicine

Qigong and Tai Chi are two of the oldest methods of mind-body medicine long known to positively affect the mind and body of the practitioner. Qigong is a many-thousand-year-old method of cultivating the energy of life using movement, breath, static postures, awareness, sound, touch, and imagery. Tai Chi is perhaps the best-known method of Qigong.

It has been estimated that in Beijing alone 1.3 million people practice just one form of Qigong every day (Tai Chi) and that in China as a whole 80 million people practice Qigong every day. So with this number of votes of confidence, maybe we in the West should wonder what these time-tested methods have to offer our self-care. Fortunately, this is beginning to happen.

According to a 2002 National Health Interview Survey, approximately 950 thousand American adults have practiced Qigong and five million Americans have practiced Tai Chi (Barnes, Powell-Griner, McFann, & Nahin, 2004). The *Wall Street Journal* called Qigong "the hottest trend in stress relief" (Weil, 2004). Dr. Andrew Weil (2004) says, "I often recommend Qigong as a relaxation method and also think it can be an important part of a well-rounded fitness program ... Plus research in Asia suggests that practicing Qigong regularly can lower blood pressure, reduce the frequency and severity of asthma attacks, promote the healing of ulcers, reduce arthritis pain and even enhance immunity (p. 1)." *Time* magazine called Tai Chi "the perfect exercise" (Gorman, 2002). The well-known author Eckhart Tolle says, "Tai Chi and Qigong will play an important role in global awakening." On *The Oprah Winfrey Show* on Friday, November 1, 2007, Dr. Mehmet Oz—Director of the Cardiovascular Institute of Columbia University Medical Center of New York and award-winning author—said, "If you want to be healthy and live to 100, do Qigong . . . Qigong reverses the aging process."

The many systems of Qigong are ancient methods of cultivating the body's vital energy, called *Qi*. They use movement, breath, posture, awareness, sound, and touch and are one part of the multifaceted system of Chinese medicine. To understand Qigong in a more comprehensive way, you must realize that just as the term *psychotherapy* is a catchall term—including many branches, such as cognitive-behavioral, humanistic, Freudian/neo-analytic, Jungian/archetypal, and transpersonal—so are there many branches of Qigong. And each branch is important to understanding the whole of Qigong.

Qigong is a multifaceted tradition that includes the following methods: (1) movement and stillness (Cohen, 1997; Ha & Olsen, 1996; Mayer, 2004a and b), (2) external emission for healing (Cohen, 1997), (3) medical self-healing (Chuen, 1999; Francis, 1993; Johnson, 2000), (4) spiritual practices (Cohen, 1997; Luk, 1972; Sha, 2003; Mayer, 2004a and b), (5) internal alchemy (Luk, 1977), (6) internal martial arts and *nei jia* (O'Brien, 2004), (7) inner power/*nei kung* (Danaos, 2002), (8) stretching/*daoyin* exercises (Kohn, 1989), (9) medical Qigong (Johnson, 2000; Sancier, 1996a and b), (10) Taoist meditation (Kohn, 1989), (11) animal forms of Qigong (Feng, 2003; Mayer, 2004a and b), (12) self-defense methods (Chia, 1986; Francis, 1998; Mayer, 2004b; Ming, 1986; O'Brien, 2004), and so forth. In common to all branches of Qigong is that, at its roots, Qigong contains a treasure-house of ways to cultivate the energy of life for a multiplicity of purposes.

Many scholars believe that Qigong began at the time of the Yellow Emperor (ca. 2690–2590 BC) when the theoretical foundation for Chinese medicine was laid. The movement of the body's energy for healing purposes probably goes back as far as the earliest humans. When ill or wounded, our earliest ancestors must have touched themselves and each other and learned movements to heal themselves, like rocking back and forth. In terms of definitive evidence, we know that Qigong practices date at least as early as 168 BC, because a chart depicting forty-four standing and seated Qigong postures with associated commentaries and prescriptions for various diseases was discovered in the King Ma tomb. As Cohen (1997) states, the term *Qigong* (work or play with Qi, the energy of life) as a therapeutic art was first used in 1936 in a work by Dong Hao entitled *Special Therapy for Tuberculosis: Qigong* (p. 13–18). But Qigong derived from Taoist methods of *daoyin* (leading and guiding the life force of the universe, a tradition with written sources that date to at the time of Taoist Master Xu Sun, who died in AD 374). However, even earlier than this, the ancient cross-cultural roots of Qigong existed in shamanic practices that formed the roots of cultures in Native America, Greece, India, Japan, and China, and of various religions, including Buddhism, Hinduism, Judaism, and Taoism (Mayer, 2004b).

Western culture was first introduced to the pain-reducing effects of Chinese Qigong in 1971 when the *New York Times* columnist James Reston had an emergency appendectomy with acupuncture needles and no anesthetic, and he felt no pain. Since that time, a wave of interest has gradually grown in investigating the wider dimensions of Qigong. The PBS special with Bill Moyers interviewing Dr. David Eisenberg introduced the Western TV audience to the use of Qi in medical treatment in Chinese hospitals. A number of well-respected authors have written on the applications of Qigong in medical settings, including Michael Lerner (1994) in his *Choices in Healing*, and Dr. David Eisenberg's *Encounters with Qi: Exploring Chinese Medicine* (1995). To date, there have been eleven international conferences reporting research results. At these conferences[8] numerous studies from China reported Qigong's positive effect on a wide variety of diseases, such as kidney disease,[9] chronic hepatitis,[10] cancer,[11] and paralysis due to stroke.[12] The problem has been that many of these studies do not meet Western research methodology standards. However, as you will see below, there are many studies in well-respected journals supporting the efficacy of Qigong with a wide variety of health problems; and the International Society for the Study of Subtle Energies and Energy Medicine (ISSSEEM) has complied hundreds of studies and papers on the uses of energy in healing.[13]

How the self-healing methods of Qigong actually create a healing response remains a matter of speculation. Researchers are still in the process of trying to determine the extent that the energy noted in many ancient healing traditions exists, or whether the healing response to Qigong is a function of hypnosis, biochemical reaction, endorphin response, and so forth.[14] This subject is beyond the scope of the purpose in this book to explore the clinical usefulness of Qigong as a complementary tool to help our health-care crisis.

Mainstream medicine often speaks in a derogatory way about alternative modalities for their lack of solidity of research. Even scholars within the Qigong community have been critical of the research standards and the political and cultural factors biasing many past studies (Palmer, 2007; Cohen, 1997). In my peer-reviewed articles on this subject, I also have been critical of Qigong research methodology standards in many cases (Mayer, 1999; 2003). The richness and complexity of Tai Chi and Qigong pose challenges to the reductionistic (causal) approach to proving efficacy (Wayne & Kaptchuk, 2007). To stay balanced—in addition to looking at the political and economic factors regarding why more research is not done in these areas—it is important for those who criticize to realize that as much as twenty to fifty percent of conventional care, and virtually all surgery, has not been evaluated by randomized controlled studies. Richard Smith, editor of the *British Medical Journal,* says, "Only about 15 percent of medical interventions are supported by solid scientific evidence ... this is partly because only 1 in 5 of the articles in medical journals are scientifically sound and partly because many treatments have never been assessed at all" (Smith, 1991, p. 798).

It is true that Qigong is not a panacea, and research in many cases is not up to modern standards. To prevent " the baby being thrown out with the bathwater," however, in my peer-reviewed research of Qigong, when I have pointed out problems in the research methodology (Mayer, 1999; 2003), I conclude these articles by writing:

Although many of the studies of Qigong practice and hypertension have methodological flaws ... which may account for some unknown portion of improved health outcome measures ... we should be circumspect before fully discounting positive effects reported in mortality rates, incidence of strokes and retinopathy (Kuang et al., 1991), and other positive outcome measurements in patients who have suffered from long-term hyperten-sion (Kuang et al., 1991; Jing, 1988; Wu & Liu, 1993), or chronic renal fail-ure (Suzuki et al., 1993). These represent significant numbers of long-term sufferers of severe hypertension. Even if methodological flaws, such as expectancy biases and placebo effects, contributed to positive results, the results need to be considered seriously in an area that has such significant health ramifications. (Mayer, 2004b, p. 132)

In addition to addressing issues about research methodology, I have tried to bring objective balance to the idealization that some have about Tai Chi and Qigong. I have addressed issues regarding transcendence of psychological issues to my Qigong colleagues (see Chapter Five); and as you will see in Chapter Fourteen, an excess of Qigong practice can even, on some rare occasions, lead to psychotic symptoms.

However, even though there are problems at times with Qigong and Qigong studies, significant research from substantial sources is beginning to accumu-late, including respected scientific journals regarding Qigong and Tai Chi's effi-cacy in helping in the areas of (1) cancer (Chen & Yeung, 2002); (2) asthma (Reuther & Laderidge, 1998); (3) chronic pain (Wu et al., 1999); (4) diabetes (Iwao, Kajiyama, Mori, & Oogakio, 1999); (5) fibromyalgia (Astin et al., 2003); Mannerkorpi & Arndorw, 2004); (6) heart rate variability (Lee et al., 2002); (7) long-term disabilities (Trieschmann, 1999); (8) neurological illness (Weintraub, 2001); (9) Parkinson's disease[15] (Schmitz-Hubsch et al., 2005; Li, 2007); (10) shin-gles[16] (Irwin, Pike, & Oxman, 2004); (11) preventing falls among the elderly (Province et al., 1995); (12) reducing strokes and increasing blood flow to the brain for subjects with cerebral arteriosclerosis (Sancier & Holman, 2004); (13) insomnia (Irwin, Olmstead, & Motivala, 2008); (14) attention deficit hyperac-tivity disorder (Hernandez-Reif, Field, & Thimas, 2001); (15) cardiopulmonary, musculoskeletal, and postural problems (Wolf, Coogler, & Xu, 1997); (16) anti-aging (Sancier, 1996a); (17) bone density issues (Chen, Yeh, & Lee, 2006); (18) immune system deficiencies (Sancier,1996b); (19) chronic physical illnesses in the elderly (Tsang, Mok, Yeung, & Chan, 2003); (20) osteoarthritis in older women (Song, Lee, Lam & Bae, 2003); and so on.[17]

When we think about the way our culture is oriented to medications rather than promoting self-healing practices, it is interesting to note a study of thirteen adolescents with an average age of fourteen-and-a-half years and a diagnosis of ADHD, who were taught Tai Chi for thirty minutes, twice a week for five weeks. The Conner's Teacher Rating Scale was used by the subjects' teachers to evaluate the subjects' behavior prior to the Tai Chi classes, during the classes, and two weeks after the classes had ended. The 28-item scale rates overall hyperactivity, as well as subcategories of anxiety, asocial behavior, conduct, dreams, and emotions. Results of the study showed that the adolescents' teachers perceived the subjects as less anxious, emotional, and hyperactive. These improved scores also remained consistent throughout the two-week follow-up period, without Tai Chi (Hernandez-Reif et al., 2001). If studies like this were borne out with larger numbers of students using Tai Chi as one of the first lines of treatment (along with better-funded counseling programs, dietary advice, and other non-invasive methods), it could provide an alternative that would avoid drug side effects and the stigma of being on medication. Also, such natural approaches could help build self-esteem and instill a message about dealing constructively with emotions rather than taking a drug to make them go away.

In the approach to Qigong offered in the following chapters, you will see how this age-old longevity technology can be integrated with Western body-mind healing methods to enhance our self-healing repertoires for everyday life.[18] Blending certain essential attributes of each these different traditions makes a more healing amalgam. Two of these attributes are the transcendent attributes of Qigong and the transmuting attributes of Western psychology and body-mind healing methods.

Some are concerned that Qigong, and other traditions of relaxation, may help a person to rise above many issues by activating an altered state of consciousness and have healing effects; but Qigong may not help a patient to work through deep-seated issues, which is a process that could produce longer-lasting healing results. In the following chapters, you will see how Bodymind

Healing Psychotherapy weaves together transmuting and transcending healing methods to resolve this false dichotomy.

I am glad that you are joining me on this journey during which you will see how Qigong and Tai Chi are key tools for creating a specific kind of altered state of consciousness that gives us battle-fatigued soldiers of the information age some vital tools for relaxation, energized empowerment, and many health-related benefits. But what is unique about this particular pathway that we are to embark upon is that you will learn how to extract the essence of Tai Chi and Qigong and use them for your health even without doing Tai Chi/Qigong movements. In terms of our goal to find Self-healing methods for our physical and mental health, you will see how these traditions come to their fullest fruition when they serve as an integral (Walsh and Shapiro, 2006; Wilber, 2000; Mayer, 2009) spoke in the wheel of integrative medicine and are combined with the transformative dimensions of Western bodymind healing traditions. As a matter of fact, you may grow to believe, as do I, that at the very center of the wheel of the medicine of the future is energy psychology. Because whether we partake in a surgical procedure or take a medication, our attitude and our energetic state affects how a treatment takes hold. Whether we call it a spoke of the wheel of integrative medicine or a place at the very center of the wheel of healing, this is the place we are about to explore . . . this is the sphere of energy psychology.

Summary of Qigong's Benefits to the Sphere of Energy Psychology

The following are some of the ways that Qigong can play an important part in adding to the sphere of energy psychology:

1. *Qigong contains useful relaxation methods.* Dr. Herbert Benson (1983) first coined the term *relaxation response,* and showed its ability to reduce hypertension and cardiac problems. Qigong fits well into the guidelines stated by a National Institute of Health Technology panel (NIH, 1996), which concluded that integrating behavioral and relaxation therapies with conventional medical treatment is imperative for successfully managing these conditions. The panel did

not endorse a single technique but stated that a variety of techniques worked in lowering one's breathing rate, heart rate, and blood pressure as long as they included two features: (1) a repetitive focus of a word, sound, prayer, phrase, or muscular activity, and (2) neither fighting nor focusing on intruding thoughts. Repetition is a key element in activating healing processes—for example, in energy psychology repeatedly tapping on points while focusing on new constructive beliefs has been related to greater treatment success rates (Andrade & Feinstein, 2004). In the Eye Movement Desensitization and Reprocessing (EMDR) method, moving the eyes repeatedly from side to side while stating constructive beliefs is believed to be integral to positive treatment outcomes. If repetition is such a key to healing why not further investigate Qigong and Tai Chi traditions—which, over thousands of years, have developed sophisticated ways to use whole-body repetition of movement, repetitive movements for isolated body parts, and repetition of sounds to promote healing.

2. *Qigong does not only activate a relaxed, altered state, it activates a "state-specific state" (Tart, 1968; Rossi, 1986) that is both relaxing and empowering.* This state is called *fongsung*, or relaxed awakeness. It can be helpful for alleviating symptoms of stress and empowering those who have deficits in the areas of self-assertiveness, those who are victims of trauma, and so forth.

3. *Qigong not only produces a relaxed state of awareness; but also in its unique way, it provides a pathway to develop qualities seen as useful by therapists who integrate meditation into psychotherapy.* Qigong and Tai Chi can reciprocally inhibit unwanted behaviors adding to Wolpe's (1958) behavioral approach; they can aid in developing an "observing self," adding to Deikman's (1982) transpersonal perspective; and they help to cultivate a "cohesiveness of self" adding to Horner's (1990) psychoanalytic methods. Qigong can help to "anchor" that state of awareness that helps to facilitate ego cohesion in maintaining one's center when meeting the emotional tides of life, adding to Bandler and Grinder's (1979) hypnotherapeutic approach to anchoring. Qigong, like many forms of meditation, can help us to develop a compassionate relationship to our life issues.

4. *Qigong traditions, particularly Tai Chi, can help traumatized patients regain a safety zone in their bodies.*

5. *Qigong adds an energy-cultivation practice beneficial to those who are depressed or suffer from sympathetic nervous system overload, such as in cases of fibromyalgia, chronic fatigue, and trauma.*

6. *The well-known relaxation and energizing attributes of Qigong have been applied to many issues that psychologists see in their everyday practices—such as insomnia, anxiety, joint problems, energy deficiency, and chronic pain.* As an everyday practice, anyone can tap on these healing benefits as has been reported in China for thousands of years before Western psychology emerged.

7. *Whereas some meditative traditions are oriented to transcendence, Qigong and Tai Chi are, for the most part, body-oriented traditions,*[19] *which cultivate a cohesiveness of self* (Horner, 1990). From an integrative perspective, the way Tai Chi and Qigong are usually practiced, they do not specifically focus on psychological issues, such as early emotional wounding and negative beliefs. However, I will put forth the case that oftentimes transformations in a person's psychological stance in life can be a result of this practice. As you will see in Chapters Five, Fifteen, and Sixteen on Bodymind Healing Psychotherapy, an approach that specifically incorporates the psychological dimension and these body-oriented practices can synergistically combine for the benefit of the whole person.

8. *Tai Chi and Qigong help those with reactive attachment styles to develop a cohesive center when the everyday issues of life assault or impinge upon one's sensibilities; and together with psychotherapy, these two Eastern disciplines may provide a bodily base for developing centered emotional expression.* (See Chapters Sixteen, Seventeen, and Eighteen.)

9. *Qigong and Tai Chi are multifaceted traditions that are not only meditative but they can also be seen as forms of hypnosis, and therefore may result in similar health benefits known to be related to hypnosis* (Rossi, 1986; Rossi & Cheek, 1988). Both have an empirically time-tested record for enhancing health for a multiplicity of health-related conditions (Sancier, 1996a and b; Pelletier, 2000).

CHAPTER TWO

Energy Psychologies: Tapping the Vital Healing Power of the Bodymind

Energy Psychology: An Einsteinian Approach to Psychology

The energy-medicine revolution is in the early stages of affecting psychology. Actually, energy has long been an important concept in psychology in the work of early seminal leaders in the field. Even in Freud's seemingly nonenergy, nonbody-oriented therapy, energy is perceived to be key to healing (Freud, 1923; 1933; 1990). Freud borrowed the term *cathexis* from the Greek to speak about the direction of energy to different zones of the body, which was a fundamental aspect of his bodily oriented psychosexual phases. In addition, Freud's notion of *libido* was a sexually focused way of talking about life energy that could be sublimated into creative and intellectual pursuits. You have likely heard the term *complexes,* which really means "complexes of aggregated energy" around some life issue. However, in modern psychology there exists a lack of appreciation for Freud's emphasis on energy and the body—perhaps because he did not specifically use energy-oriented or body-oriented methods in his therapy, despite that they underlay the foundation of his seemingly intellectual psychoanalysis. And his clinical treatment methods, in line with the prevailing worldview of his era, were cognitive, nonbody-oriented, talk therapy methods.

There have also been a number of other authors who have spoken of the importance of integrating the energetic dimension (Reich, 1970; Lowen, 1975;

Seem, 1989; Requena, 1989) and Chinese medicine (Hammer, 1990) into psychology. In their broadest reach, I believe that all forms of psychotherapy have energy psychotherapy unconsciously embedded in their methods; because, for example, in cognitive psychotherapy new beliefs create new energized life pathways, and in Freudian approaches, working through old stuck psychodynamics liberates libidinal energies.

Just as there has been a shift from a Newtonian to an Einsteinian approach to medicine, there is now a growing "Einsteinian approach to psychotherapy and behavioral health care," which specifically and consciously puts energy at the forefront of what composes, transforms, and heals the psyche. We now know that matter is a form of energy and that harnessing the power of energy has vital, peaceful uses in the external world, as well as in the world of medicine. Likewise, the psyche is composed of energy, and harnessing its power and using it to bring vitality, peace, and healing to our inner worlds is an equally important endeavor.

There is a new growing field called "energy psychology." Already, it has many publications[1] and a national organization, the Association for Comprehensive Energy Psychology (ACEP), with a membership in 2008 of more than 1,000 members from a wide variety of health professions, including approximately thirty-nine medical doctors. Cofounded in 1998, by David and Rebecca Gruder and Dorothea Hover-Kramer, ACEP opened to membership in the spring of 1999.

The Origins of Energy Psychology

Just as the founding of psychology was inappropriately credited by some to modern researchers like Wilhelm Wundt, a similar issue exists in the arena of energy psychology. Credit for the founding of energy psychology is given to a modern psychologist named Roger Callahan, the originator of Thought Field Therapy. Callahan built upon the work of psychiatrist John Diamond (1979), who integrated the acupuncture meridian system and muscle testing from applied kinesiology to assess the flow of life energy through the meridians (Goodheart, 1964). Callahan believes that emotional disturbance is caused by "perturbations in the thought field" and that accurate diagnosis is necessary to "unlock" these perturbations. His approach uses applied kinesiology for assessment and algorithms involving tapping acupuncture meridian alarm points along with his proprietary Voice Technology method to treat psychological conditions. These approaches led to meridian-based therapies, which often claim instant cures of a wide variety of psychological problems, including phobias (Callahan, 1985; Nims, 2002); and anecdotal and early positive research evidence lends support to some of these claims (Andrade & Feinstein, 2004). Differentiating how and whom these methods work for is one of the next steps that needs to be taken for this branch of energy medicine to be better accepted by mainstream approaches.

In this early stage of energy psychology's evolution (Kuhn, 1996), there are a wide variety of bases for what various psychotherapists see as defining energy psychology. What some view as essential, other energy psychologists may not find beneficial or important. As you will see below regarding muscle testing stemming from applied kinesiology, some energy psychologists use it and some do not. Likewise with tapping algorithms, there is wide divergence regarding its usefulness, clinical efficacy, and importance. In the pursuit of validating research, one should keep in mind that psychotherapy is an art as well as a science, and that subjective and objective are both important parts of the whole spectrum of research (Jonas & Levin, 2000).

Breadth of the Field of Energy Psychology

There is a wide range of psychological methods under the umbrella of what is now called *comprehensive energy psychology*. One such method is the popular Emotional Freedom Technique (EFT) developed by Craig (2004)—who does not think the order of treatment algorithms really matters and who does not claim, like Callahan, that his EFT derives from diagnosis. Other energy psychology methods, including the Tapas Acupressure Technique (Fleming, 1996), Seemorg Matrix method (Clinton, 2002), and Hover-Kramer's biofield methods (Hover-Kramer, 1996; Hover-Kramer & Shames, 1997), rely on other major energy systems, such as chakras and biofields.

Tapping and Other Treatment Methods

Some energy psychotherapists use an elaborate series of acu-points called *algorithms* to treat various disorders (Callahan, 1985; Craig & Fowlie, 1995); others say that just one point is needed (Gallo, 2002, p. 36). Some use these algorithms or cognitive restructuring in conjunction with other methods, such as eye movements (Craig & Fowlie, 1995; Benor, 2008). Some energy psychology methods do not use tapping: Nims uses a *cue* to produce energetic shifts (as cited in Gallo, 2002, p. 79), Clinton's Seemorg Matrix method (2002) holds chakras, and Diepold advises touching and breathing as the preferred method (as cited in Gallo, 2002, p. 18).

Muscle Testing as a Form of Assessment

There are energy psychology methods that use muscle testing as a key method of assessment (Gallo, 2000), and others that do not use muscle testing, such as the Tapas Acupressure Technique (Fleming, 1999), the negative affect erasing method (Gallo, 2000), and the Emotional Freedom Technique (Craig & Fowlie, 1997).

Energy Psychology: Integrated with a Wide Range of Therapies

Though there are those who look at energy psychology methods as stand-alone treatments, the majority of those who describe themselves as energy psychotherapists integrate their methods with a broader base of psychological methods and traditions. For example, energy psychology methods are being integrated with many forms of therapy, including transactional analysis (Lammers, 2002), Adlerian psychology (Wheeler, 2002), Eye Movement Desensitization Reprocessing (Hartung & Galvin, 2002), and hypnosis (Gross & Ratner, 2002; Pulos, 2002). Energy psychology is also being integrated with some aspects of cognitive (Craig & Fowlie, 1995) and psychodynamic (Nims, 2002, p. 81) therapies. Dr. Dan Benor (2008, in press) has created an integrative method, which he calls WHEE—an acronym for Wholistic Hybrid of Eye Movement Desensitization Reprocessing—and the Emotional Freedom Technique (EFT).

Energy Psychology in Medical Settings

Energy psychology has been integrated as a behavioral health-care tool in medical settings for phobias of medical devices, such as needle phobias; fears of dying; highly stressed caregivers; chronic pain; pediatric disorders; cardiac care; surgical phobias; and so forth (Green, 2002). In a broader definition that includes Qigong, energy psychology is being used to treat patients who are suffering from hypertension, chronic pain, insomnia, etc. (Mayer, 1997b, 1999, 2003, 2007. As mentioned in Chapter One, Dr. Mehmet Oz and Julie Motz use energy psychology methods to prevent organ rejection in heart replacement surgery at Columbia Presbyterian Hospital in New York.

Scope of the Field

To get a sense of the points of both agreement and controversy in the field, a survey was conducted, at the Fifth International Energy Psychology Conference held in May 2003 in Phoenix, of 265 participants who identified themselves as energy psychology practitioners with a substantial base of experience. The professional affiliations of those who participated included approximately ten percent psychologists; ten percent social workers; forty percent mental health or marriage, family, and child counselors; three percent physicians; six percent nurses, five percent other licensed health-care providers; and twenty-six percent unlicensed counselors. Approximately sixty-five percent considered energy psychology their primary, or one of their primary, psychotherapeutic modalities; thirty-five percent considered it secondary to another modality (Feinstein, 2004b).

In the survey, thirty-five percent agreed that there are "effective" and "ineffective" points. Thirty-five percent felt that virtually any subset of the acu-points typically used within energy psychology could bring about the therapeutic effect, and thirty percent were in the middle or offered no opinion. Identical percentages were found in relationship to the importance of the order in which the points were stimulated, with thirty-five percent feeling that it mattered and thirty-five percent feeling it did not matter.

Forty percent felt that energy checking (presumably with muscle testing) is a critical tool in energy psychology, thirty percent felt it is not, and thirty percent were in the middle or offered no opinion. Sixty percent believed that energy checking could accurately assess the state of a meridian, less than one percent disagreed, with the remainder saying they were in the middle or did not know. Fifty percent believed that energy checking could also yield reliable answers to questions that go beyond the immediate meridian response, ten percent disagreed, and forty percent were in the middle or offered no opinion. Twenty percent felt it was important in a reasonable proportion of cases to assess and treat the specific meridians involved in the problem, twenty percent did not, forty percent were in the middle, and twenty percent offered no opinion.[2]

In summary, there is a large range of opinion within the field of energy psychology about what constitutes the field and which treatments are best at which times. It is in this sense that the field of energy psychology is in a preparadigmatic phase (Kuhn, 1996), as is the research of discovering which methods work best with which people.

The Emotional Freedom Techniques

There are a wide range of energy psychology methods. Perhaps the most popular is Craig's Emotional Freedom Techniques, often referred to in the singular as the Emotional Freedom Technique (EFT), that combine many different energy psychology methods. The following is the basic "recipe" for EFT as cited in the *EFT Manual* (Craig, 2004; Feinstein, 2004a, p. 27):

1. **The Setup:** While continuously rubbing the sore spot on the chest (upper left or upper right) or tapping the Karate Chop point (SI-3), repeat this affirmation three times: "Even though I have this_____, I deeply and completely accept myself."

2. **The Sequence:** Tap about seven times on each of the following energy points while repeating the reminder phrases at each point*. Here, I list only the EFT Eight Point Treatment Chart (Feinstein, 2004,a p. 27):
   EB (Beginning of the Eyebrow) = BL-2 (Bladder Meridian)
   SE (Side of the Eye) = GB-1 (Gall Bladder Meridian)

UE (Under the Eye) = St-1 (Stomach Meridian)

UN (Under the Nose) = GV-26 (Governing Vessel Meridian)

Ch (Between Chin and Lower Lip) = CV-24 (Conception Vessel)

CB (Collarbone) = K-27 (Kidney Meridian)

UA (Under the Arm) = SP-21 (Spleen Meridian)

* In Craig's full method other points are also used: BN, Th, IF, MF, BF, KC (see Craig's EFT Manual [2004]).

3. **The Nine Gamut Procedure:** Continuously tap on an acu-point on the back of the wrist called *the gamut point,* where the bones of the little finger and ring finger meet (acu-point TW-3) while performing each of these nine actions:

(1) eyes closed, (2) eyes open, (3) eyes down right, (4) eyes down left, (5) roll eyes in a circle, (6) roll eyes in other direction, (7) hum two seconds of a song, (8) count to five, and (9) hum two seconds of a song.

It should be noted that Gary Craig seldom uses the Nine Gamut procedure anymore; he prefers shorter protocols. Variations on, and intricacies of, practicing the basic protocol can be seen on his Web site at www.emofree.com.

4. **The Sequence Again:** Tap about three times on each of the energy points listed in step two above, repeating the "reminder phrase" at each point; that is, EB, SE, UE, UN, CH, CB, UA, BN, TH, and so forth.

As do many current mind-body health practitioners, Craig has his patients assess their subjective units of distress (SUDS) level before and after treatment. This serves as an "objective / subjective" method of measuring change.

Energy Psychology Research

Many of the leaders in the field of energy psychology, such as David Feinstein (2004), Donna Eden (1998), and Fred Gallo (see Gallo, 2002, for a good overview of leaders in the field), are part of this movement that is stretching psychology's limits and bringing the body and energy back into a field that once placed an overemphasis on mind and participated in the mind-body split. Additionally, there is a growing research base that lends credence to the efficacy of some or many of its methods.

As Feinstein (2008) points out in his article, one of the ways to gain confidence in a early proposed therapy is to look at doctoral dissertation research. Three dissertations that have investigated the efficacy of energy psychology procedures found positive treatment outcomes—two based on systematic observation of individuals who received treatment and a third based on a controlled experiment. The first, using such objective measures as standard anxiety inventories, demonstrated significant improvement in forty-eight individuals plagued with public speaking anxiety, after just one hour of treatment with Thought Field Therapy (TFT). Following the treatment, the subjects reported decreased shyness and confusion and increased poise and interest in giving a future speech. Treatment gains were still present in four-month follow-up interviews (Schoninger, 2001). A second dissertation followed twenty patients who had been unable to receive necessary medical attention because of intense needle phobias. They also showed significant immediate improvement after an hour of TFT treatment and in one-month follow-up interviews (Darby, 2001). A third dissertation investigated the effects of TFT on self-concept with twenty-eight subjects who presented with a phobia. Two self-concept inventories were administered a month prior to the treatment and then two months after the treatment. Again, the TFT treatment reduced the phobias substantially; and in this study, significant improvement was also found in self-acceptance, self-esteem, and self-congruency two months after the treatment. A wait-list control group of twenty-five subjects did not show improvement (Wade, 1990). (See www.innersource.net for David Feinstein's *Energy Psychology Interactive* CD, which includes a video of acrophobia—the phobia of heights.)

As the emerging field of energy psychology has been incorporating tapping, touch, and other energy-healing methods into psychotherapy (Gallo, 2002), it is beginning to investigate the efficacy of energy-based, psychophysiological approaches in a more scientific manner. One controlled study was conducted in Brazil by principal researcher Joaquin Andrade, MD (Andrade & Feinstein, 2004). Over a five-and-a-half-year period, approximately five thousand patients— diagnosed at intake with an anxiety disorder—were randomly assigned to an experimental group (involving imagery and self-statements paired with manual stimulation of selected acupuncture points) or a control group (involving cognitive-behavior therapy [CBT] and medication). Ratings were given by independent clinicians who interviewed each patient at the close of therapy—at one month, three months, six months, and twelve months. The raters made a determination of complete or partial remission of symptoms or no clinical response. The raters did not know if the patient was in the experimental or control group. At the close of therapy sixty-three percent of the control group were judged as having improved and ninety percent of the experimental group were judged as having improved. Fifty-one percent of the control group was judged as symptom free and seventy-six percent of the experimental group was judged as symptom free. At one-year follow-up, patients receiving acu-point treatments were less prone to relapse or partial relapse than those receiving CBT and medication as indicated by the independent raters' assessment and corroborated by brain imaging and neurotransmitter profiles from a sampling of the patients.

Brain mapping revealed that subjects whose acupuncture points were stimulated tended to be distinguished by a general pattern of brain-wave normalization, which not only persisted at the twelve-month follow-up but also became more pronounced. In neurotransmitter profiles with generalized anxiety disorder, acu-point stimulation was followed by norepinephrine levels falling to normal reference values and low serotonin levels rising to more healthy levels. Parallel electrical and biochemical patterns were less pronounced in the CBT medication group. In a related pilot study by the same team, the length of treatment was substantially shorter with energy therapy and related methods than with the CBT and medication (mean = 3 sessions versus mean = 15 sessions). For further information, see www.innersource.net.

One problem with using brain-wave research is that at this early stage in understanding the individual variations and meanings of activation of different centers in the brain, the cautious observer cannot determine with certainty the validity and reliability of the results (Carey, 2005).

Because the Andrade study was initially envisioned as an exploratory in-house assessment, not all the variables that needed to be controlled in robust research were tracked, not all criteria were defined with rigorous precision, the record keeping was relatively informal, and source data was not always maintained. Nonetheless, the studies all used randomized samples, control groups, and blind assessment. The findings were so striking that the team decided to report them. More detailed reports of some of the studies are being prepared for submission to scientific journals. If subsequent research corroborates these early findings, it will be a notable development because a combination of CBT and medication is currently the established psychological standard of care for anxiety disorders. Since tapping is just one of the methods of Qigong, it will be interesting to see what happens when the wider range of Qigong methods are examined with more sophisticated research protocols.[2]

Brain research shows some promise in assessing efficacy of energy psychology treatment methods. A study by Swingle, Pulos, & Swingle (2000b) examined the changes in brain activity using an EEG. The patients with successful outcomes who were treated for phobias after a car accident showed increases in brain amplitudes related to mental quiescence (increases in slow 3–7 hertz brain waves in the occipital region), whereas those who reported immediate improvement but did not sustain improvement on three-month follow-up showed trends opposite to those clients who sustained improvement. In another study by Swingle (2000a), children diagnosed with epilepsy were treated with Emotional Freedom Technique and after two weeks of daily in-home treatments, they experienced a significant reduction in seizures accompanied with improved EEG measures.

Use in Disaster Relief

Any new discipline trying to gain acceptability must prove itself in many spheres. In this light, it is interesting to note the use of energy psychology in treating trauma victims in Kosovo. Over the past six years, Carl Johnson, PhD, a clinical psychologist retired from a career as a post-traumatic stress disorder (PTSD) specialist with the Veteran's Administration has frequently traveled to the sites of some of the world's most terrible atrocities and disasters to provide psychological support based in energy psychology methods.

In an article in a journal published by the Institute of Noetic Sciences, it was reported that the first 105 people treated in Kosovo by Johnson and his colleagues were followed for eighteen months after their treatments (Feinstein, 2006a). Commenting on Johnson's research, Feinstein (2008) says in his updated article in the journal *Traumatology*:

The 105 people treated during Johnson's first five visits to Kosovo, all in 2000, had each been suffering for longer than a year from the post-traumatic emotional effects of 249 discrete, horrific self-identified incidents. For 247 of those 249 memories, the treatments (using TFT) successfully reduced the reported degree of emotional distress not just to a manageable level but to a "no distress" level ("0" on a 0-to-10 "Subjective Units of Distress" scale, after Wolpe, 1958). Although these figures strain credibility, they are consistent with other reports (see below). Approximately three-fourths of the 105 individuals were followed for 18 months after their treatments and showed no relapses—the original memory no longer activated self-reported or observable signs of traumatic stress (Johnson, Mustafe, Sejdijaj, Odell, & Dabishevci, 2001).

Refer to the aforementioned article (Feinstein, 2006a; 2008), for a more complete description of Dr. Johnson's work, poignant case illustrations, and graphs of the research results. Johnson made nine trips to Kosovo between February 2000 and June 2002. His later visits were as much to train local health-care providers in TFT as to treat additional patients. He also received follow-up information on approximately three-fourths of the initial 105 people treated, primarily from two physicians who participated as translators in the initial treatments and who continued to care for the individuals who received the treatments. According to Feinstein's article (2006a, 2008) and Johnson et al. (2001), once a patient's memory had been cleared of its emotional charge, it remained clear. The initial treatment had proven a potent and durable healing in all cases. The physicians did eventually ask Johnson to see two of the patients a second time, and their problems—similar though less intense than the original memories—were treated. Dr. Skkelzen Syla, the chief medical officer of Kosovo (the equivalent of the U.S. surgeon general), stated in a letter of appreciation:

Many well-funded relief organizations have treated the post-traumatic stress here in Kosovo. Some of our people had limited improvement but Kosovo had no major change or real hope . . . until we referred our most difficult trauma patients to [Dr. Johnson and his team]. The success from

TFT was reported to be 100% for every patient (as cited in Feinstein, 2006a, p. 19).

When we hear stories like those about the work of Dr. Johnson, we may wonder how generalizable these results are. In addition to the Kosovo data, various other personnel of disaster relief organizations have reported positive results in Rwanda, Africa; New Orleans; and with tsunami victims. In each case, when a team went into a disaster area, local observers in positions of authority offered strikingly positive postdeployment assessments, most often with invitations or appeals for return visits. Pierre Llunga, PhD, the director of the El Shaddai Orphanage in Rwanda and university professor, wrote to the TFT Trauma Relief Team members who worked with the orphanage, "Our life has been changed in a better way."

Likewise, all three of the local organizations in New Orleans that had invited the TFT Trauma Relief Team to work with people following Hurricane Katrina requested additional treatment and training from the team. Dwayne Thomas, MD, chief executive officer of the Medical Center of Louisiana at New Orleans, sent a letter of appreciation to members of the TFT Trauma Relief Team about a month after their first visit to New Orleans. He wrote, "As you know, our staff has been through (and continues to experience) a significant amount of primary and secondary trauma. We have offered staff many different interventions . . . the overwhelmingly positive response to the [TFT] therapy was a welcome and delightful surprise for us all."

Charles Figley, PhD, founder of the Green Cross and a leading figure in trauma treatment noted that, "energy psychology is rapidly proving itself to be among the most powerful psychological interventions available to disaster relief workers in helping the survivors, and as well as the workers themselves" (as cited in Feinstein, 2006a).

Questions have been raised by psychologists in the media about whether going into the field with unproven treatment methods that have not been scientifically examined can produce harm. This is a legitimate concern; and it is not easy to produce rigorous research when a therapy team goes into an area where a disaster has recently struck, particularly when the team is traveling to a culture with which the team is unfamiliar. The number of variables needed to be controlled for scientific research is extensive, and opportunities to set up stringently controlled research conditions are highly restricted. For more information about the use of energy psychology in disaster relief, see https://energypsych.org/article-feinstein4.php.

Another question about generalizability of energy psychology relates to how broad-based the types of positive treatment effects are. It is known that Eye Movement Desensitization and Reprocessing (EMDR) similarly began with impressive results with post-traumatic stress patients (Shapiro, 1995); the positive results of the method later showed that it was effective with other syndromes as well. From this, and other evidence, we know it will take time, and further research, to determine the extent of energy psychology's efficacy and generalizability.

One important criterion, before the mental-health field is willing to accept a new experimental method, is to examine new procedures in professional journals; and articles are beginning to appear in many reputable journals. A study published in the *Journal of Clinical Psychology* examined whether the effects of energy psychology procedures were due to placebo; and it explored the question of how much improvement could be gained in a single session with individuals who volunteered to receive help with irrational fears of insects or small animals, including rats, mice, spiders, and roaches. The energy psychology approach was compared with a relaxation technique that uses diaphragmatic breathing. Significantly greater improvement was found, based on standardized phobia scales and other measures, in the group that received the energy psychology treatment. On follow-ups, six to nine months later, the improvements held (Wells, Polglase, Andrews, Carrington, & Baker, 2003). A study conducted at Queens College in New York to see if these findings could be replicated produced markedly similar results (Baker & Siegel, 2005). The Wells EFT study (Wells et al., 2003) brings energy psychology past the threshold formulated by the Division 12 Task Force of the American Psychological Association for establishing EFT as a "Probably Efficacious Treatment" for specific phobias (Feinstein, 2008; Chambless & Hollon, 1998, p. 11). Other studies are in progress.[3]

Research on Tapping Acu-points: Do Specific Points Matter?

With preliminary evidence suggesting that the procedures used in energy psychology are more effective than relaxation training in the treatment of phobias, a next logical question is whether it matters which points are tapped. Is there something about simply tapping the body that has a curative effect, or is there really something unique about the points that were identified in ancient China? In response, the evidence is mixed. An early investigation of this question suggested that in treating forty-nine people with height phobias, the patients who tapped the traditional points showed significantly more improvement than those who tapped placebo points (Carbonell, 1997). In a subsequent study published in the medical journal *Anesthesia & Analgesia*, treatments that involved stimulating acu-points were applied by the paramedic team after a minor injury and were compared with treatments that stimulated areas of the skin that are not recognized acupuncture points. Again, the treatments that used the traditional points were more effective, resulting in a significantly greater reduction of anxiety, pain, and elevated heart rate (Kober et al., 2002). A third study used a randomized, controlled, double-blinded design in treating thirty-eight women diagnosed with clinical depression (Allen, Schnyer, & Hitt, 1998). The researchers compared the use of acupuncture points, during twelve treatment sessions over an eight-week period, specifically selected for the treatment of depression with acupuncture points, also during twelve sessions over eight weeks, usually used for other ailments, and with a waiting-list control group that received no treatment. Following the acupuncture treatments, fifty percent of patients who received the depression protocol showed no sign of the disorder, while only twenty-seven percent of the patients in the other two groups experienced relief of their symptoms. Following the initial clinical trial, the women from the other two groups were also administered the depression treatment over an eight-week period. Seventy percent of them experienced a drop in depressive symptoms, with sixty-four percent showing complete remission according to DSM IV criteria. These findings suggest that targeting the proper points was an important ingredient of the treatment.

A fourth study, however, did not detect a difference between tapping traditional points and tapping nonacupuncture points in treating fear—though both tapping procedures proved more effective than no treatment (Waite & Holder, 2003). While serious questions have been raised regarding some of the conclusions reached by the authors of this study (Baker & Carrington, 2005), there is also clinical evidence suggesting that stimulating certain points not identified in traditional acupuncture may have therapeutic effects. While this is an area where further study is clearly needed, research in China suggests that the stimulation of many of the traditional acupuncture points—with their lower electrical resistance and higher concentration of receptors that are sensitive to mechanical stimulation—produces stronger electrochemical signals. Many acupuncture points are also believed to have specific effects, such as increasing serotonin levels and strengthening or sedating the energy flow to a particular organ.

For more information on research on energy psychology see www.energypsych.org, www.innersource.net, and www.emofree.com.

The Benefits and Problems with Energy Psychology

Tapping Points

In Chinese medicine there are many ways to activate acu-points—needling, electrical acupuncture, pressure, tapping, heat, light touch, circling, and by intention. We have mentioned that there is a divergence of opinion among energy psychologists regarding bringing meridian-based tapping into psychotherapy. There is research that points in the direction of these tapping methods being clinically useful in many cases (Andrade & Feinstein, 2004). There has also been much speculation as to why tapping works when it works. Alongside the Eastern perspective that tapping meridians activates the energetic rivers of the life force in our bodies, one plausible Western explanation is that tapping helps to break up energy fixations; and as Freud put forth, fixations are one of the major impediments to mental health. It makes intuitive sense that tapping may facilitate the breaking up of fixations. In particular, when integrating the somatic dimension into a modern psychology, which has otherwise relied on mental solutions to psychological blockages, we can posit that integrating the tapping of the body may add needed energy to help get people out of habitual ruts. In addition, it should be remembered that tapping is not usually done alone in energy psychology, but is done while addressing negative cognitions and beliefs by saying such phrases as *even though I am____, I can still love and accept myself.* This statement originally came from Callahan to treat *psychological reversals*, which was TFT's explanation of self-sabotage. Others in the field have expanded this phrasing to such ways as *even though this problem is currently ruling my life, I choose to be patient while I discover new and surprising ways to overcome it.* Using transformative cognitions like these helps to honor what I later describe as the *transcendent/transmuting dialectic.*

Even though Dr. Francine Shapiro, the EMDR method's originator, does not consider herself an energy psychologist and she emphasizes information reprocessing as the key to EMDR patients' successes, her work can be viewed as a form of energy psychology. Dr. Shapiro (1995) suggests that neuronal bursts caused by eye movements may be equivalent to a low-voltage current and therefore responsible for synaptic changes. She says, "It may be that the repetitive action of any ... alternative stimuli—or even repetitive bursts of attention generates such a current. The shifting of the synaptic potential of the neural networks that include the dysfunctional material may cause the information to undergo progressively more processing with each set, until it arrives at an adaptive resolution" (p. 316). Others hypothesize that EMDR's positive research results are based in part by reenergizing neural pathways in, among other areas, the orbital frontal cortex by breaking up old patterns of fixations there. In a similar way, perhaps tapping on meridian points breaks up fixations in these channels and clears pathways allowing life energy to flow naturally.[4]

Among the various rationales for tapping is a behavioral psychology explanation. One of the foundations of modern behavioral self-control strategies is Wolpe's (1958) theory of reciprocal inhibition. Wolpe, a behavioral psychologist, hypothesized that various maladaptive patterns would extinguish if they could symbolically occur in the presence of an incompatible response, such as relaxation. Psychologist Jim Lane believes that EFT's tapping method reduces central nervous system hyperarousal to provide rapid desensitization of triggers and depotentiates limiting cognitive beliefs along the lines of reciprocal inhibition.[5]

The reciprocal inhibition point of view leads to using tapping while the patient focuses upon, or says, words related to the old negative cognition, dysfunctional state or belief, that is, "tapping away" the old dysfunctional belief. This is believed to send deactivating signals to areas of the amygdala that regulate emotional arousal (Feinstein, 2006c, p. 2).

However, since the field of energy psychology is still in an early phase regarding techniques and theoretical frameworks, other theoretical frameworks with differing methods of application that serve the same purpose as tapping currently exist. For example, for those who favor the viewpoint that the purpose of various energy psychology methods—including tapping, humming, and eye movements—is to anchor new states of awareness, they would apply these methods while focusing upon, or stating, a new life-enhancing belief. Deactivating stuck energy versus anchoring new beliefs do not need to be mutually exclusive theoretical frameworks or treatment methodologies. Further research is needed to determine which theoretical viewpoints coupled with which treatment methods work best for which issues.

There is neurophysiological theoretical support for physical explanations of the merit of tapping. Dr. Ruden (2005) presents a neurobiological hypothesis that tapping stimulates the release of various neurotransmitters that regulate moods, such as glutamate, serotonin, and GABA. He hypothesizes that tapping stimulates glutamate release and promotes affect activation and that following the tapping a combination of serotonin and GABA are released, which prevents the restoring of the fear response by unlinking the conditioned stimulus to the unconditioned fear stimulus pathway. Dr. Goodheart reports that tapping on the left side of the head along the temporal sphenoidal line around the ear fosters an acceptance of such positive statements as *I am worthwhile*, while tapping on the right fosters an acceptance of such negativepositive statements as *I am not worthless*. He speculated that by tapping on these sites, the filtering system is temporarily disengaged, allowing the assimilation of desired messages (as cited in Gallo, 2002, p. 47).

On the other hand, there are a variety of energy-based psychotherapists who do not consider tapping to be useful and report non-beneficial or detrimental results. Dr. Asha Clinton, the founder of the Seemorg Matrix method (2002), found that in her clinical experience "tapping on points jangled some of my clients and increased their anxiety and fear; we discovered that holding each chakra in turn by contacting it with the center of the clients palm seems to produce a deeper, more peaceful, more thorough treatment. This has become the preferred, though not the only method" (p. 95). Clinton not only holds chakras that are out of balance, but she also has patients simultaneously touch other chakras that can aid the out-of-balance chakra. Nims (2002), after practicing Callahan's method for many years, found that tapping was not necessary and that verbal or nonverbal cues were just as effective, if not even more so. Furthermore, John Diepold (2002), another leader in the energy psychology movement, says that he developed the touch and breath method to move away from tapping because he found: "Colleagues using Thought Field Therapy reported that patients sometimes made statements about tapping that reflected criticism or discomfort, ... such as *This is silly. This looks stupid. I can't do this in public ... It hurts if I tap too hard. Tapping distracts me.*" These types of responses "compromised compliance with follow-up treatment and homework. Additionally some patients who are victims of abuse either refused to tap or took tapping as an opportunity to hurt themselves" (p. 20).

Another issue is that acupuncture, and the wider Chinese medical traditions in which it is embedded, has a wider knowledge of points oriented to a patient's ideographic (unique) condition, as assessed through pulse and tongue diagnosis. Energy psychologists should be open to drawing further on that knowledge base as treatment protocols are established. Because an acupuncturist would not necessarily use the same points used by an energy psychologist to heal various disorders, the question arises: has energy psychology discovered a shorthand method that could be a major step forward in helping the evolution of energy-based healing traditions? In supporting this position, we would need to include the research on understanding how the mind *(placebo effect*, better called the *belief effect)* has been shown in meta-analytic studies to be responsible for approximately fifty-five percent of cures (Rossi, 1986, p. 15–19). So, we can imagine how adding the psychological dimension to tapping just a few well-chosen points could create powerful healing effects.

DISTRACTION

Another major concern that clinicians have about tapping is that it may temporarily distract/dissociate patients from their issues, thereby preventing a longer lasting "working through" of psychological issues. One way to measure whether this is the case is through longitudinal research; that is, examining how long a patient's reported changes last. From the Andrade & Feinstein study (2004) and from brain change studies (Swingle et al., 2000b), the research points to many patients' maintaining long-term changes over time as a result of tapping and many of EFT's broader methods. As discussed earlier, there are plausible theoretical reasons as well as a neurobiological basis for the positive results (Ruden, 2005). Further examination is needed of such research methodology issues, some of which will be addressed below.

Though there are probably degrees of truth in all viewpoints regarding the advantages and disadvantages of current tapping techniques, Bodymind Healing Psychotherapy (BMHP) prefers, as a first line of treatment, to activate "the energy of the core Self" through a variety of other methods. In addition to the issues listed above, my concern from a psychological viewpoint is that the number of points touched in various algorithms may lead to an obsessive dependence on points rather than on the "real Self" to produce change.

QIGONG AND TAPPING

As an ancient sacred wisdom tradition, Qigong has much to add to modern discussions on touch and tapping, because Qigong is a method of cultivating the energy of life through a variety of means—one of which is touch. In addition, since Qigong used various methods of touch and tapping for thousands of years before modern energy psychology took on some of these methods, it is reasonable to think that Qigong might have something to add to our knowledge.[6] See Chapter Six for more discussion on how self-touch of various points on the body is an important part of Bodymind Healing Psychotherapy and Psychospiritual Postural Anthropology in treating anxiety disorders.

Qigong has a wide range of touching and tapping methods. In Master Lam's (1999) book about Yi Chuan healing (my home Qigong tradition), he discusses touch in relationship to the different elements—fire, earth, metal, water, and wood. To exemplify: in the Yi Chuan system, fire energy presses and withdraws suddenly like a plunger unblocking a drain; earth involves slow circling movements; metal touch flows from surrounding tissues to the place where it is needed (metal is an inward movement like a caravan closing in on itself for protection against hostile outer forces); water energy places the hand over an injured spot and makes sustained vibrations downward, as if sending signals inward to the skin, muscle, and bone; and wood energy moves outward from the center.

So, once a more fully developed paradigm of psychological energy healing is created, we can begin to wonder what conditions will be best served by energy psychology's stimulating touch method of tapping. It makes intuitive sense that it may be best in situations where increased energy is needed; for example, in a case of depression. Whereas, in certain cases of hypertension, tapping touch may be too activating rather than self-soothing.

The wider Chinese medical tradition incorporates Qigong in its range of treatment methods along with acupuncture, herbs, and touch methods, such as *Tui Na* and acupressure. The Chinese tradition often prescribes Qigong movements so that a patient will have self-healing methods to use between sessions and for health maintenance in general. In its broadest definition, *Qigong* means "cultivating the energy of life" and includes self-touch of points in a variety of ways. I remember from an acupressure certification program that my instructors would talk about applying more pressure for deficiency conditions and using softer touch for conditions of excess.[7] As clinicians integrate the verbal/cognitive dimensions of energy psychology into their practices, further research will be needed regarding which type of touch is best suited for different conditions, rather than having a "one-size-fits-all" touch protocol.[8]

While in this early phase of energy psychology's development, it would be beneficial to draw from the empirical tradition of Qigong, and its accumulated wisdom, to find the most healing movements and places to self-touch in order to enhance energy psychology's healing repertoire.

Muscle Testing

Muscle testing is the common way of describing one of the assessment methods of applied kinesiology, first developed by George Goodheart (Frost, 2002), and now it is used by a variety of health professionals, such as chiropractors. The muscle test of applied kinesiology is conducted by having a patient resist a practitioner's applied force to a target muscle. The theory is that organ dysfunctions, allergies, and so forth are accompanied by a weakness in a specific corresponding muscle. Some energy psychologists now use muscle testing to test various aspects of a treatment's effectiveness; that is, whether a given psychological intervention has cleared a psychological issue or negative belief.

Though not all energy psychologists use muscle testing, myself included, there is a body of research that points to the validity (Perot, Meldener, & Gouble, 1991) and reliability (Frese, Brown, & Norton, 1987) of this technique. However, other studies do not support the validity or reliability of muscle testing as a diagnostic test (Haas, Cooperstein, & Peterson, 2007).

Various questions and concerns have been raised about muscle testing as an assessment tool. There is, for instance, a difference in the amount of pressure that is required to test whether an indicator muscle locks following a statement the subject believes to be true, as contrasted with a statement the subject believes to be false. Further, just because a subject believes something to be true does not mean that it is necessarily true. Also, because subtle energies are involved and if the mind influences subtle energies, then the practitioner's and the subject's beliefs, expectations, and hopes must be prevented from skewing the outcome if the test is to be accurate. Firm conclusions cannot be drawn from the research and many of the most-respected energy-oriented practitioners emphasize that energy testing is as much an art as it is a science (Durlacher & Scott, 2002).[9]

Some of those who use muscle testing have raised questions that simple changes in language can affect the test (Monte, Sinnott, Marchese, Kunkel, & Greenson, 1999). Even experienced clinicians report inconsistent results, raise questions about the intentionality of the muscle tester, have concerns about incongruence between the subject's rational and emotional response to some stimulus, and raise issues about how conscious or unconscious "experimental bias" can creep into results and create confounding variables (Durlacher & Scott, 2002; Wiseman & Schliz, 1997). Some energy psychotherapists who use muscle testing use it not as an objective method of assessment, but more like an attunement experience to train the intuition of the therapist and patient.

Borrowing a muscle-testing method used in chiropractic and physical therapies to test and clear muscle and organ imbalances and applying it to psychological clearing has advantages and disadvantages.[10] For high-hypnotizable people (Wikramasekera, 1998), an experienced physical change in muscle strength along with a new cognitive shift helps to support the belief that change has taken place; and because the placebo (belief) effect is so powerful, this may augment the actual creation of change. On the other hand, there are differences in the process of change in a muscle as compared with the change of an embedded psychological issue.

Regardless of the validity of muscle testing, there can be problems taking a procedure well suited to one sphere and transferring it to another. The muscle-testing method originally came from the chiropractic and applied kinesiology professions, and differences exist between the world of musculature and the realm of the psyche. Though a good masseuse or bodyworker may be able to loosen a blocked muscle in a few minutes, many psychological issues take a working-through process over time, a *titration* (moving back and forth into and out of the energy complex) that needs to be tested by the fire of life and worked through in the alchemical chamber of relationship.

Take, for example, a person who has an intense social phobia of approaching members of the opposite sex and has a powerful energy psychology session during which he or she feels an awakened sense of confidence. Just because the person now has a positive muscle test when he or she states the belief of *I have cleared all of the psychological issues that stand in the way of my being fully confident as I walk up to a new person*, it does not mean that belief will stand the test of time. The muscle test confirming such a belief can be misleading and create false expectations.

In the Bodymind Healing Psychotherapy (BMHP) approach to energy psychology we do not use muscle testing due to a variety of reasons. In addition to my not having sufficient training in this method, not being inclined in this clinical direction, and having the aforementioned reservations, I am also concerned that muscle testing can potentially set up transference problems in depth psychotherapy. For example, a patient may develop an expressed or unexpressed trust issue with his or her therapist. The patient may wonder if the therapist is pressing harder because he or she wants a certain outcome. Even if this is not true, the suspicion may influence trust in subsequent therapy. For example, for low hypnotizables (Wickramasekera, 1998) this may be more of a factor than for high hypnotizables. For high hypnotizables it places reliance on an outside agent (the tester) or a body part (a muscle) and takes the patient away from reliance on his or her own emotional core. More research is needed to validate these hypotheses and to determine for whom muscle testing works, and for whom it may create problems in a psychotherapeutic relationship. Some of the transference issues involved with doing ethical energy work in a therapeutic context are addressed in the book *Creating Right Relationships* (Hover-Kramer & Murphy, 2006). BMHP favors using a SUDS scale (subjective units of distress scale) for an objective/subjective measurement of treatment results because it directs the patient to his or her emotional core and it helps to develop the hermeneutic (Warnke, 1987) of exploring inner knowing.

BODYMIND HEALING PSYCHOTHERAPY'S PERSPECTIVE ON MUSCLE TESTING

BMHP prefers, as a first choice in assessment methods, to use the body's felt sense. By allowing words and images to arise from this felt sense and resonating them back to the body to find a fit, the resultant hermeneutical process helps a person to discover an inner knowing and uncover his or her own unique felt meaning of a life issue (Gendlin, 1962; 1978). This seems to be more psychologically congruent with a self-empowering psychotherapeutic process. So many people in our culture have *alexithymia* (difficulty putting feelings into words), or more psychodynamically put, have a problem "differentiating their affects." Thus, when a change does or does not take place after a given psychological intervention, rather than testing a muscle for confirmation, I favor an approach that allows patients to tune in and "inwardly search" (Bugenthal, 1978) for their own new state of being, drawing from the center of themselves. This promotes development of affective states.

A Tai Chi Perspective on Muscle Testing

Finally, because BMHP draws much of its knowledge from the Qigong/Tai Chi traditions and these traditions teach that the primordial Self is most developed when awareness is brought to one's center-line *(axis mundi)*, the training is to de-emphasize putting awareness and emphasis on the muscles. Muscle testing in this regard moves contrary to the Taoist principle of cultivating the center in the belly (Tan Tien) and the center-line. So, we see how the principle of depth psychology concerning developing and putting awareness on one's emotional core is more closely aligned with the Taoist Tai Chi practice of putting awareness on the center of oneself physically and spiritually.

On the other hand, all healers have their own specific tools that work for them—so for those who are inclined to use muscle testing, I hope the above discussion will add to the dialogue as the field explores the issues concerning which techniques are most helpful in facilitating the transformative process for different types of people.

Quick-Fix Mentality

Many energy psychology methods claim instantaneous results (Callahan, 1985; Nims, 2002), or results that are "usually permanent" (Craig & Fowlie, 1997, p. 33). In addition, there are many initial studies lending support to the effectiveness of energy psychology with certain issues, such as anxiety (Andrade & Feinstein, 2004), phobias (Callahan, 1985), trauma (Feinstein, 2006), post-traumatic stress, (Feinstein, 2006a; 2008), and so forth. According to Andrade and Feinstein (2004), energy psychology seems less effective with conditions that have a strong biochemical etiology, such as major endogenous depression, psychosis, bipolar disorders, personality disorders, and dementia.

Generally speaking, BMHP prefers as a working model, the *practice model* versus the *quick-fix model*. It is the experience of most patients and most psychotherapists that although the process of transmutation from psychotherapeutic inner work sometimes moves forward in leaps and bounds and often provides transformative felt shifts, it is more helpful to think of change as an ongoing process. For example, with a case of public-speaking phobia, there are many methods that can bring a person back to the state-specific state of consciousness that was experienced in a transformative moment in therapy. Some of these methods include inner work uncovering psychodynamic roots, working with various cognitive psychotherapy methods, and finding anchors (whether from energy psychology or other hypnotic anchors). However, this most often requires the use of a "re-membering" process when past triggers get reactivated. In this respect it is important to distinguish between psychological first aid and long-term healing (Feinstein, 2006c). Furthermore, pushing the idea of instant cures can lead to shame in those who do not have such positive instantaneous results, and it can lead to false reports to please the therapist, thus resulting in the so-called *halo effect*.

Though it is very fitting with our modern pharmaceutically-oriented culture, where managed care measures cost savings by claims of "instant cures," BMHP asserts that the preoccupation with quick cures are often antithetical to true lasting change and healing that comes over time from the "working through" process. From a Taoist perspective, not trying to change, can activate change.

We need to be circumspect as we look at instant cures in order to determine how much the healing is due to real, lasting change versus a halo effect that occurs through hypnotic induction. For example, in one demonstration of instant cure that I witnessed at a conference, a well-known leader in the field said to a woman reporting change in a major issue, "not only has that changed; but while we changed that, I also affected 1,370 other related issues." Because most people in the audience were caught in that hypnotic, authority-laden group consciousness that often surrounds leaders, no one challenged this authority figure. Unable to believe my ears that the leader was serious, I asked one of his most ardent followers, "Was this leader kidding?" He replied, "Yes, I know, I've tried to get him to tone down that type of thing."

It should be noted that spontaneous remissions and miraculous cures are possible and have been reported at many healing places with a number of legitimate healing modalities, whether it be Lourdes in France, John of God in Brazil, Olga Worral, and so forth (Benor, 1992; Weil, 2004). So, it should not be a surprise that such occurrences could take place through an energy psychology approach.

A variety of issues still need further examination. What creates physical versus psychological cures? What types of psychological issues are most affected by energy psychology, and of those, which are most likely to have a quick healing take place? For example, what is the difference in quick-healing results between using energy psychology methods with core life issues and with a simple phobia? Also, the repeatability of cures is certainly a desired goal at the forefront of a Western scientific paradigm; but in the Einsteinian era of quantum principles, sometimes the healing of one person by a given healer may not be repeatable for another person. This is not a reason to discard the method. The reasons that contribute to an individual's healing are multifaceted, including the power of the so-called placebo effect.

A practice model is inherent in Qigong practice and in the BMHP approach to psychotherapeutic change. In subsequent chapters you will read examples from the last few years of my clinical practice in BMHP that confirm for me that quick, lasting results from some energy psychology and BMHP methods are possible; but as well, I have often found that long-term depth psychotherapy is required to produce lasting change, particularly with core life issues. Toward this end I use the ten levels of BMHP (see Chapter Five), which includes traditional psychotherapeutic methods, energy psychology techniques, Qigong, and symbolic process methodologies.

The Depth of the Energy Psychotherapy Traditions

Certainly those in the energy psychology field are aware that there exists an older tradition of energy psychology. Many energy psychologists make reference to such traditions as Chinese medicine and Hindu Chakra systems. As a matter of fact, another name often used for energy psychologies is *meridian-based psychologies,* thus showing their oriental origins. The common use of acu-points along the meridian systems in energy psychology further indicates its connection with ancient sacred wisdom traditions, like acupuncture.

One intention of this book is to expand the foundation of energy psychology—to root it more firmly in the ancient sacred wisdom traditions that I believe best represent its foundations. Also, in the following chapters, I will show how symbolic process traditions and other tools of depth psychotherapy can add vital ingredients to the healing methods of modern energy psychology and can add to an integral Bodymind Healing Psychotherapy.

Political Problems with the Founder of Modern Energy Psychology

A problem with basing the efficacy of energy psychology on the foundation of Roger Callahan's work is that he has had some political problems with the American Psychological Association (APA), which has had unfortunate effects on the growth of this approach.

One issue is that Callahan claims his Voice Technology method (VT) cures virtually all psychological problems with ninety-eight percent effectiveness (according to a personal communication by Dr. Larry Stoler, past president of the Association of Comprehensive Energy Psychology). In addition, the training in Callahan's VT method is extraordinarily expensive—he charges $100,000. At the current time, the APA is not giving continuing education units (CEUs) for training in energy psychology in part due to its association with Dr. Callahan's work; however, continuing education courses have been approved on a case-by-case basis by the mandatory continuing education accrediting agency for licensed psychologists (MCEP) in California. As the field of energy psychology continues to be broadened and put on a more comprehensive base, and its efficacy is more firmly established, hopefully the APA will reconsider the value of giving CEU's to psychologists who want to learn more about well-founded energy psychology approaches.

One promising new development is that the flagship journal of the APA, *Psychotherapy: Theory, Research, Practice, Training,* has accepted an article from Dr. David Feinstein (2008), called "Energy Psychology: A Review of the Preliminary Evidence." With articles like Dr. Feinstein's getting exposure in the mainstream psychological press, it may be that energy psychology will become more recognized, and more continuing education courses will get approval from various credentialing organizations so that more health professionals can make up their minds about the value of various energy psychology methods. I feel honored that the continuing education courses that I offer, which incorporate elements of energy psychology, have been among those approved by MCEP.

Research Methodology Issues

1. *Generalizability of Results:* Who are the people who do and do not respond to these methods and why? Rossi (2002) wrote:

> Whenever a new and numinous method or psychosocial belief system is introduced, it will usually be able to boast a number of fast converts who will report marvelous results. It is likely that this immediate positive experience comes from highly suggestive five to ten percent of the general populations who have a special talent for mind–body accessibility and healing. Only later, when the larger proportion of the population that does not have such talent complains of lack of success, does the novelty numinosum neurogenesis effect lose its psycho-genomic potency. (p. 194)

In order to examine how generalizable a treatment method is, researchers examine selection biases and dropouts from treatment of people and in studies that report positive effects. For example, are the people from groups where the group energy creates "the weekend effect" (an effect where workshop participants get a transformative experience that does not last)? Are the people for whom the treatment "instantly works" highly susceptible? Or do they tend to cluster in particular personality categories as measured by standard psychological tests? Are the reported successes in groups and in individual sessions from those who are highly hypnotizable? (This could be measured by using one of the standard measuring scales of hypnotic suggestibility[11] with those who report positive results compared with those who drop out of treatment or who do not report success.) All of the above issues relate to the generalizability of energy psychology methods.

Answering Rossi's question is still a work in progress for energy psychology. As time moves on and increasing numbers of patients and ordinary people claim success, the efficacy of energy psychology methods gain credence. Reports of trauma victims in disaster areas who cannot be said to have prior special talents in mind-body healing methods and reports and studies of successful patients drawn from the general public add weight to countering the concern about the generalizability of energy psychology methods.

2. *What are the long-term, lasting results of these methods?* This type of research is called *longitudinal research.*

The Andrade and Feinstein (2004) study is one initially positive indication in support of the maintenance of continued long-term (longitudinal) treatment results for patients in their research. One study of the Emotional Freedom Technique (EFT) examined workshop participants, before and after the workshop, and found a significant decrease (P > 0.0005) in all measures of psychological distress at a six-month follow-up (Rowe, 2005). There are various research methodology issues with studies of this nature; for example, the workshop participants may have been operating under a halo effect, which can create a bias due to a desire to validate one's workshop experience; and groups of this nature may have a selection bias that is not representative of the wider population or clinical population encountered in mental-health practices. In a study by Wells et al. (2003) on the effectiveness of EFT versus abdominal breathing in the treatment of animal phobias, the results indicated that a thirty-minute EFT treatment produced significantly greater improvement, and this improvement was maintained for six to nine months. Though these studies are promising regarding the lasting effects of certain energy psychology methods, further research and replications of these studies are necessary to make definitive conclusions.

Studies from other journals also point in the direction that energy psychology results appear to last over time in some other specific cases; for example, in cases of acrophobia (Carbonell, 1997), blood injection injury phobia (Darby, 2001), and trauma (Diepold & Goldstein, 2000). Swingle et al. (2000b) reported results of two treatments of EFT for PTSD symptoms and found significant positive changes in brain waves and stress symptoms at a three-month follow-up. For more on issues involving research, see Gallo's (2004) review of some of this literature (Gallo forthrightly acknowledges that these studies are not from peer-reviewed literature and are lacking in sufficient research design). In fairness, it should be mentioned that a double standard is being applied when a short-lasting treatment is expected to produce long-lasting results in order for that method to be worthwhile. As Gallo (2004) points out:

> It is interesting that the same level of criticism is not invariably raised when a psycho-pharmacological study demonstrates that a benzodiazepine or a beta-blocker is able to relieve anxiety or deter a phobic response. Follow-up studies would seldom support the effectiveness of the psychotropic in relieving the phobia or anxiety disorder over time, after the agent has been discontinued. Nonetheless, the ability of a treatment to afford even temporary relief is considered acceptable by the medical community and as far as the general public is concerned.

As mentioned above, we need to be mindful of the potential detrimental effects that the expectation of one-time cures can have on patients. A primary concern in the field of psychology is whether such claims may lead to shaming people whom the methods do not work for, or lead to a halo effect through over-reporting positive results. One variable to consider in measuring the success of a treatment is to measure dropouts from treatment. In some energy psychology studies, this is not a reported variable. I suggest that such data be systematically reported in the ongoing evolution of research in the field in order to determine what kinds of people drop out from treatment and for what types of people the treatments work.

3. *Do energy psychology methods seem do meet the test of believability on the face of it?* This is called *face validity;* that is, does this method really measure and produce the changes that it claims?

The experience of most clinicians supports the belief that a working-through process is usually necessary to create change. Although sudden shifts do occur, and transformative experiences do happen in therapy, a compulsion to repeat old patterns ("repetition compulsion") often emerges as old habits reemerge. Thus a method that claims or implies instant results that last without practice over time meets with skepticism concerning its face validity. This does not mean the method is not valid, it just means that the method fights an uphill battle against human experience. Certainly there are times that instant, long-lasting transformation occurs; but the job of research is to examine for what types of people, with what conditions does this change maintain over time with or without continuous application of the treatment methods.

Toward a Comprehensive Energy Psychology: Bodymind Healing Psychotherapy

It is one aim of this book to widen the foundation of the existing field of energy psychology by incorporating a deeper substructure to support the edifice of this emerging field. I propose that integrating Qigong (known to be one of the five branches, or some say, the very roots of Chinese medicine), depth psychotherapy, and symbolic process approaches into energy psychology will contribute to not only the greater field of psychotherapy but also to our current bodymind health crisis (Mayer, 2007).

In the following chapters, you will see how different elements of the bodymind healing traditions can add to the energy psychology tradition in some of these specific ways:

- *Going Beyond Mechanistic Approaches: Experientially Based Anchoring Methods*
  As you will see in Chapter Sixteen, Bodymind Healing Psychotherapy (BMHP) favors, as a first line of treatment, the use of a patients' own gestures at the moment that a felt shift takes place in order to anchor state-specific subpersonalities involved in that change. Though tapping is used in BMHP, an approach is favored that uses points that are metaphorically congruent with meanings known to, and agreed upon, by the patient. For example, if I suggest that a patient tap on his or her chest (acu-point CV-17) to anchor a state of being with the heart, its meaning is clear to the patient. You will be able extract from these case examples how your everyday gestures and points on the body can activate the healing energy of your primordial Self to anchor new life stances to change old entrenched patterns.

- *Emphasizing the Meaning of Points*
  In energy psychology when the patient is instructed to tap on various points, the meaning of those points is not usually discussed in detail. Bodymind Heal-

ing Psychotherapy proposes that "meaning" is a key healing and energy-acti-vating agent, and it is a significant component of activating "the mind-body trance state." For example, you will see in Chapter Sixteen how discussing the meaning of the Karate Chop point, and its association in acupuncture theory with activating the yang meridians associated with the back of the spine, helps a patient to develop a metaphorical "spine." One can think of explicating the meaning of acu-points to patients as a method of further enhancing the placebo effect, thereby potentially increasing the positive ele-ments of hypnotizable effects or simply empowering the patient with a sense of being included as a partner in understanding the deeper meanings of his or her treatment. By including the patient, it helps create a connected under-standing, rather than a disconnected state where only the therapist holds the esoteric knowledge of the deeper meaning of the points. As you are work-ing on your own, you can get a book—such as Michael Gach's *Acupresssure Potent Points* (Bantam, 1990)—to find the meanings of various acu-points on your body to empower your self-exploratory journey, whether you are in psy-chotherapy or not.

- *Adding Breath to Touch*
Diepold (2000) proposes a "touch and breathe" method as an alternative to tapping. This coincides well with the acupressure and Qigong methods of treating conditions of excess. As an addition to this approach, I propose a circle, stop, breathe, and feel method to be incorporated with energy psy-chology, particularly in cases involving conditions of excess—such as high stress and hypertension (particularly with hypertension based in the Chi-nese category of "excess liver Qi rising"). I originally learned the circle, stop, and feel method from Yi Chuan Qigong Master Han Xinyuan, in 1976 as part of our Standing Meditation Qigong training. I introduced it into my own Standing Meditation practice and to my students in the 1980s to help prevent stagnation of Qi. I learned that this method was also part of the touch methods of "polarity therapy" developed by Dr. Randolf Stone, when I was introduced to this method of self-touch by Kozoko Onodera, director of the Polarity Therapy Center of Berkeley in the late 1970s. When I was

trained at the Acupressure Institute of Berkeley in 1990, I found that this was a basic method of acupressure training. From the early 1970s to the mid-1990s, I began to introduce these methods gradually as an adjunct to my psychotherapy and behavioral health practice.

Hidden in the circle, stop, and feel method is an activation of the *wuji* state (defined as the void, the mother of Qi), which is central to the altered state induced by static forms of Qigong practice. In the realm of touch, and in Qigong/Tai Chi practice, the process of stopping after the circling can induce the practitioner into the wuji state, and the circling movement helps to activate the Qi. Whether it is through self-touch or practicing Tai Chi/Qigong, in moving from circling to stillness and back to stillness, the practitioner repeats the cosmogenic creation myth of Tai Chi—moving from "nothing" and stillness to movement, and back to stillness. The beauty of this simple movement is that elaborate conceptualizations are not needed and the movement has the potential to accomplish this wuji state when done properly. If difficulties arise in inducing this altered state, when practicing self-touch or Qigong movements, other aspects of the BMHP methods can be introduced to transmute issues that are in the way.

- *Adding Depth Psychotherapy to Energy Psychology*
The tradition of depth psychotherapy has not been sufficiently incorporated into energy psychologies. In the following chapters, you will see how symbolic process traditions, a key element of depth psychotherapy, can be integrated into energy psychology.

- *Moving Beyond Imagery: The Felt Kinesthetic Sense of the Rivers of Qi.*
In Chapter Four, you will see how BMHP's methods contain ways to combine imaginal traditions with the long-known rivers of Qi in the body through the use of breath and movement.

My Goal

As a presenter at energy psychology conferences, I envision my purpose is to define further the roots of energy psychology as not having derived from any modern researcher, but from the ground of ancient sacred wisdom traditions and depth psychology. The particular roots of the bodymind healing energy psychology tradition that is the subject of this approach are those that are grounded in cross-cultural traditions of postural initiation and various ancient symbolic process traditions, including mythology, alchemy, and astrology. The following chapters will show how a deeper connection between the field of energy psychology and these traditions, particularly Qigong, can help reconnect modern psychology with primordial wisdom and practices that honor our psychological ancestors. Most important, my aim is to help modern people empower themselves with Self-healing tools to alleviate our suffering from the difficulties of modern life, the human condition, and from deep-seated psychological wounds and issues.

CHAPTER THREE

The Ancient Roots
of Energy Psychology

Once upon a time a stream passed through many different kinds of terrain. It had its falls over great cliffs and its twists and turns, but it enjoyed the adventure of traveling alone. It had acquired considerable skills in overcoming barriers, but one day it reached the sands of the desert and found that as fast as it ran into the sand, its waters disappeared. It was in an "existential crisis," suffering from feelings of emptiness, stagnation, dryness, and being cut off from the circle of life.

The stream was convinced that its destiny was to cross the desert, and yet there seemed to be no way. Then a hidden voice from the sands whispered, "The wind crosses the desert, and so can the stream. By hurtling in your own accustomed way you cannot get across. You will either disappear, or at best, you'll become a stagnant marsh." You must allow the wind to carry you over to your destination by allowing yourself to be absorbed in the wind."

This idea was not acceptable to the stream. After all, it had never been absorbed before. It didn't want to lose its individuality. And, once having lost it, how was the stream to know that it could ever be regained? The sands replied, "The wind performs this function. It takes up water, carries it over the desert sands, and then lets it fall again. Falling as rain, the water again becomes a river."

"How can I know that this is true?" "It is so, and if you do not believe it, you cannot become more than a quagmire, and even that could take many, many years; and it certainly is not the same as a stream." "But can

I not remain the same stream that I am today?" "You cannot in either case remain so," the whisper said. "You are called what you are even today because you do not know which part of you is the essential one."

When the stream heard this, certain echoes began to arise in its thoughts. Dimly it remembered a state in which it—or some part of it, had been held in the arms of a wind. With this thought the stream let go for a moment, and lo and behold, it started to rise up. It was scary—as if the essence that it had identified with for a long time was evaporating away. But this awe-filled evaporation process did indeed bring an experience of a deep, long-forgotten part of its identity.

As the stream continued to rise up with a feeling of elation, memories of its long journey alone began to coalesce. The stream remembered how it had fallen from its home in the clouds after early wounding in its life, and had withdrawn to an isolated life, bound by the banks of the river of duality. With this depressing realization it noticed its form change into a dark cloud. Remembering all the time spent lost from its connection with all things, the stream felt very sad.

With this awareness, tears started to roll down its face. It noticed that the tears fell in the form of rain, down to the sands below, beginning the process of watering new seeds, which would eventually grow into flowers.

The stream realized that the cycle of its journey had not been meaningless. It appreciated the cycle of creation and learned something from every part of it. At this moment the stream was filled with electricity as it appreciated the cycle of aloneness and togetherness, merging and separating. Lightning and thunder filled the heavens as the stream felt the wholeness of its essential nature.

—Michael Mayer
Adapted from "The Stream and the Sands" in *Tales of the Dervishes* by Idries Shah

The Age-Old, Broader Traditions of Energy Psychology

There are a broad, unfathomably deep number of traditions of energy healing and energy psychology that go back to ancient times. Actually, Western medicine is one of the world's only healing traditions that does not utilize these concepts. Due to our mechanistic bias, we seek answers to questions about our health and disease in physical structures, biochemical processes, and atomized parts. In ancient traditions a human being is seen as comprising more than a physical body. In the age-old yogic tradition, for example, the energy of consciousness manifests in successively denser forms, determined by its energetic frequency, culminating in physical tissue (Rama, Ballentine, & Weinstock, 1976).

In Chapter One, I spoke of the inner energy crises in terms of physical depletion in our technologically active, 24-7 culture. Though our media may focus more on the outer energy crises, and the search for sustainable solutions for our depleted fossil reserves, there is an equally insidious inner energy crises of "battle-fatigued soldiers" of the information age and the nineteen million Americans suffering from depressive disorder (Dunn, Trivedi, Kampert, Clark, & Chambliss, 2005) who reach for pills and extra cups of coffee in order to restore depleted internal reserves. The answer to this multifaceted energy crises is not in any one branch of the tree of human knowledge . . . the quest to live a life filled with our vital energy requires a broader and deeper journey into the roots of human culture, and our Selves.

How do we tap into the source of energy that is within us, and all around us, when our vital force is depleted? Over the eons, ancient sacred wisdom traditions have found many ways to activate the energy of life. It is crucial for our health and our lives that we, too, draw from these age-old roots. Just like it takes gas to move a car, so it takes energy to move a stuck or depleted human being to a new place.

Among the age-old traditions that enable the psyche to move to new places are bodymind-oriented traditions, such as methods of postural initiation (Goodman, 1990; Mayer, 2004b)—like yoga (Rama et al., 1976; Shearer, 1982); meditation (LeShan, 1974); sacred forms of dance (Tomio, 1994); methods of self-touch (Gach, 2004); touch by others (Brennan, 1990); and a variety of ancient sacred wisdom traditions stemming from the mystical core of all religions and symbolic process traditions. As these pathways are combined with modern bodymind healing methods, they can join hands to help heal the inner energy crises of modern times. These traditions do more than just help restore energy to the depleted; they are at the core of "healing" in the deepest sense of the word. The earliest energy psychology was created to bring the energies of the life of the individual human soul back into balance. These age-old esoteric psychological traditions believe that many human disorders start in the energies at the archetypal level—from, for example, the human tendencies to hold anger, be frustrated by unfulfilled desires, be anxious about not living up to our own or other's expectations. These traditions believe that disorders manifest in the human mind and are incarnated in our bodies in areas of increasing levels of energetic density, that is, these imbalances then manifest in the musculature and finally the spine. From this perspective, life is looked at as a school for learning how to deal with these issues, and then returning to the source of creation for renewal.

Finding the way to return to the source of creation, and to thereby renew ourselves, has been a central subject in cross-cultural mythology (Eliade, 1965). Each different tradition has its own way of returning to the source of the healing energy of the cosmos. For example, in the Taoist tradition it is believed that prior to creation, the void (or the mother of Qi, *wuji*) existed, from that was born the two (Tai Chi), then the five elements, and from there was born the myriad of things. Therefore, in Taoist practice, when a person gets lost in the myriad of things, he or she repeats the creation myth in reverse and returns through various practices (such as Tai Chi) to the mother of Qi, and is then bathed in the womb of life energy found in static forms of meditation (Mayer, 2004b). In particular, the first and last Tai Chi nonmovement is a static form of meditation, which is meant to lead to the initiate's dissolving into a wuji state. In the Greek tradition, this was called a *catabasis*, meaning a "reverse birth," and was enacted by the initiate being drawn, feet first, into a cave, where a transfiguring underworld journey then took place. For the initiate this catabasis process reportedly included learning to see human souls as stars, waiting for a transformative dream before exit was allowed, and recovering laughter (Meier, 1967, pp. 100–112). In cross-cultural shamanic traditions, the "loss of soul" was treated by a shamanic journey (Eliade, 1964; Ingerman, 1991). An important element of many such traditions is how to keep connected to "sacred space" after returning to the "real world." A Native American shaman might keep his eagle feather or a sacred pipe or a shield of his medicine animal as a power object to remind him of his journey to the "other world."

Hypnotic Anchors and Ancient Sacred Wisdom Traditions

And so God says to us, "Make for me a holy place so that I can dwell inside you.

Yes, it is possible to stay connected with me at all times in all places, even as you engage in the life of the world."

—Rabbi Shefa Gold
Commentary from the Old Testament[1]

In modern hypnotherapeutic parlance, *anchors* (Bandler & Grinder, 1979) are used as cues to bring back healing states of consciousness. Think of an anchor as a weighted object dropped by a boat over a hidden treasure; when the anchor is put down and a storm blows the boat off course, the anchor brings the boat back to the desired spot to recover the treasure. In hypnotherapy, an anchor brings a person back to a treasured, "state-specific state of consciousness" (Tart, 1968; Rossi, 1986); this experience can be kinesthetic, visual, auditory, or olfactory (Bandler & Grindler, 1981).

Ancient energy psychology has a treasure-house of such anchoring methods that go back to ancient times, long before hypnotherapy coined the idea. Many centuries before current energy psychology introduced the idea of using humming a song as part of the Nine Gamut process (Craig & Fowlie, 1995) to balance the brain, songs were used in ancient sacred wisdom traditions to heal. Found within the deeper mysteries of the Jewish tradition, there are songs to help heal virtually every psychological malady.[2] For example, one orthodox

Jewish man whom I was working with was suffering from severe negative thinking and resultant depression. Among other aspects of our depth psychotherapy, he found that singing the song "This Too Is for the Good" (*Gam Zeh Tovah*) was helpful in countering negative cognitions when they arose. When he sang this, he experienced a felt shift from a negative constricted feeling into a bodily felt sense of openheartedness.

As I spoke about in the previous chapter, Bodymind Healing Psychotherapy's approach to energy psychology holds a practice model as its basic stance, rather than it holding a one-time fix model. Within this model, both transcendent and transmuting songs have their place. For example, the Jewish song that honors the oneness of all life (*shama*) is used to enter into a transcendent altered state whereby one arises from the differences and oppositional elements of life to "re-member," and get back in touch with the oneness of all creation. On the other hand, as "soul music" teaches us, and other traditions know as well, it is oftentimes most helpful to choose a song that goes into the pain and transmutes it. For example, one female patient, who had just lost a long-term relationship and did not know how she could ever put her life back together again, found herself singing Tom Petty's "I'm Free Falling" in the shower. In conjunction with our longer-term therapy work together, she used this song to identify with everything in the universe that falls, is freed up to create new realities, and survives. This became her anchor when she was in the midst of her deepest pain. It helped to remind her—along with the "cognitive restructuring" we did (see Chapter Five)—that like the seeds of an oak tree falling to the ground, life goes on.

Body-based (kinesthetic) anchors have also been used by a variety of cross-cultural traditions for anchoring altered states. Long before energy psychology used tapping of points to facilitate transformation, Christians tapped their bodies, using the sign of the cross, to anchor their connection with Jesus. Interestingly, the specific points tapped in the sign of the cross (the third-eye point [GV-24.5], the heart [CV-17], and the lung points [LU1]) are sacred energy points according to pagan and oriental traditions. Though Christianity derived the points of its cross from older pagan traditions, it holds these traditions in low regard and oftentimes observers do not complete the lower part of the bodily cross by tapping the belly. Perhaps this is to bring forth the transcendent state of consciousness they wish to emphasize, while eliminating the lower connection with the earth point in the belly. This can be juxtaposed to those traditions, such as the Taoist tradition, that emphasizes tapping on the power center of the belly (Tan Tien); a tradition like this is therefore, in this respect, more aligned with what are commonly described as "God immanent" traditions.[3] God immanent traditions emphasize how the sacred is manifested in all creation—the earth and the body.

In the Jewish tradition *Tefillin*—small leather boxes containing the sacred pathway of the Jewish holy book the Torah—are wrapped over key points on the body as prayers are said or sung. The points on the body where the boxes are placed, where knots are tied, and even where the leather thongs are wrapped are key points for healing and opening spiritual states of consciousness (Schram, 2002). For example, the place where the Tefillin box sits on the forehead (Governing Vessel, DU-24) is referred to in acupuncture literature as the Spirit Court, which is said to calm the mind, to balance the spirit, and to treat mental diseases. The place on the occiput where the Tefillin knot is tied is called Wind Mansion (DU-16) in Chinese medical literature and is widely used as a treatment for both concentration and memory and to treat dizziness, stroke, aphasia, and headache. The places where the leather thongs of the Tefillin are wrapped create pressure at key acupressure points, such as the point on the wrist called Ghost Heart (Lu-9)—in acupuncture literature, this point is recommended to treat agitation and is reported to be calming to the mind. Dr. Schram (2002), a researcher who is familiar with both acupuncture and Tefillin wrapping says, "regardless of the belief system behind the procedure, it seems clear that putting on Tefillin is a unique way of stimulating a very precise set of acupuncture points that appears designed to clear the mind and harmonize the spirit" (p. 8).

In ancient sacred wisdom traditions, not only are specific ways of sensing the body used to activate and anchor altered states, but so are auditory and visual representational systems used for such purposes. In these traditions, one of the key ways that the energies of the lost soul were brought back into balance was through listening to a story, visualizing its landscape, and identifying with its characters.

The most primordial imaginal method of introducing new states of consciousness and balancing our human psyches is found in the process of dreaming. Almost every night, built into the human organism, our inner dream weaver tells us a story that has the potential to bring us back into balance, if only we can assimilate the message being sent. Thus, it says in the Talmud (the Jewish interpretive text of the Old Testament) that "a dream left not interpreted is like a letter left unopened." A key element of depth psychotherapy is to help a person interpret these messages from the unconscious (Freud, 1899; Jung, 1974; Hillman, 1975; Gendlin, 1986) and use the images in the dreams to anchor new ways of being.

As you will see, symbolic process methods and imaginal traditions are like waking dreams (Watkins, 1984) that can help a person change his or her life stance. From a hypnotherapeutic viewpoint, these are primarily visual anchoring methods that bring a person to state-specific states of consciousness associated with new states of awareness.

Depth Psychology, Ancient Sacred Wisdom Traditions, and Energy Psychology

The term *depth psychology* was initially coined by the Zurich psychiatrist Eugen Bleuler (*Tiefenpsychologie*) "in order to indicate that Freudian psychology was concerned with the deeper regions or hinterland of the psyche also called the unconscious. Freud himself was content just to name his method of investigation . . . psychoanalysis" (Jung, 1953, p. 259). Whereas, Bleuler wanted to shift attention from taking things apart to seeing them in depth, and to establish a different ground that was less scientific and more metaphysically philosophical; and he proposed *depth psychology* as the "appropriate" name for psychoanalysis (Hillman, 1979, p. 24).

Bleuler's different ground was not a new ground. Modern psychology is replete with incidents of taking concepts from older traditions and insufficiently honoring their historical roots; that is, in academia it is said that psychology was founded by Wilhelm Wundt in his laboratory in Leipzig, Germany; and it is said that energy psychology was founded by Roger Callahan. But as you will see, modern psychology and energy psychology derived from older traditions. Similarly, depth psychology had roots in an older tradition first tapped upon by Greek philosopher Heraclitus, who brought together psyche, logos, and bathos (depth). With Heraclitus, the image of depth was designed to throw light on the outstanding trait of the soul and its realm (Snell, 1969). Heraclitus's famous quote of "You could not find the ends of the soul, though you traveled every way, so deep is its logos," led those who followed this path of psyche to the realm of symbols and mythology. Freud, as one who followed this path, took many of his early core concepts from mythology—for example, his well-known Oedipus complex, and the death principle of *Thanatos*. Jungian analysts are the theorists best known for tapping on this older tradition of "soul making" (Hillman, 1975, p. 67) by taking psychology down into the underworld realm of Hades more than into the transcendent upper realms symbolized by Zeus (Hillman, 1979b, p. 27). Many Jungian analysts, along with other therapists from different backgrounds, use symbols, imaginal methods, and stories as their key tools to gain access to these depths.

The depth psychologist often uses storytelling from the treasure-house of symbolic process traditions to open a patient to new awareness. For example, using the last mystery play of the ancient world, *Amor and Psyche* (Neumann, 1956), the therapist might mention how a woman needs to learn to say no as did the character Psyche, when the lost souls in the river Styx begged her to give up the coin she needed for the ferryman, Charon. Thus Psyche could complete her journey to and back from the underworld. Or for a man with similar problems with boundaries, the therapist might refer to *The Odyssey* (Houston, 1992) and how Odysseus wisely put wax into his ears and tied himself to the mast of his ship, whereas the sirens' songs drew his men to jump off the ship to their death onto jagged rocks. Symbolic stories enable sensitive listeners to transform old, deeply rooted patterns and shift their energetic state.

A wealth of symbolic process and imaginal practices can be found in so-called mystery religions, initiatory traditions (Campbell, 1978; Hall, 1988; Kingsley, 1999; Steiner, 1973; Matthews & Matthews, 1986), and as part of cross-cultural mythologies (Neumann, 1954; Eliade, 1964). Symbolic process healing methods were a fundamental part of the earliest prereligion called *shamanism* (Eliade, 1964; Campbell, 1988) and were part of the repertoire of the world's religious leaders (Schure, 1977). Metaphors deriving from chemical/metallurgic processes (Edinger, 1985; Eliade, 1956) or from celestial bodies (Rudhyar, 1970; Mayer, 1984) were used to help individuals see how their own transformative processes could be aided by connecting with the symbolic energies of the wider whole of which we are a part. These symbolic process traditions formed the early foundation of modern depth psychology (Jung, 1957–1970; Hillman, 1975; Meier, 1967). Additionally, these traditions showed that the link between symbol and transformative energy was part of this foundation.

You may be asking yourself why there is all this talk about symbols in a book on energy psychology. For those who doubt the connection between symbol and energy, remember that Dr. Jung defined an archetypal symbol as an "energy potential." With his psychology defined as a depth psychology, and an archetype defined by Dr. Jung as an "energy potential," this energy-oriented approach to symbols lays the foundation for an untapped, depth energy psychology. And Qigong can supply some of the keystones and building blocks....

Qigong and Creative Visualization: Anchoring Healing Altered States

Long protected by the Great Wall of China, Qigong is one of the oldest among these intact traditions that delineates a wide spectrum of methods for energy healing. My viewpoint is that one main purpose of these traditions is to aid in the process of anchoring with state-specific, sacred altered states of consciousness. The postures and movements of Qigong and Tai Chi that are proposed in this book offer both body-based and visual ways of anchoring these primordial states of consciousness to individuals in need of a new life stance.

Many ancient sacred wisdom traditions provide transpersonal anchors to help connect people to specific healing states, which I like to call *transpersonal state-specific states of consciousness*. I use the term *transpersonal*—as did Dane Rudhyar, one of the first people to use this term in 1930—to refer to the movement of divine energies "beyond" the ego, but also to refer to a descent of spiritual energy "through" the person (Rudhyar, 1975, p. 38). For example, Hebrew letters in the

Kabbalah are taught to denote transpersonal state-specific states of consciousness (Suares, 1973; 1976) as represented by particular sounds (that is, *B* denotes a grounded state corresponding to the number *2*, whereas *M* brings forth a more soothing melodic state); particular yoga postures bring forth openings to specific healing states; and similarly, each Tai Chi/Qigong posture represents a transpersonal state-specific state of consciousness that can bring people into an altered stated beyond their everyday life stance. As well, the Tai Chi/Qigong postures can bring on specific needed healing states. For instance, the Bear Walking posture evokes a state of grounded power (Mayer, 2004b, pp. 126–129).

Those who practice Standing Meditation Qigong *(Zhan Zhuang)* in postures, such as Standing like a Tree (illustrated in Chapter Twenty-one), have a method whereby "rootedness" can be cultivated. In the approach to energy psychology that follows, you will see how specific Standing Meditation Qigong practices can be adapted to "treat" different bodymind psychological states in our everyday lives.

Typically in Standing Mediation Qigong practitioners are advised to stand with their weight over the Bubbling Well points (K-1), located slightly forward of the center of the ball of the foot. But there are also "prescriptive" methods to help initiates "shape-shift" into stances that can be helpful to balance specific, off-centered aspects of their way of being. For example, for the practitioner who is overly aggressive, the sifu may suggest that he or she adapts to bring the center-line a bit further back; if someone is held back in his or her way of being, the sifu may suggest that he or she shift his or her awareness more forward. We can all, with greater awareness of our postures and stances, experiment with shifting our stances and our energetic states in our everyday life.

Tai Chi/Qigong: A Rosetta Stone of State-Specific, Healing Altered States

Just as the Rosetta Stone, discovered in 1799, gave us access to the ancient realm of Egyptian language and ways of seeing the world, Tai Chi/Qigong is a "Rosetta Stone" that provides us access into the healing, altered states of consciousness of ancient Taoist/Buddhist/shamanic traditions of postural initiation.

Similarly, we can think of each Tai Chi/Qigong posture as part of a healing alphabet. Alphabets contain the keys to open state-specific domains of experience. The English alphabet opens a different domain of experiencing the world as compared to the Egyptian hieroglyphics or the Hebrew alphabet (Suares, 1973). Right-brain alphabets open another kind of state-specific realm; rock and roll music opens a different domain from Indian ragas. Likewise, each posture in the "alphabet" of Tai Chi/Qigong can form and induce different transpersonal state-specific states of consciousness. As the right-brain language of music can help us attune to and play with these specific healing, soothing universal vibrational frequencies and rhythms, so can Tai Chi/Qigong.

Those who practice Tai Chi Chuan for many years may discover how each Tai Chi posture has four different levels of healing purpose: healing, spiritual unfoldment, self-defense, and shape-shifting your life stance (Mayer, 2004b). Those who are introduced to the two-person, self-development exercises called "push hands" or "joining hands" know that these practices help bring healing, balance, and states of equilibrium to those who are trained in this art. In the Tai Chi "joining hands" practices, which I call "cultivating the Golden Ball" (Mayer, 1994b, pp. 172–180), the initiate learns how to yield to one's partner; flow where there was rigidity; respond with nonreactive no-force to an impinging and assaultive force from another; bounce another off of the sphere of his or her body *(fajing);* and counter his or her instinctual sympathetic nervous system fight, flight, or freeze tendencies. As Master Ha teaches it, we learn how not to collide with and how not to separate from another . . . not a bad practice to transpose metaphorically to everyday life.

One of the greatest secrets of this alphabet is that it is not the letters themselves that contain the greatest treasures of the language but the space between the letters. In music the notes are fundamental, but the silence after the notes is one of the gifts of this language. Likewise in Tai Chi/Qigong, the space between the movements is key—the quality of stillness between the movements and the state of relaxation that one carries into the movement is a fundamental aspect of this right-brain language. Also, the images that are behind the movements (letters) are a fundamental aspect of this language. This "alphabet" of Tai Chi/Qigong postures can be applied to the psychotherapeutic setting, (Mayer, 2007), and it can give energy to our everyday lives.

Imagery: The Missing Element in Qigong's Definition

Life is not measured by the number of breaths we take,
but by the moments that take our breath away.

   —Anonymous

Qigong is usually defined as "work (*gong*) with the energy of life (*Qi*)," and it is associated in popular culture with practices that synchronize movement and breath. In addition, *Qigong* is usually defined as a "...a many-thousand-year-old method of cultivating the energy of life through breath, movement, posture, touch, sound, intention, and awareness." However, this definition leaves out a key element: Qigong also includes the cultivation of the energy of life through imaginal methods. This addition is not a new idea, but it is nevertheless frequently left out in popular conceptions of Qigong. Yet it is a part of most teachers' presentations of Qigong practices.

   In virtually all facets of Qigong, the use of imagery is key. For example, in animal forms of Qigong, practitioners are taught not only to imitate the physical movements of a given animal but to focus their intention on imbibing the spirit of that animal and imagine that they are the animal, while moving and while still. In standing like a tree, one can visualize having roots to develop rootedness, and imagine swaying and circling in the wind to develop flexibility and prevent the stagnation of Qi. The depth of an initiate's practice of developing rootedness is then tested by the master teacher who pushes on the initiate in order to test what he or she has cultivated rootedness *(sili)*, that is, to see if the imaginal has become real. Furthermore, in Taoist Qigong Meditation (often called Taoist Internal Alchemy), static Qigong postures are combined with various visualizations to cultivate energy and to heal the body and mind (Kohn, 1989; 2001; Luk, 1972; 1977). For example, practitioners imagine mixing fire and water to balance the internal elements of their physical and mental states.

   In Qigong, one important addition to modern guided imagery traditions is that visualizations are mixed with somatic practices. For example, practitioners may do more than just think about adding water to the imbalance of excess fire in their body, they may swallow saliva (Luk, 1977); and on the exhalation, imagine and feel the saliva descending to the belly (Tan Tien)—this reduces excess fire and increases parasympathetic nervous system relaxation. In general, Qigong is a buried treasure-house containing ways to bring balance and healing to the human body through visualizations on the elements of life and by providing practitioners with pathways to spiritual unfoldment and to cultivate the energy of life. Practitioners thereby have ways to activate their inner alchemy in the process of learning to become "adepts of the elements."

I believe that imaginal traditions, such as storytelling, myths, and imagery are forms of Qigong and that even when the body is not explicitly mentioned, these traditions help us to cultivate the energy of life.

By combining imaginal traditions and Qigong, a pathway can be opened to find the energy of life that the gods hid in our inner biocomputers at the mythic beginning of time. In this sense Qigong is not only a tradition of working with our breath; but when combined with its imaginal roots, it leads us to moments in life that "take our breath away."

Storytelling as Qigong and Trance-Formation

Regarding the use of storytelling to activate our Self-healing energy, review the old Sufi teaching story "The Stream and the Sands" at the beginning of this chapter. This story is a good example of how storytelling can be a form of Qigong (cultivation of the energy of life). At a moment of existential despair when we are feeling isolated or disconnected from our purpose in life, if we hear a story like this, a "trance" may be induced that helps us remember how we have become constricted by our identification with the narrowing banks of the stream of life or have become separated from others and from the spirit of the universe from whence we came. Maybe the story helps us get in touch with how its part of the experiment of human evolution to feel such separation so that we can manifest the individual destiny of our separate selves. Or maybe it helps us remember that we pay a price when we forget the bigger picture of how we are, in truth, children born from, and for, the wider universe. When we lose sight of these messages, we run into the desert of life. A story like this can open our consciousness to remember our wider selves; and for sensitive listeners, it may bring about a change in our body's energy. So, a "trance-formation" induced by story (Bandler & Grinder, 1981), or by Qigong, can create a "transformation" of our Selves and our vital energy.

A story like this can open us to an experience of oneness with all of life, which is a fundamental purpose of many cross-cultural spiritual traditions. There are many paths that can lead us to this state of oneness. For example:

- Sacred songs are used to enter this state, such as the singing of Jewish *Shama*, which honors and helps us to merge with the oneness of life. In the Kabbalah, this state is called *Ain Soph*—the origin of the energies of the archetypes (*Sefirot*) of creation.

- In esoteric psychology, astrological symbols are used to help us realize how our personal identities are formed from the energies of the universe (Rudhyar, 1970). This may help us reconnect with the wider whole of which we are a part (Mayer, 1984).

- Taoist Qigong physical practices along with accompanying visualizations are meant to activate *wuji*, a return to the void, the mother of Qi.

- The Native American who listens to the creation stories of the tribe and their descent from the animals and forces of nature and experiences the interconnectedness with "all of his or her relations" in life—the trees, four-legged ones, the insects, the earth, and *Wakan-Tanka*, the Great Mystery behind the energy of the universe.

- Buddhist meditation practices facilitate a letting go of the attachment to the individual, isolated ego; and such sayings as *the sky and the palm of his hand are the same in the mind of the Buddha* refer and lead the practitioner to the path to find this state of consciousness.

These are all cross-cultural "dissolving practices," which help the listener to let go of the experience of the separate Self and merge with the source of the energy of life. The story of "The Stream and the Sands" is the Sufi imaginal induction into this energetic state of dissolving into the source of the stream of life, entering into the stream of life, and returning again to its source. This back and forth play of life helps to induce the astute listener into a state-specific state of consciousness that opens up a wider universe of meaning and its energetic manifestations.

Stories, Myths, and Fairy Tales Used to Help Heal Archetypal Issues of the Human Condition

Imaginal traditions contain multifaceted tools for cultivating the energy of life, psychologically and spiritually. In the storytelling and symbolic process traditions listed above, the listener is induced into a transpersonal energy state that can be helpful in expanding his or her spiritual horizons. Other types of storytelling and symbolic process traditions can heal more specific issues, like certain blocked archetypal issues of the human condition, including being different or being narcissistically demanding of attention. In all these cases, it is the bodily energy/image dialectic that is key to healing.

Mythological stories in general (Larsen, 1990; Heuscher, 1974), and the stories of Greek mythology in particular, have been used as methods of transforming our relationship to the archetypal issues of life (Neumann, 1956; Kerenyi, 1951; Barring & Cashford, 1991; Mayer, 1993). I discussed earlier how the stories of *Amor and Psyche* and *The Odyssey* function this way. In more modern times, psychologists like Bruno Bettleheim (1977), with his *Uses of Enchantment*, and hypnotherapists like Milton Erickson (Zeig, 1985) have also used stories to heal archetypal issues of the human condition. Though they did not mention energy per se, as listeners we know that it is fundamental to the experience of hearing a transformative story to feel a shift in energy, along with a shift in consciousness. A basic fact of the deeper dimensions of human experience is that images, myths, and stories activate energy in us, as does physical exercise.

Remember back when you were a child and one of your parents told you a story. As my father read me "The Ugly Duckling," I remember feeling a sense of energy rushing through the core of me for I, too, was different like the ugly duckling, and my differences now had meaning. A sense of strength came into my body where before there was a debilitating sense of doubt about my differences.

When parents tell their whining children the story of "The Boy Who Cried Wolf," a receptive child may put some reins on his or her incessant crying-out for attention. Stories and symbols have the power to transform energetic states, and create new worlds of possibilities. In the Gospel of John in the Bible, the connection between the power of the Word and story is known to be associated with creating new beginnings: "In the beginning was the Word, and the Word was with God, and the Word was God." Likewise, hypnotherapists who are adept in the use of stories know that physiological correlates accompany the opening of consciousness that occurs when a story is heard (Achterberg, 1985); also, they know that this bodymind shift that takes place has the capacity to create new realities (Zeig, 1985; Wallas, 1985).

If while listening to a story, we could use sensitive instruments to examine our neurochemistry, we surely would be able to measure a healing biochemical change. And if we had instruments that were subtle enough to measure our Qi, we might be able to detect a qualitative or quantitative change in our energy state after hearing a meaningful story. This goes along with Oschman's (2000) contention that the whole body is electromagnetically linked through the fascia and connective tissues, in such a way that it forms an undivided energetic matrix.

Expanding the Sphere of Energy Psychology: Qigong, Imaginal Traditions, and Shape-Shifting

...The path to heaven doesn't lie down in flat miles. It's in the imagination with which you perceive this world, and the gestures with which you honor it.

—Mary Oliver
Winter Hours

Milton Erickson (1948/1980), the master hypnotherapist and storyteller, has shown that stories, words, and images create an altered state of consciousness within which the patient can reorganize his or her inner psychological life. He says, "It is this experience of re-associating and reorganizing our own experiential life that eventuates in a cure of bodymind symptoms, not the manifestation of responsive behavior which can, at best, satisfy only the observer." (p. 38)[4]

Those who think the field of energy psychology consists simply of tapping meridians, muscle testing, and so forth are taking too narrow a view of this age-old, multilayered fertile field. It has long been known—at least since the time of the temple of Aesclepius (from the end of the sixth century BC to the end of the fifth century AD)—that energy is key to healing. Energy is not just the energy of our body, but also the energy of the universe. This energy can be activated through a wide variety of methods. Some of these energetic pathways lying in the lower layers of our psychological/archeological dig are physical exercise, tapping, touching, moving like the animals, standing like a tree, self-soothing, loving, dissolving practices, and the power of the energy of symbols and stories to heal.

A carefully chosen image or story has the capacity to shape-shift us into new life pathways, by changing our life stance and opening us to a wider sphere of possibilities than our old entrenched patterns. When hearing the story of "The Boy Who Cried Wolf," the incessantly demanding child may experience a shapeshifting into a more self-contained state. Listening to "The Ugly Duckling," an inadequate, collapsed-chested person who is ashamed of his or her differences may experience his or her bodymind change into a stance of confidence. When hearing the story of "The Stream and the Sands," the alienated person who lacks purpose may begin to be transformed into an energetic state filled with a sense of connection to the wider whole of which he or she is a part. Just like physical stances in the tradition of postural initiation (Goodman, 1990; Mayer, 2004b) can shape-shift us into new life stances, so can images, symbols, and stories.

These age-old shape-shifting traditions have two poles, or two rivers, that become one to the aware observer. One polar end of the continuum uses imagination to heal the soul (Hillman, 1975). Here, by speaking the metaphors of life, the adept of this language uses the elements of life to heal.[5] We have just seen how the seemingly nonenergetic concept of symbols is a significant method of activating energy (as when a story, such as "The Stream and the Sands" is told). At the other end of the continuum are bodily energy traditions rooted in age-old shamanistic practices—for example, the internal martial arts tradition, Qigong, Tai Chi, and Taoist alchemical meditations. These psychophysiological, imaginal healing traditions are cross-cultural and cross-temporal and existed in various forms in such places as Native America, India, Asia, and Greece (Goodman, 1990; Tomio, 1994; Kingsley, 1999; Mayer, 2004b).

One of the first scholars to speak of "the imaginal," and who coined the phrase *imaginal realm,* was the French philosopher Henry Corbin (2001). In his study of Sufi and Persian texts, he discovered that in these literatures there was believed to be a realm that existed above our ordinary three-dimensional consciousness. Students of Corbin's work summarize his view of the imaginal this way:

> While some aspects of the imagination are clearly contrived, these texts suggest that there is also a place in our imaginations where things are "real," in the sense that they are not being "imagined" by someone, but are images that have some kind of integrity or existence on their own. Thus the imagination appears to have two aspects: one intentionally fabricated; the other presents itself to us intact. Corbin used the term "mundus imaginalis" (imaginary realm) to differentiate between the "imaginary" (i.e. something equated with the unreal or with fantasy) and the "imaginal" (i.e. a world that is ontologically as real as the things we see or touch or know intellectually). . . . In Corbin's view—and that of archetypal psychology—the images that come from the mundus imaginalis are a reality in some dimension other than the sensible and intellectual dimensions that we are most familiar with and have been taught to value and respect. (Frenier & Hogan, 2006)

The Physician's Energy Staff: Co-optation and Denigration of Aesclepius

Why have traditions of energy psychology and energy healing not been more incorporated into Western healing and psychotherapy? Though storytelling is commonly used in modern psychotherapy, when stories are told, the energetic component of their ability to heal is not often explicitly recognized. And with body energy practices, they are usually placed out of the realm of psychotherapy or are often viewed with denigration.[6] There are some justifiable, modern reasons for viewing energetic traditions with caution—with some cases of psychotic breaks being caused by the "Primal Scream" type of therapies in the

1970s. But there are more deeply rooted historical reasons for the resistance to incorporating energetic methods into modern psychotherapy and behavioral health care.

The central symbol of Western medicine is the staff of the Greek god of healing, Aesclepius, with a snake winding around it. This image speaks to us in timeless metaphorical language about how, at the core of healing, the movement of energy winds up and around the spine.

Why is the very thing that the staff of Aesclepius symbolizes so ignored and devalued by the medical profession that adopted it? In the fifth century AD, the early Christian emperors, such as Theodosius II, destroyed the Aesclepian temples. When I led two trips to Greece in the 1990s, our group visited various temples in Epidaurus, Acrocorinth, and Athens and saw statues with cut-off arms, legs, and heads scattered all around these temples—the violent remnants of the battle against paganism. The rubble that now lies in place of edifices to Aesclepius, the "god of healing," serves as a potent symbol for the destruction and denigration of ancient holistic methods of healing.

Whether the symbol of Western medicine is on an ambulance or in a doctor's office, when we look at the snake winding up and around a staff, we may not realize that this symbol was co-opted from the temples of ancient Greece. The emerging Western civilization took the symbol because the Asclepiads were revered in the Mediterranean world for their healing abilities—to take the power of that symbol added to the respect of the "new medicine." It would be lopsided to discount some of the scientific advances that have grown since the time of this old, empirically tested approach to healing—such as polio vaccines and many surgical advances including organ-replacement surgery, heart bypass and valve replacement surgeries, sterilization of medical equipment, and so forth. However, we might also wonder what was lost from the old traditions that were co-opted. In our modern culture that looks down on the ways of our ancestors, sometimes a visit to our grandparents yields an archeological treasure-house of valuable knowledge that helps us in the present. Can this ancestral knowledge help us on our quest to find answers to the modern health-care crisis?

The temple of Aesclepius was the first holistic healing center of the Western world, where surgery was performed and a gymnasium was provided for exercising. The central symbol of Aesclepius symbolizes the old tradition of energy healing. Hands-on healing was an integral part of the treatment as shown by the fact that Aesclepius's teacher was Chiron, the derivative of the modern word *chiropractic*. We do not know exactly what Aesclepius's training regimen was; however, we may surmise from Chiron living in a cave and his name being associated with a race of centaurs (half man/half horse) that perhaps he transmitted teachings of animal movements to Aesclepius. As part of the tradition of holistic healing in the temple, an Aesclepian priest would often send a patient to the Dionysian theater as a treatment. There, he or she would put on a mask (*personae*, the origin of our word *person*); this was one of the early derivations of modern psychology's psychodrama. We might also wonder whether animal movements were prescribed as part of the cure; for example, a shy or depressed person may have been told to put on the garb of a lion and act out that part in a play. Some say it that the word *catharsis* derived from this Dionysian theater at the temple of Aesclepius. Honoring the importance of the world of images, dream incubation was a fundamental part of healing here. When a patient had a healing dream, the Aesclepian priest would take this as a sign that a healing had taken place and that it was time for the patient to leave the temple. Thus, Sigmund Freud (1899, 1965) was not the first to use the interpretation of dreams as a key to psychological healing.

The early Christians waged a battle against worship of the old deities, like Aesclepius, in their attempt to promote the belief in one God and Jesus as his only son who had miraculous ability to heal. The Aesclepian temples threatened the belief that Jesus, as son of "the one and only God," was the only one who could bring back people from the dead. But myths of Aesclepius say that he also succeeded in raising the dead, such as Glacous, the son of Theseus. In addition, Aesclepius was also attributed with miraculously restoring eyesight to people who were blind from birth and curing the lame and paralyzed.[7]

Denigration of the snake seems to be built into the myths of our modern Western culture. In the Old Testament, it was the snake that tempted Eve into "original sin." One hypothesis for why the snake was devalued is that it was associated with the sexuality and promiscuity of the old goddess religion. According to Merlin Stone (1976), the snake was vilified to stop the sexual practices of the followers of the goddess religion who mated with men out of wed-lock as they participated in snake-dancing rituals. The Israelites, and the tribe of Levites in particular, wanted to be able to determine the identities of their children, which could not be done if the orgiastic practices of goddesses were followed. Thus, came the establishment of a monogamous religion, centuries of sexual repression, and an ethos that constricted, denied, or transcended the body. Some of the remaining effects of these historical roots are easy to identify, such as women in the Victorian era dressed in corsets. Other factors are subtler and form an unconscious part of our everyday Western culture that is cut off from the body.

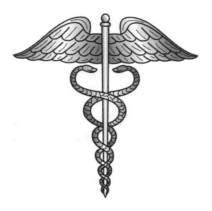

The right way to wholeness is made up . . . of fateful detours and wrong turnings.

It is a "longissima via," a path that unites the opposites in the manner of the guiding caduceus, a path whose labyrinthine twists and turns are not lacking in terrors.

—C.G. Jung
 Psychology and Alchemy

Figure 2. The Double Snake

Modern civilization is living in the karmic rubble of Aesclepius's disjointed body. Our mythos of worshipping one God up in the heavens has disconnected us from the premodern belief in the West and from the Eastern-influenced belief that our feelings and our own body's energy is sacred and needs to be valued in every-day life as "a pearl of great price."[8]

In pre-Christian traditions, images of the snake were associated with healing. Whereas Aesclepius's snake is depicted as a single snake winding around a staff, an even older image of the caduceus of Thoth in Egypt, or Hermes in Greece, shows a double snake winding around a staff. Many meanings are associated with the double snake. Some say that Hermes's healing came from being able to ascend to the heavens, as well as being able to guide others on the path to the underworld (Pedraza, 1977). Because symbols are, by their nature, expansive in nature, no single fixed meaning can be attributed to them; only in the individual process of interpretation can we find their meanings.

The Double Snake: The Mental Image/Body Energy Dialectic

I like to think of the symbol of two snakes winding around a staff, the caduceus of Hermes, as representing two healing powers: the activation of bodily energy and the use of imagery. These have long been known to be important healing powers that wind up the staff, or spine, of ancient healing methods. We can give ourselves poetic license and imagine that the Aesclepian single snake symbol of holistic healing unifies these two snakes of bodily energy and image.

The idea of the interrelatedness of bodily energy and symbolic image is a center post of the psychology of Dr. Carl Jung who said, as mentioned earlier, that symbols are "energy potentials." A key element of Jungian psychotherapy is to get in touch with the power of a symbol, and thereby transform energy, which leads to a change in an old pattern of behavior. From the earlier discussion of "The Stream and the Sands," "The Boy Who Cried Wolf," and "The Ugly Duckling," you have read that image and stories are connected with activating energy and inducing shape-shifting. Toward the end of Dr. Jung's life, he changed his idea that archetypes were psychic, meaning "of the mind," to archetypes being *psychoid*, that is, of the mind and body. It is this conceptual shift that provides the foundation to build a depth-oriented energy psychology.

In Volume VIII of his collected works, Dr. Jung (1960) addresses a key concept of his depth psychology, that archetypal image and instinct represent two ends of a continuum (pp. 211–215). Using the analogy of a spectrum, he spoke of instincts being related to the infrared end of the spectrum of healing, and imagery being related to the ultra-violet end of the healing continuum. In BMHP'S approach to energy psychology the instinctual end of the continuum is represented by the primordial traditions of the body, including Qigong, breath work, and so on. The imaginal dimension of healing comes from symbolic process modalities.

Why bring the body into the equation when our intention, our symbols, and the images themselves have such transformative power? The answer to this question is that there is a difference between visualizing a river and swimming in one; there is a difference between imagining we are exercising and actually moving our bodies. In internal martial arts training, a common combined physical and imaginal practice is to imagine that you are being attacked in order to increase energy and proper alignment of physical postures. Most of us do not need a scientific analysis to differentiate the neurochemical distinctions between just imagining and combining the imagination with a physical practice . . . we can sense the difference.

The question of which should be at the forefront—the mind (intention, symbols, and images) or the body—has been a matter of controversy in the mind-body healing professional community. At one conference I attended, Dr. Larry Dossey was the keynote speaker; and at a banquet with about a hundred tables of leading-edge healing practitioners, he spoke on the theme, following up on several of his articles (Dossey, 1992; 1994), that it is time to go beyond energy psychology and see that "intention" is the key to psychological healing. I raised my hand and somewhat shyly came to the microphone. Thinking about my twenty-five years of training in the Yi Chuan, where I learned the value of integrating intention and energy, I asked, "Is not to split energy and intention a false dichotomy?" I continued, "If the two were not intimately connected why, in the research of Dr. Bernard Grad in his experiment at McGill University (Gerber, 1996, p. 78) with various subjects holding and intending to send healing energy to barley seeds in water, did depressed people (with low energy) suppress plant growth and nondepressed people have significantly better results in facilitating plant growth?"

In a banquet room of about five hundred people, there was dead silence. Dr. Dossey paused while pondering for what felt like a full sixty seconds. He then did something that made me respect him even more than I had before, he said, "I don't know the answer to your question; but I'm gong to think about it." At the next conference where Dr. Dossey and I were both presenting, I ran into him and jokingly reminded him who I was, "Remember me? I'm the heckler they send to harass you and ask impertinent questions at all the conferences." He laughed and invited me to sit with him at dinner. We then discussed issues about the roots of modern bodymind healing, during which time I told him how my practice in Yi Chuan Qigong over the last twenty-five years had led me to the experience of these two streams joining.[9]

As an answer to the questions I posed to Dr. Dossey, the practices in the approach to energy psychology that follows in the next chapter will demonstrate how the two rivers of energy and intention can be better partners in healing. Each of us may find an inclination in our work to focus on one or the other; but like the yin-yang symbol of the Tao, a colored dot of energy is in the half circle of intention, and the opposite colored dot of intention is in the half circle of energy.

The spectrum of symbolic process inner work when combined with the body, involves a continuum that moves from stories/images with no explicit body dimension integrated into their use, to bodily traditions with no use of images. It should be noted that even with no explicit body dimension, the power of story affects the felt experience of the body; and when a person does a somatic practice, the mind is affected.

CHAPTER FOUR

Combining Qigong, Imagery, and Breathwork: Practices to Activate State-Specific Altered States

The symbols of the self arise from the depths of the body.

—Carl Jung

In the prior chapter, you read that the body (and the body's energy) is "in the mind of" imaginal traditions. Similarly, the mind is a vital component in traditions of the body. Not only do words and images have the capacity to put us into trance but also so do postures and movements of the body. Explicitly combining visualization traditions with the age-old knowledge base of Qigong can add to the bodymind's ability to promote psychoenergetic healing.

Following the theme of the wisdom of the story at the beginning of the preceding chapter, "The Stream and the Sands," the practices that follow are age-old methods of initiating us into the experience of being like the stream—letting go, evaporating, and dissolving into the winds of spirit. These practices are oriented to help us return to the energy from whence we came, thereby reclaiming our birthright to remember the experience of what it is like to be "light-er."

Each of the following practices emphasizes a different part of the experience of activating these energies. There are many ways to experience Qi—through activating the power of the mind, through feeling it in our hands, through movement, and through the breath and the relaxation response. In truth, these aspects all operate together; but because of our different proclivities and "representational systems,"[1] different people may have an easier time focusing on one over the other. Each of the following rivers provides a different way to merge into the ocean of Qi (wuji), which the Taoists believe is the source of life's energy.

These practices create trance states, or altered states of consciousness, that can open us to the experience of transcendent energies and thereby facilitate the creative reorganization of the psyche. From the Taoist practitioner's perspective, they provide keys that open the doors to Qi—the domain of state-specific transcendent altered states of consciousness.

House of Five Doors: Bodymind Doors to Opening Energy Trance States

To illustrate the importance of combining the mental/imaginal dimension with the body, and the body with the mental/imaginal dimension, the rest of this chapter outlines various doorways to healing trance states. The five following methods serve as a protointroduction to Bodymind Healing Qigong and illustrate how Qigong (cultivating the energy of life) can be done with or without moving the body. Starting with a breathing practice, there are then four other "doors" that blend image and body, with increasing emphasis on the body:

1. *Activating the River of Life through Microcosmic Orbit Breathing*

2. *Experiencing the Light of Qi: Using a Candle*

3. *Introductory Exercises for Experiencing the Qi: The Energy Ball between Your Hands*

4. *Intention and the Direction of Qi: The Interface between Imagination and Energy*

5. *Rocking Back and Forth to Create a Healing Trance: Tai Chi Ruler*

I. Activating the River of Life through Microcosmic Orbit Breathing:

Microcosmic Orbit Breathing is the method referred to in *The Secret of the Golden Flower* (Wilhelm, 1931, 1963). It was long used in secret Taoist initiatory training to achieve such a deep sense of relaxation that it was reported "to help one return to being like a fetus again." It was claimed that when done properly, this breathing technique could help people regain their youthfulness and vibrancy and that in practicing it, people could experience golden energy radiating from their bodies and become like a golden ball or a golden flower (Wilhelm, 1963).

As you practice this method, be open to notice how it changes the way you experience yourself along with any changes in energy that you feel. The steps of Microcosmic Orbit Breathing (Wilhelm, 1963; Cleary, 1991) are as follows:[2]

- *Begin by focusing on the breath moving up the spine, arising from a point at the bottom of the spine at the perineum, (the Huiyin point between the anus and the genitals). Feel this as a natural rising (as an inflated helium balloon naturally rises up to the sky) rather than as a forced inhalation. Then imagine the breath coming over the top of the head (to the Baihui point), where the lines of the ears meet at the top of the head, the "soft spot" on a baby's head.*

- *While you are doing this practice, the tongue touches the large indentation in the upper palate behind the front teeth, connecting two of the major meridian lines in the body. The one up the back, the Governing Vessel, is called the Du or the Tu Mei; the one going down the front of the spine, the Conception Vessel, is called the Ren or Jen Mei.*

- *On the exhalation, focus on the breath coming down the front of the body until it reaches the belly (Tan Tien) and feel the pause after the out-breath.*

- *The length of the breath that is associated with the cultivation of Qi is called long-breath. To find it, imagine that your exhalation is like a tire that has a slow leak in it and someone is sitting on the tire. This can be differentiated from short-breath that is like a blow out in a tire. Long-breath builds Qi and gives us a grounded yet light feeling. Traditionally, Qigong/Tai Chi teachers will not describe this breathing method, and they tell you to just breath naturally because they want to you to discover this treasure internally, from your own inner work. Long-breath is a natural exhalation through the nose that is not really through the nose; it is more deep and internal, sinking down the front of the spine (Ren channel) to the belly (Tan Tien) in the very core of you. If you force the breath out of your nostrils trying to expel a bug caught there, this will be short-breath. Long-breath is deep, smooth, nonforced, calming, and generates a relaxed force (fongsung); however, though it generates a strong internal force, if you put a feather in front of your nose it would barely move, or it would not move at all. (Long-breath is also an entryway into "reeling silk" practices—one of the secrets of cultivating Qi with Tai Chi movements that are syn-chronized with the breath.)*

- *After the Qi has sunk to the belly (Tan Tien) through your exhalation, a natural pause for a few moments in the cycle of breathing occurs and the movement of the Qi continues down to the perineum. (Some people like to count the length of the exhalation and the pause and notice that the number of both naturally increases as repeated cycles of the Microcosmic Orbit Breathing take place, and that they become increasingly relaxed. As you experience the sinking of the Qi, you will notice the pause after the exhalation will be longer than the pause after the inhalation. It is not helpful to be given a suggested number by your teacher, such as breathe in to a count of five, pause one, breathe out eight, pause five, because then you will try to replicate that externally imposed number rather than find your own natural process of deepening.) From here, the inhalation naturally arises for a new cycle up the cen-ter of the back (Du channel).*

- *If at first you have a hard time feeling the energy, do not try to force it. You might try to imagine it as water by visualizing a waterfall pouring down from over the top of your head, then flowing down your body like a river as you exhale. If you feel blockages hampering the water from moving down the body, do not try to force it through. Instead, continue to breathe and imagine the constriction to be an ice-block that will melt in time by the gentle warming of the waters by the sun. As the breath comes down to the belly, imagine that you are coming to a still pool or a calm sea where you can come to rest. Feel your river expand as it meets and dissolves into the sea.*

In many forms of meditation, breath is a primary object of focus, and images like the sea can aid the experience of meditation. The sea is an apt metaphor for representing the mind: on the surface it tends to be choppy, with waves of thought or emotions taking us in one direction then the next, subject to the whims and rough weather of the outer environment. In meditation in general, and in Microcosmic Orbit Meditation, as you breathe for a while, you may find your jumpiness settling down. Beneath the waves of the sea of life, you find a calmness in the sea deep below. There are still currents deep below the surface of the ocean, but they have a different quality than the ones on the surface.

Discovering or returning to a calm place beneath the crosscurrents of life is one theme shared by many forms of meditation. All forms of meditation induce state-specific states of consciousness (Rossi, 1986; Rossi & Cheek, 1988; Tart, 1968) that have their own unique attributes. What is unique in this Taoist alchemical breathing method is the particular ways in which it combines the focus on the breath, particular body parts, energy, and imagery. Each adds a vital component to the whole, with a multiplicity of purposes:

Specific Healing Attributes of Microcosmic Orbit Breathing

- EXHALATION AND SINKING QI: REVERSING THE SYMPATHETIC NERVOUS SYSTEM'S FIGHT, FLIGHT, OR FREEZE RESPONSES

According to ancient Qigong empirical research, focusing on the out-breath and the pause after the out-breath helps to "sink the Qi." According to modern bodymind health-care practitioners, it is used to reverse sympathetic nervous system overload and induce a parasympathetic nervous system relaxation response. When we are afraid, the instinctive fear response induces us to hold our breath, our energy rises, and energy goes out to our extremities as our bodies get ready for fight or flight. Microcosmic Orbit Breathing can help to reverse the fear response by using a breath that emphasizes letting go, and by focusing on energy traveling down the inner center-line to the belly.

- FOCUS ON THE BELLY

By bringing awareness down to the belly, we return to the center of ourselves, the place where our umbilical cord connected us to our mothers. We thereby metaphorically and organically connect ourselves with the protective center of ourselves. Considered by the Taoists to be the center of the body, the Tan Tien is located approximately three fingers' width beneath the navel and inward toward the center of the body. This zone is also sometimes referred to as the Sea of Elixir *(Qi Hai)*. In *Merriam-Webster's Collegiate Dictionary*, the word *elixir* is defined as "a substance held capable of changing base metals into gold." Regardless of the objective truth of these esoteric claims, many who practice focusing on their bellies while meditating report different types of ideas rising to the surface of awareness about their lives—ideas that seem to come from a deeper place. From a psychological perspective, using a metaphor of changing lead into gold enhances the psychic intention and the state-specific state of consciousness to open such transformational potential.

- ### THE CENTER-LINE OF THE BODY—THE CONCEPTION AND GOVERNING VESSELS

The notion that particular parts of the body or meridian lines have their own inherent power is a supposition of empirically tested Chinese medicine. Some recent research has shown that particular meridian lines activate parts of the brain not activated by sham needles. Such a study using an MRI showed that needles inserted into particular points on the Bladder meridian, not on the bladder, activated parts of the brain associated with the bladder (Cho et al., 1998).

The meridian lines focused upon in Microcosmic Orbit Breathing travel up and down the spine and are known to be among the most important meridian lines. So, we might expect that placing our attention on these meridians may have more impact than other areas of the body on which we could focus.

- ### IMAGINAL METHODS HIDDEN IN MICROCOSMIC ORBIT BREATHING—THE SEA OF ELIXIR, THE GOLDEN FLOWER, THE GOLDEN BALL

Imaginal methods are also used in this classical practice. The practitioner visualizes the breath going up and down the spine and uses descriptive metaphors, like the Sea of Elixir, the Golden Flower, or the Golden Ball. As mentioned earlier, these images may increase one's propensity to enter into an altered a state of consciousness. I have added to the classical method of Microcosmic Orbit Breathing the practice of imagining the exhalation turning into a river and allowing the image of the river to merge with the sea in the belly (see Chapter Five, the River of Life practice).

- ### CIRCULAR BREATHING

The circular breathing pattern of the "microcosmic orbit" makes intuitive sense regarding its healing import. Some breathing methods focus on rapid in-and-out breaths while forcing the breath up the spine, visualizing the breath as a square pattern, or holding the breath after the inhalation. Here, in the Microcosmic Orbit Breathing method, we have a circular breathing pattern that flows up, down, and around the spine. From the perspective of Taoist Qigong, this emphasis on circular, rather than linear or square, facilitates a return to the more primordial and circular realm of womblike existence. It makes sense that this type of breathing would be a good balancing method for a culture like ours, which has the tendency to be linear, square, fast-paced, and oriented to bringing energy straight up to the head.

While presenting a workshop on the East Coast, I heard a radio program during which a breath expert suggested "square breathing." Compare for yourself how you feel with the rounded methods and metaphors of Microcosmic Orbit Breathing and which works best for you.

Microcosmic Orbit Breathing: A Center Post of Bodymind Healing

In many of the chapters that follow, you will learn how you can use Microcosmic Orbit Breathing to deal with various psychophysiological issues, including chronic pain and anxiety. In the next four practices, see how this type of breathing adds to the trance state of combined imaginal and body-oriented methods.

Some support regarding the healing power of Microcosmic Orbit Breathing comes from a preliminary study by Dr. Leonard Lascow (1998), who is doing groundbreaking research in exploring the effects of different states of consciousness and intentionality on tumor cells. In one of his comparative studies of biological responses to different intentions, he discovered that focusing intention on the phrase *return to the natural order and harmony* produced a thirty-nine percent inhibition in tumor cells. The intention of unconditional love neither stimulated nor inhibited cell growth, and Microcosmic Orbit Breathing produced a forty-one percent inhibition (Lascow, 1998, p. 306).

Though Dr. Lascow's experiment showed that Microcosmic Orbit Breathing affected these cells more than other methods did, there are many aspects of the research methodology that were inadequate for substantial claims to be made. For example, we do not know whether in a larger sample of subjects, some people would find different types of breathing to be more or less effective. It would be interesting to expand upon the type of research. Regardless of the comparative scientific merits of each type of breathing for different people in different circumstances, from a purely experiential viewpoint, the specifics attributes of this type of breathing, the particular metaphors used with this method, and the focus on the center-line of the body could intuitively be expected to produce a powerful type of meditative response.

Macrocosmic Orbit Breathing

Macrocosmic Orbit Breathing expands on the breathing method above (Huang, 1974). On the exhalation, instead of going down to the belly (Tan Tien) or the perineum, the practitioner allows the breath to descend all the way to the ground, by experiencing the breath going down through the bottoms of the feet (Kidney-1). From a synthesis of various sources, I developed a practice that further extends the imaginal dimension of this breathing exercise (Luk, 1972; Huang, 1974; Schafer, 1977; Ulansey, 1989). Have you ever, on a starry night, been fixated on the Big (or Little) Dipper, sensing there must be some mystery and magic to its existence that you wish you could draw from? If so, try this method:

> On your next inhalation, imagine the breath going all the way up the spine, out the top of the head (Baihui), to a star above your head; on the exhalation send the breath down to the central core of the earth. Then imagine that you are becoming an axis mundi (Eliade, 1959) as you imagine your spine aligning with the earth's axis and becoming the central axis that unites heaven and earth. As you align with the pole star above your head, picture the rest of the Big Dipper; and on your exhalation, imagine its bowl spilling loving energy from the universe and your heart.

In this practice your bodymind becomes aligned with the macrocosm, the spiritual energies of the wider universe. Once again, in Macrocosmic Orbit Breathing the focus is on the breath; but the imaginal dimension adds to its transpersonal healing power. I like to call this breathing method Full Extension Breathing, due to the breadth of what it encompasses.

2. Experiencing the Light of Qi: Using a Candle

This practice emphasizes the imaginal door to a trance state by using a Qigong exercise with no Qigong movement. Here, we see how the integration of other dimensions—Taoist breathing methods, classical hypnotic types of verbal instructions, a spiritual viewpoint of letting go and being nonattached—all come together to enhance the felt sense of energy as we identify with, and visualize being, a candle. It is classically reported that the experience of activation of Qi is like activating the light of the human energy field.

Sit in a dark room with a candle as your only source of light. Notice your breath coming in and going out through your nostrils. Find a long-breath, as in the previously mentioned practice. Imagine breathing light into your heart on the inhalation and out from your heart on your exhalation. Imagine that you are this candle, and the glow around it is the glow that is around you. Practice this combination of visualization and breathing for about five minutes, or longer if you are so inclined.

Practice with an attitude of doing no-thing, that is, not trying to do anything, not trying to have any experience in particular, but just waiting to experience what arises from being with your breath. If nothing happens, you might imagine that the candle has a living consciousness that knows it will take a long time for you to find the way. You simply have not yet become one with it, and loving and letting go are sometimes difficult for us all to do. The candle has compassion, for it knows from direct experience what it means to have its light extinguished. Maybe it is that awareness of losing and rediscovering light that enables the candle's compassion to fill the dark space of your room with its gentle glow. Though sometimes you have constricted and forgotten to breathe, and the loss of oxygen has made you lose your light, relighting it has always been just a breath away. On one of your exhalations—whether it will be now or tomorrow or even sometime when the candle is not lit—you may let go and remember and experience this again, knowing the eternal candle is always lit and emitting loving kindness, even when you forget that it is there.

Identification is one of the primal psychological mechanisms. Called *imprinting* in the animal kingdom, it can be seen when a young bird instinctually follows and imitates its mother; and if a human appears at a key developmental period, the young bird does the same with that person. In the human kingdom, a young child identifies with his or her parent's behaviors and gradually introjects those ways so that they become integral parts of the Self. We take on the attributes of those who we identify with.

Identification is one of the primary means of creating an altered state of consciousness that promotes healing. It has long been known in cross-cultural shamanic literature that healing is induced by having a person identify with an element of nature with which he or she is out of balance. In Native American shamanic methods of "soul retrieval," the spirit of the eagle is called forth; and through identification with the farthest seeing bird, the spiritually lost individual may be lifted above current life problems and find his or her vision restored in the process. Healing by identification is rooted in the idea set forth in the Upanishads, "By seeing oneself in all beings and all beings in the self, enlightenment is found." According to ancient philosophy, all elements of the universe are contained in the Self, such as fire, water, earth, and air.

Modern hypnotherapists use identification with the elements of nature to create a healing trance state. From the above exercise, you may have experienced the mind's ability to activate the felt experience of the glow of light—the energy called Qi. Is this an illusion? There are many examples of using imagery to heal (Rossi, 1986; Achterberg et al., 1992). In the Simonton Cancer Clinics, the person suffering from cancer identifies with the pictures of the healthy white blood cells (macrophages) that surround and attack the cancer (the T and B cells). This significantly activates the healing response of the body-mind (Lerner, 1994, pp. 163–166). It would be interesting to do a scientifically controlled experiment studying what happens to cancer cells, or to the immune system in general, when one meditates on various different objects of nature, including candlelight.

3. Introductory Exercises for Experiencing Qi: The Energy Ball between Your Hands

While the above exercise emphasized the visual channel to activate Qi, this next static Qigong exercise emphasizes the kinesthetic channel to activate Qi.

Find a comfortable sitting posture. In Taoist Qigong it is often suggested to place both feet flat on the floor and sit on the edge of the chair so that your back is straighter. Sitting in this way is an energetic improvement on the half or full lotus positions where some Qi is blocked in the legs. For three to five minutes, notice your breathing becoming longer and deeper; notice the pause after the out-breath and how your in-breath arises from that pause. Once you feel a state of calmness, with your palms facing each other, place them about six to eight inches apart, in front of your heart, forming an imaginary ball. Remember when you were a child and open to playing games? Pretend that you can feel a magnetic field in your hands. As you try to pull your hands apart, the magnetic field slightly inhibits their expansion. Next, try to press your hands together. Again, imagine that your hands are two, opposite-poled electromagnets that have a hard time coming together.

You may begin to feel the ball of energy that inhibits the hands from coming together, and the electromagnetic force that prevents them from pulling apart. This can happen the first time you try this exercise, or it may take a few days, weeks, or months of practice.

In the tradition of hypnotherapy, the idea of "natural magnetic forces" of our bodies is used for bodymind healing (Rossi & Cheek, 1988, pp. 38–42). Whether we want to think of this sense of energy as real or imagined, the state of consciousness we enter can be used to draw forth our healing resources. In the Taoist tradition, Qi is held to be as real as physical matter.

If while doing the above exercise, you experienced a feeling of energy or relaxation, imagine this feeling spreading through your body as you let go on your exhalation—through your arms; trunk; pelvis; and finally, legs and feet. Eventually you may find that energy will move to a particular part of your body just by thinking about that part of your body and allowing your exhalation to move through it. For example, do the above exercise with your hands on your thighs faceup or facedown. Just focus your intention on one hand and notice what sensations develop in that hand. Maybe you will feel it tingling, growing warmer, more relaxed, or more energized. Eventually you will develop confidence in your mind's ability to focus healing energy.

The hands are a very powerful tool used through the ages to promote healing (Brennan, 1990). In a study reported in *T'ai Chi* magazine, Luke Chan (1995) reports on a Qigong clinic in Zhining, Qinhuangdao Province, China, where Dr. Pang Ming, a Western and traditional medical doctor, combines technology from the West with Eastern healing methods.[3] At his clinic Qigong masters place their hands over, or on, patients who have cancer, while the cancers are viewed on an ultrasound screen (pp. 34–35). Usually in his method of *Chilel* (called *Zhineng Qigong* in China), a wuji state is activated by linking with the love and compassion of the "10 million" fellow practitioners worldwide. This may add to the power of the trance state and perhaps to nonlocal field effects. Chan, one of the best-known teachers of this method, reports witnessing bladder cancer disappear in a matter of minutes while a Qigong teacher worked on a patient; he has a videotape of the process.[4] It will be interesting to see whether such reports will prove valid when put through the scrutiny of modern scientific observers. For now, we can use the reports to add to the activation of a positive mental set. If when we try and do not succeed to activate Qi for our own healing purposes, we need to be careful not to judge ourselves and create constriction in the rivers of our Qi. Instead, we should view our psychospiritual practice as one that involves patience, nonattachment, and an opportunity to explore the healing potential of Qi.

4. Intention and the Direction of Your Qi: The Interface between Imagination and Energy

It has long been known that imagination creates changes in consciousness and the body. Less known is the fact that by combining breath with imagery, the experience of energy and its healing effects can be amplified and directed within the body.

> *As a personal experiment, try using Microcosmic Orbit Breathing and imagine a stream coming down the front of your body as you exhale. Then imagine that the river of breath goes down to your left thumb. Do you notice any different sensations there, such as tingling, warmth, and so on? Then imagine that the river is flowing to your right thumb. Do you notice the sensations shifting to the other thumb?*

For those who have doubts about the ability to focus energy and think it is just a "head trip," it is interesting to note that Dr. Basmajian, a physician and scientist, published an article in *Science* magazine providing evidence that human beings could learn to voluntarily control a single cell (as cited in Achterberg, 1985, p. 199). When very small electrodes that could measure electrical activity of a cell were inserted into a motor nerve cell, and auditory feedback was given to the person when that cell would fire, the person could quickly learn to fire it at will.[5] Though Basmajian's study shows us that there is evidence that human beings can learn to voluntarily control the electrical activity of a single cell, such power should be used cautiously. Be careful not to focus too much on an area that is in need of healing, because there is often already an excess of energy in that place. It is better, as discussed more fully in Chapter Seven (discussion of The Yin-Yang Balancing Method), to focus on the river of Qi that moves through that blocked area than on the spot itself. Trust that the overall energy in your bodymind can in time restore balance; and instead of focusing on the inflamed area, I recommend focusing on the belly (Tan Tien), on the heart, or on the opposite side of the body to promote balance. Most important, remember to try not to use force. And remember that it is not you who is doing the healing; it is the loving energy of the universe that heals you.

When I was told by Sifu Ha to practice Standing Meditation for one hundred hours over a few months, I (as did many other students of this art) began to experiment with my imagination, intention, and the resultant shifts of energy that coincided with these shifts in awareness. This tradition is called the Yi Chuan, which uses the mind or intention to enhance the cultivation of our relationship with the elements of the universe. But we need not immerse ourselves in a Chinese tradition to experiment with such states of awareness. In *Healing with Love* (1998), Dr. Leonard Lascow indicates that he has similarly experimented with how different states of awareness effect healing. For example, he has conducted some initial experiments comparing different state-specific states, such as letting go of desires, focused intention, and Microcosmic Orbit Breathing. His preliminary research, that was cited earlier, showed the ability of Microcosmic Orbit Breathing was able to affect cancer cells (p. 306). And if you should doubt the ability of love to heal, you might want to read the study reporting that rabbits that were touched and shown affection developed less arteriosclerosis than those fed the same poor diet and were not touched and loved (Nerem, 1980).

The important point is not to discover which laboratory experiments work the best in general; but instead, when you need a shift in consciousness, to discover for yourself which practices work best for you. One of the major themes of this book is that when we change our intention we shape-shift into a different state of consciousness, which brings on correlating psychophysiological changes.

Throughout this book you will learn how the combined use of intention, breath, and awareness has created healing results for many of my patients. For example, in Chapter Seven you will read about how the combination of Macrocosmic Orbit Breathing, visualizations, and Qigong were able to help a woman, whose leg had been crushed in a car accident. They eliminated her need for pain medication and reduced and eliminated her pain. Additionally, in Chapter Sixteen, you will review how a woman in psychotherapy was helped to stand up to a dominating, overbearing father by using a Tai Chi stance where she simultaneously set a boundary and also expressed a welcoming intention. Shifts of intention help us to shape-shift and draw from the universal archetypal energies to heal our life issues.

5. Rocking Back and Forth to Create a Healing Trance: Tai Chi Ruler

Finally, bodily oriented Qigong movement exercises have their own state-specific attributes. In the exercise below, not only be aware of how just doing this practice activates a trance state but also notice how adding the particular imaginal exercise enhances the experience of Qi. Along the lines of recent brain research discussed in Chapter Eight, it could be hypothesized that activating the meaning centers of the brain—the amygdala, cingulate cortex, and so forth—adds to the experience of energy and the ability to enhance bodymind healing.

To explore your healing resources, in a standing or sitting position, place your hands around your ball of Qi and begin to rock back and forth, which is illustrated in the Tai Chi Ruler practice, Chapter Twenty-one. The rocking motion activates the healing response, as a mother instinctively knows when she rocks her infant when he or she is upset. Rocking back and forth soothes and heals. Blind people also intuitively do this movement to activate their Qi. Rocking back and forth activates energy by alternately filling and emptying the opposite poles of yin and yang. Magnetic fields and piezoelectric effects are generated this way; and if we are sufficiently relaxed, we will find the magnetic field where yin and yang play, and we will go into trance. To do the moving Qigong movement called Tai Chi Ruler:

> Put your right foot slightly in front of your left foot. The left foot should be at a forty-five-degree angle. Both knees are always bent. As you rock forward onto the right foot, hold the ball of Qi and integrate movement with the exhalation. Make sure your center-line does not go over your right foot. As you rock forward, the ball is relatively close to the body and moves down to the area of the belly. As you rock forward, exhale, and pause. Imagine returning stress or toxic energy to the earth, which welcomes it as fertilizer. As you rock back into your left foot, the ball rises up with your in-breath. The ball rising on the inhalation is farther out from the body than it was on the downward arc of the exhalation. Along with the in-breath, imagine drawing in healing energy from the earth, until your hands, still in the shape of the ball, arrive at the level of the shoulders. The front of your right foot has risen on the in-breath, with the heel still on the ground. If your back foot is at a forty-five-degree angle, you will naturally feel a stretch in your lower back. This area is called the Ming Men, which is an important gateway of vital energy. Continue with your exhalation, moving your hands back downward. Next, for balance, switch the position of the two feet so that the left foot is forward and the right one back.

This exercise is excellent for combining imagination and movement to activate a trance state. Use it to practice healing a particular part of the body. (Remember, as with all exercises, do not to use them as a substitute for medical attention if needed.) These movements form part of a traditional Taoist exercise system called Tai Chi Chih, or Tai Chi Ruler.

The idea of "the ruler" implies that this method is a way to take measure of the day or of our internal universe—to feel the measure of the quality of the ball of energy we carry with ourselves today. We can imagine that we hold the earth itself in our hands. What kind of earth do we want—a peaceful one or an uptight, rushing, anxious one? Through the exercise of Tai Chi Ruler, we practice finding the felt sense we desire, and having "the whole world in our hands."

With a little practice, we may begin to experience the ball rising by itself along with our breath. Hypnotherapists conceptualize such a state as one of arm levitation or hand signaling; and they use such a trance state to promote bodymind healing (Rossi & Cheek, 1988, pp. 39–46). Whether we want to conceptualize this as a trance state or as an experience of Qi, the spiritual technology of ancient Qigong practice may lead us to feel as if we are in a tub of water that goes up to our shoulders. As happens when we are in water, our hands float up to the surface with no muscular action needed. Taoist texts say that this is one of the signs of Qi—a sense of movement that happens by itself, with no effort, like floating up in water. We can create a Taoist hypnotherapeutic healing induction as we rock back and forth in the Tai Chi Chih tradition:

If you just experienced the transformation of the air into water, can you allow the gravitational force of the water to carry your stress or disease downstream to the earth below as your hands move downward, or will it float away up to the sky as you let go and your hands rise upward?

There is a depth of healing potential in this movement. In more advanced training with this method, we discover how when the toe is raised the lower back is slightly pushed back, "filling the hollow." Thus, this practice is a good preventative medicine for lower-back problems. This movement is also a secret method for reversing the normal fight, flight, or freeze response of the body. Normally, when we are attacked, the sympathetic nervous system brings the energy up to the head and extremities as the fear response of the body kicks in. Here, we follow the response upward with our hands as we inhale; but at its peak, we bring the energy down to the lower back (Ming Men). Then we draw the energy downward with our exhalation as we let go. As we discussed in the Microcosmic Orbit Breathing method, we sink our energy to the belly (Tan Tien); but here, the Qi is grounded even more by integrating hand movements and body posture. No wonder this method is being used in trauma trainings by the world-renowned psychiatrist Bessel van der Kolk in his training of trauma therapists.

We should all be armed with the full spectrum of bodymind and symbolic process modalities for the benefit of activating our primordial energies to heal ourselves.

Beyond Qigong as Qigong Movements: Activating the Core Energy of Our Being

All of the Qigong practices in this chapter, whether they involve using imaginal processes or using the body, activate healing energy at the core of our being. When someone thinks about medical Qigong, they may think about many movements with captivating names, like Dragon Rises to the Heavens, Healing the Internal Organs, or Raising and Lowering Qi with Heavenly Palms. But the activation of Qi may be a simpler thing. I remember in one of my medical Qigong trainings, many students, including me, were looking forward to learning loads of new moves from world-renowned medical Qigong Master Sat Chuen Hon. He began the workshop stating that Western medicine focuses on curing disease and that Chinese medicine is not disease-focused. Instead, Chinese medicine focuses on restoring equilibrium to the whole system. He took out a Ping-Pong ball, dented the ball, and then asked the assembled group of health professionals, including Western doctors and nurses, what to do to cure the dent. One person recommended that we poke a tiny hooked needle into the dent to pull it out. Many people offered suggestions while Master Hon made a seemingly unrelated request: "Can someone please get me a cup of tea?" Meanwhile, another medical professional suggested that we take the needle and go into the other side of the Ping-Pong ball to push out the dent that way.

A few moments later, the meaning of Master Hon's request became apparent: he put the Ping-Pong ball into the tea, and the ball expanded back to its original state. He continued his lesson and said, "By surgically operating on the Ping-Pong ball, you may have temporally cured it, but you also may have irreparably damaged it. By increasing heat and using natural elements as a first resort, we can facilitate the healing of the Ping-Pong ball and ourselves." Then he continued with his lecture about how, through cultivating the essence of a human being's vital energy and expanding it from the center, many diseases on the periphery of the body can be healed. He discussed the natural balance of fire/heat and water/cool in the body and how one key principle of healing is how to re-create balance when these forces are in disharmony.

Virtually all Qigong masters would agree that the best way to activate "the Ping-Pong ball" of our life energy is to practice Standing Meditation. As Sifu Fong Ha puts it, "It is Standing Meditation Qigong that best fills our Qi bank accounts."

However, there are many ways to go to the center of our Selves and find our inner heat, and there are many ways to find our ability to cool ourselves down when we are overly active. Qi may certainly come from physical exercises, like Qigong; but the energy of life also comes from the center of our Selves when we are in the state of imagining. Activating our Qi through guided imagery methods can help us transmute blocked mind-body issues as we identify our dysfunctional beliefs and work through the issues that create the "dent in the ball of our lives."

Transcending versus Transmuting Your Psychological Issues

The methods delineated thus far in this chapter have been transcendent methods; that is, they activate healing energy that helps us to rise above life's problems. Some experience this as taking a bath in the source of life's energy, adding weight to the Taoist claim in *The Secret of the Golden Flower* (Wilhelm, 1963) that Microcosmic Orbit Breathing practices lead to an experience of the Sea of Elixir. These methods provide an introduction to the continuum of practices that aid in the cultivation of the transcendent energy of life for body-mind healing. They provide the building blocks for other methods, introduced in subsequent chapters, that are transmuting in nature and enable the specific working through of psychological issues that encumber the free flow of our vital life energy.

CHAPTER FIVE

Bodymind Healing Psychotherapy: The Psychology of Shape-Shifting

The history of science is rich in the example of the fruitfulness of bring-
ing two sets of techniques, two sets of ideas, developed in separate con-
texts for the pursuit of new truth, into touch with one another.

—Robert Oppenheimer
Science and the Common Understanding

A New Origin Myth for Psychology

All things have an origin myth, and this origin myth determines to a large extent the way that each thing is seen ... and its destiny. When we say America was discovered by Columbus, we view our destiny in a different way than when we say America was discovered by Native American peoples. The Columbus myth leads to a justification of manifest destiny ... After all, Americans who believe in manifest destiny have then rationalized that at the very roots of the form-ing this country was the right to expand the territory, just as Spain expanded its territory, in keeping with the will of our founders. On the other hand, if we put Native Americans at the origin of our creation myth, then we will be reminded of how this country needs to make decisions based on how our chil-dren will fare seven generations from now.

The same is true for psychology. When I was in my master's degree pro-gram in the early 1970s, as part of my training to become a psychotherapist, I learned the myth that psychology began in the laboratory of Wilhelm Wundt in Leipzig, Germany, in 1879. This leads to a research orientation toward seeing psychology's purpose. Many psychotherapists learn that psychology began with

Sigmund Freud, and his psychoanalysis. This leads to understanding that the purpose of psychology is "analysis."

There is a magical, incantational, hypnotic power that results from the myth of the origin of any phenomena. That creation myth puts us into a trance.

If we want to expand our horizons about psychology, we can look into the etymology of psychology's origin myth and break out of our induced trance of believing what we have been told that *psyche* means "mind." This narrow view leads to a vision and destiny different than what the Jungian analyst James Hillman (1975) tells us in *Re-visioning Psychology*. He points out that the word *psyche* is derived from the Greek and means "soul," and he and other scholars tell us that the soul is metaphysically comprised of the elements fire, earth, air, and water (p. 127). According to this viewpoint, psychology is not just about the study of mind; it is also about other elements of being, such as fire (the energy of our Selves), earth (grounding our Selves through body methods), air (yes, of course, mental/cognitive methods are important, and so is the breath), and water (feelings are a key, as is developing the ability to modulate appropriately the watery, affective dimension of life). This definition gives us room to expand the narrow range of modern psychology and connect the substance of the Self[1] with ancient sacred wisdom traditions.

What is the origin myth that has become "psychology"? Each different ancient sacred wisdom tradition opens a pathway to a different terrain. A psychology based in the imagination does not take any of these as the true origin. Literalization leads to a myopic psychology that betrays the breadth and depth of the human experience. For example, if we journey upstream to psychology's origins, where astrological language is spoken, in that linguistic terrain a couple's judgment about his or her partner's flakiness might be spoken of in terms of a difference between their differing essences of earth and air. We do not need to "believe in astrology" to speak this way, excite the imagination, and open a door to psychological healing (Mayer, 1984). Or if we saw mythology as psychology's origin, we might use ancient Greek mythology and the art of storytelling as our valued ancestral tools of psychological healing to transform the way people look at their problems (Mayer, 1993). Then when an employee is getting ready to ask for a raise and is frozen in fear, he or she might invoke the image of the Perseus-like quest not to get turned into stone by looking into the face of Medusa (the boss.) The mythic implements that Perseus used might come in handy, such as the reflective shield that Perseus was given by Athena; for indeed reflecting upon what is really so scary can bring wisdom to reverse the fight, flight, or freeze response. Some have suggested that alchemy is psychology's father and that its rich metaphors for the various phases of the metallic and psychological processes for turning lead into gold should be used for the soul's journey of self-healing (Edinger, 1985).

Regarding the origins of energy psychology, the Kabbalah of the Jewish tradition, one of the earliest forms of energy psychology, talked about how the energy of the universe that is expressed in the archetypes of the tree of life comes from *ain soph* (the void, the source of creation, similar to the Chinese concept of wuji). If we looked at the Jewish tradition as the origin of psychology, we might hear songs in addition to talking coming out of therapists offices. Because in the Jewish prayerful *davening* tradition (rocking back and forth while praying), there are songs to help virtually every affliction, such as loss of faith (*Gam Ze Tovah*, meaning "this too is for the good") and being unable to deal with the darkness of life (the original shepherd's song from the Old Testament *Mizmor David* that King David sang, and now from the New Testament verbally incanted as *The Lord Is My Shepherd*). Other Jewish sacred songs help the *davener* to dissolve into the love of the universe and connect with the source of life's energy. Singing chants and songs from ancient sacred wisdom traditions can add to other psychological inner work similar to the way that energy psychology traditions use humming to help heal the modern day psyche.

Likewise, if we go beyond the cultural biases of a Western psychology to find the roots of humanities' interest in transforming the psyche, we would find helpful methods in Buddhism. Buddhism contained a tradition of postural initiation that combined "dissolving" practices and working with the *klesas* (emotional issues) on the path to psychospiritual health (Tomio, 1994). Not just in Buddhism but also traditions of postural initiation and energy healing are part of a worldwide cross-cultural river system of healing the psyche in Greece; Native America; India; and in China, in its tradition of Qigong (Kingsley, 1999; Goodman, 1990; Tomio, 1994; Mayer, 2004b). These traditions can be of aid to our psychological processes. In particular we will see how among the deep, lost rivers of ancient psychological knowledge, the ancient mythologies of shape-shifting contain metaphors for using the imagination to aid the process of psychological transformation.

Combining somatic practices, such as Qigong, with these cross-cultural, shape-shifting healing methods can help us to heal our relationship with our primordial Selves. Just as Dr. Eugene Gendlin takes the essence of what makes therapy work in any system and gives this method to people, we, too, are reformulating the essence of the ancient roots of psychologically transformative practices to help to guide our journey into the broader and deeper ranges of a fertile psychological terrain.

The Marriage of Psychological and Energetic Approaches to Bodymind Healing

Bodymind Healing Psychotherapy can be defined this way: In order to help a patient face the challenges of everyday life, a therapist must be able to weave together psychological theories and healing methods that fit the unique person and moment. Practicing the art of psychotherapy also requires transcending methodologies in order to meet a person in that place of raw humanness where contact is made with the deep source of one's being. In this spirit, Bodymind Healing Psychotherapy draws from traditional forms of psychotherapy, energy psychology, bodymind and symbolic process approaches to healing, hypnosis, psychoneuroimmunological research, and ancient sacred wisdom traditions.

In the previous chapter, you explored how the streams of Qigong and imaginal processes can merge into a bodymind healing Qigong to enhance each tradition's healing effects. In this chapter you will see how Bodymind Healing Qigong (BMHQ) stands as a center post within the terrain of an integrative bodymind healing technology for our everyday lives. We will broaden the imaginal/somatic dialectic to include transmuting as well as transcending methods and then show how a wider range of depth psychotherapeutic methods can make an energy psychology that uses Qigong part of our everyday mode of healing ourselves and bring "soul" to our lives (Hillman, 1975).

The Most Profound Qigong Is Following Your True Life's Path

People say that what we're all seeking is a meaning for life. I don't think that's what we're really seeking. I think that what we're seeking is an experience of being alive, so that our life experiences on the purely physical plane will have resonances within our own innermost being and reality, so that we actually feel the rapture of being alive.

—Joseph Campbell

People usually associate Qigong with those graceful, healing movements you see people doing in the park. But a less well-known truth is that the most profound Qigong, the deepest way to activate the energy of life, is to follow your true life's path, unencumbered by distorted psychological issues. These issues, a natural part of the school of human life, make us notice them when they encumber the flowing river of life in our bodies, minds, and relationships with others. It is these issues that send us on healing journeys for psychospiritual growth, soul making, and finding the source of healing. Qigong, in its narrowly defined sense of using movements synchronized with breath, is just one way to restore balance and energy to our out-of-balance lives.

As discussed earlier, some of the origins of psychological healing can be found in traditions of energy psychology. Hillman (1975, 1976) differentiates *psyche* from the word *pneuma* or spirit, which has a more transcendent meaning. One classical idea about the psyche was that it was considered to be composed of the energies of the elements of the universe, such as fire, earth, air, and water (Rudhyar, 1970; Hillman, 1975, p. 127).

The earliest energy psychology in the West was created to bring the energies of the unique human soul back into balance. This was done through storytelling and the use of other symbolic process (also called imaginal) methods to help change one's way of being and way of seeing the world (Neumann, 1954, 1956; Campbell, 1978; Eliade, 1958, 1964; Edinger, 1985; Rudhyar, 1970; Jung, 1957–1970; Houston, 1992; Hillman, 1975; Kingsley, 1999; Schure, 1977; Steiner, 1973; Mayer, 1984, 1993). I call this imaginal, somatically based, and energetic path, a "'trance-forming' of one's life stance" (Mayer, 2004b).

The Center Post of Bodymind Healing Psychotherapy: The Transcending/Transmuting Dialectic

Call the world if you please the veil of soul-making. Then you will know the purpose of the world. Can't you see how necessary it is to have a world of pains and troubles to school the intelligence and make it soul.

—John Keats

In the prior chapter, you read about Bodymind Healing Qigong symbolic process methods that were transcendent-oriented, and I explained how these methods can activate a healing energy that helps us to rise above life's problems and take a bath in, what may be experienced as, "the source of life's energy." I hope you had an experience like this with Microcosmic Orbit Breathing, imagining you were a candle, holding an energy ball, directing energy with intention, or rocking and visualizing healing energy in the Tai Chi Ruler exercise.

Here, and in the chapters that follow, you will see how "transmuting traditions" can be blended with "transcending traditions" for an integrative mind-body energy psychology. Transcending and transmuting dimensions refer respectively to whether healing methods are used to rise above or to work through a life issue. Modern psychologists have long been trained that by using spiritually transcendent methods, the transmutation of psychological complexes will not occur but will be bypassed and then reappear the next time an associated trigger touches off the complex. It is the viewpoint of BMHP that dichotomizing between transcendent and transmuting needs of the patient in psychotherapy is a function of the Western dualistic mind. Such dichotomization does not do justice to the holistic spirit of healing in the deepest sense of the "perennial philosophy" (Huxley, 1970); nor, as you will see, does it meet the healing needs of an integrative energy psychology.

In his book on psychotherapy and alchemy, Dr. Edinger (1985), the well-respected Jungian analyst, discussed how there is both a time for rising above in the alchemical container of psychotherapy, and a time for descent into the dark places that need to be traveled. The time for rising up to the top of the alchemical container is called *sublimatio*. In the preceding chapter, we saw some methods for rising up in the container of life to feel our unity with the water of life (exemplified by the story of "The Stream and the Sands"). Metaphors, in general, move us to connect with the wider whole of which we are a part; and, as well, they can have both transcendent and transmuting dimensions. There is also a need in depth psychotherapy to transmute the base substances of the psyche. This requires a descent into the *negredo*, the "dark stuff," where the base matter, the "lead," of the psyche is submitted to various alchemical operations and "turned to gold."

Greek mythology can be seen as a coded language, using images of the gods/goddesses and their stories as pathways for describing how to heal the psyche (Hillman, 1975; Kerenyi, 1979; Barring & Cashford, 1991; Mayer, 1993). In this sense we can look at the gods/goddesses of the earth as symbolizing practical ways of dealing with life, divinities of the sky as symbolizing transcendent pathways, and the underworld divinities as transmuting transformative paths. And so it is in psychotherapy—there are times for practical interventions, times for transcending, and times for transmuting.

Bodymind Healing in Everyday Life: A Full-Spectrum Approach to the Image/Body Energy Dialectic

When I was training master's level students in a psychotherapy program in the 1980s, I taught a course called Symbolic Process Approaches to Psychotherapy for five years. In that class, and in the prior chapter, I discussed how I borrowed from Carl Jung's idea of a spectrum of instinctual and symbolic processes. From this I showed how symbolic processes modalities could be integrated with body-oriented practices, such as a Taoist breathing method and Qigong movements. In that course, which later became one of the foundations of BMHP, I delineated these four dimensions of the spectrum of symbolic process work:

1. **Directive or nondirective dimensions:** refers to whether the therapist or the patient comes up with the images.

2. **General or ideographic dimensions:** refers to whether the method is unique to the individual.

3. **Transcending or transmuting dimensions:** refers to whether the symbols are used to rise above or work through a life issue.

4. **Body-oriented or image-focused:** refers to the somatic or imaginal orientation of a healing method.

We can think of the components of these four dimensions of the spectrum of symbolic process methods not as fixed opposites, but rather more like a Taoist yin-yang symbol—with a black dot of yin in the white yang half circle, and the white yang dot in the black yin half circle. A portion of each quality resides in its opposite end of the spectrum. This metaphor can help us realize that these are fluid rather than fixed separate categories. For example, using this kind of Chinese nondualistic thinking, we can see that (1) a directive, therapist-guided symbolic process method often constellates a patient's own spontaneously arising, nondirective imagery; (2) a general archetypal theme can transform an individual's life issue, and an individual's personal imagery may become an archetypal teaching story for others; (3) a transcending tradition—such as a breathing method—may evoke the transmuting of psychological issues, and the transmuting of a long-standing pattern may help one to breathe a relaxed sigh of relief, which can lead to a transcendent state; and (4) body-oriented traditions evoke images, and imaginal traditions evoke affective states in the body.

As we keep in mind the Taoist yin and yang symbol, various types of symbolic process traditions will now be delineated, serving as a heuristic device to be used in a noncategorical way.

The Full Spectrum Symbolic Process Methods of Bodymind Healing Psychotherapy

Bodymind Healing Psychotherapy (BMHP) contains a full-spectrum approach to the continuum of mind-body uses of different symbolic process modalities combined with certain body-based energy practices. The full-spectrum symbolic process approach looks like this:

1. *Fairy tales, myths, and teaching stories from the world's ancient sacred wisdom traditions (Directive, transcendent, general/archetypal, and imaginally oriented)*

   Using fairy tales, myths, and stories to promote psychological healing are powerful tools (Larson, 1990; Bettleheim, 1977; Mayer, 1993). In the previous chapter, I showed how classic fairy tales, like "The Ugly Duckling" or "The Boy Who Cried Wolf," have the power to change consciousness and create an energetic shift. We saw how the teaching stories from the world's sacred wisdom traditions, such as the story of "The Stream of the Sands," are another example of a directive symbolic therapeutic method of psychospiritual healing.

2. *Transpersonal Hypnosis (Directive, ideographic, transmuting, and imaginal)*

   I used this term transpersonal hypnosis in my symbolic process classes in the early 1980s to describe a therapist-directed, storytelling method I developed that was meant to add to the field of hypnosis an emphasis on connecting patients with the wider whole of which they are a part. This method draws upon the elements of nature to facilitate healing and has both imaginal and somatic components. Some of the somatic healing components involve focusing on the breath and constellating bodymind blockages related to life issues by using the River of Life practice. Transpersonal hypnosis uses Dr. Gendlin's body-oriented Focusing method (Gendlin, 1978) to transmute these bodymind blocks by creating a felt shift as healing meanings emerge from the body's felt sense.[2]

   BMHP's method of transpersonal hypnosis is illustrated in Chapter Nine regarding its use in psychotherapy for addictions, and in Chapter Nineteen for working with writer's block and encumbrances to the creative process. In Chapter Nineteen you will see specifically how transpersonal hypnosis uses symbols of the elements of nature to connect us to the healing power of the wider whole of which we are a part. After all, the very definition of symbol derived from the word sym-bolon, which referred to a stick that was divided in half to symbolize and serve as a token receipt of the sale (Edinger, 1972). Just as these sticks were reminders of a greater unity, symbols today help to reconnect us with the wider whole of which we are a part.

3. *Bodymind Healing Qigong Methods (Directive, general, transcending, and body-oriented with imagery)*

In the preceding chapter, I introduced various Bodymind Healing Qigong (BMHQ) methods and showed how they could help to enhance transcendent imaginal traditions. In the following chapters, you will see how many of the practices of BMHQ can enhance behavioral health treatment and depth psychotherapy. Breathing methods, postures, acupressure self-touch, and Tai Chi and Qigong movements, when appropriate, can be incorporated to aid the treatment of anxiety (Chapter Six), chronic pain (Chapter Seven), trauma (Chapter Eight), hypertension (Chapter Eleven), and so on.

4. *Activating the River of Your Life (Directive and nondirective, general and ideographic, transcending and transmuting, and imaginal oriented with use of the body)*

This method will be introduced later in this chapter and is one of the core methods of BMHP. Using a combined directive and nondirective method, the therapist directs the patient to the river of his or her breath and suggests the visualization of a river in the body. But then, unique images arise nondirectively from the patient's unconscious as he or she focuses on body blocks that are in the way of the river's flow. This method combines Taoist Microcosmic Orbit Breath, visualization, and Gendlin's Focusing. It combines transcending and transmuting, directive and nondirective, as well as body and mind.

5. *The Mythic Journey Process (Directive and nondirective, ideographic and general, transmuting, as well as imaginal and incorporating the body)*

This method is a combined directive and nondirective method in which people can create their own stories using imagery and body-oriented tools in order to create a transformation in their life myth and life stance. The Mythic Journey Process helps people create a waking dream as they tap into the creative source of the inner "waking dream-weaver" from where healing images arise. I developed this process in the early 1980s to be a body-oriented, active imagination process (see Chapter Twenty).

6. *Dreams (Nondirective, ideographic, transmuting, and imaginal)*

Finally, dreams are one of the most important parts of symbolic process work. They give us a glimpse into a nondirective approach created by "the master of symbolic process"—our unconscious mind. As used here, *nondirective* is not really accurate because, in fact, we get a glimpse of direction from a transpersonal source. Once we begin to enter into interpretive dialogue with "the genie" in dreams, we may find ourselves in a state of inspired awe, as we question what is meant by the images.[3] Dream interpretation is a significant element of depth psychotherapy and of BMHP. As in the Aesclepian temples, dreams give a sense of when therapy is coming to a close, as you will see in the next chapter with the case of the graphic artist who has a dream of a flower tattoo. Most important, dream images contain transformative energy potential and, in accordance with the thesis of this book, they allow us to shape-shift into other ways of being when we "gestalt" the dream, that is, become its characters. There will be some examples of how dreams play a part in BMHP in the next chapter on anxiety/panic.

Shape-Shifting, Metaphors, and Psychological Transformation

Human beings, in our deepest essences are "shape-shifters." We are elements of creation: fire, earth, metal, water, and wood. We are empty space, as modern physics shows us. Qigong practices show us how to change our life stances by becoming like a tree, or moving like a silk worm reeling silk, transforming our identities with the lightness of Being that can be as colorful as that of a butterfly. And if current research is accurate, when we shape-shift into the appropriate element for the occasion, and return to our primordial Selves, natural health is restored and we live younger longer.

—Michael Mayer, PhD
Secrets to Living Younger Longer: The Self-Healing Path of Qigong, Standing Meditation and Tai Chi

One of the deepest symbolic process methods stemming from cross-cultural mythologies and ancient initiatory paths is *shape-shifting*. This archetypal concept lies at the roots of the earliest "psychology" and uses transfiguring metaphors to describe the process of psychological transformation. Oftentimes the process of transfiguration was expressed in terms of a change from a human form to an animal form. In fairy tales, like "Beauty and the Beast" or the "Frog Prince," the characters were transformed from a human being into another form as a punishment for some transgression; then a loved one came to the rescue to shape-shift the human being back to his human form. In Chinese folklore the Monkey King learns to shape-shift into seventy-two different forms, learns to fly, does battle with demons, and even challenges the gods as he learns lessons about his arrogance (Shepard, 2005). Greek mythology is filled with rich metaphors of such shape-shifting—as when Circe turned intruders on her island into swine, Athena transformed Arachne into a spider for challenging her as a weaver, and Artemis transformed Acteon into a stag for spying on her in her bath. In European legends human beings shape-shift into werewolves and vampires. "Almost every culture around the world has some type of shape-shifting myth" (www.en.wikipedia.org/wiki/shapeshifting). As I have pointed out throughout this book and I have discussed extensively elsewhere (Mayer, 1993), those who see myths with a psychological eye understand that these stories hold keys to using the imagination to aid the process of psychological transformation.

Long before modern clinical hypnosis and Western bodymind healing research existed, there were traditions that helped a person heal by assuming postures of stillness and using the imagination. In shamanic literature shape-shifting into different postural forms is linked to becoming all things—animal and human. In the Pacific Northwest, it is told this way:

A Native American fisherman paddles his kayak into an unknown bay. As he walks, exploring into this untouched new territory, he hears uproarious laughter and cautiously follows the sound until it leads him to the mouth of a cave. After carefully creeping through a great cavern, he sees, gathered around a great roaring fire, animals of all varieties, large and small, playing a game that makes them laugh from the depths of their different souls. The game is "shape-shifting" and they are embodying the postures of different forms, then changing into those forms. The fisherman is in awe as the animals turn into human form, and the human turns into animal forms. (Gore, 1995, p. 14)

This story symbolizes the cave of our everyday lives where we shape-shift from one state of consciousness to another, fueled by the fire of our intention. The power of shape-shifting from one stance to another to break fixated life stances and activate the healing power of "the universe of possibilities," was known in many ancient cultures. In ancient Greece, Epimenides—an initiate of this tradition—was said to have slept in a cave in Crete for years and used "rituals demanding patience, involving watching animals and following them in their movements" (Kingsley, 1999, p. 215). He was called to Athens to heal people from a plague. In Epidaurus in ancient Greece, where Western medicine originated at the world's oldest holistic healing center, shape-shifting into another identity was one of the essential elements of healing rituals. The Aesclepian priest would advise the sick to go to the Dionysian theater. Instructions were given to play a particular part in a play, or to wear a mask so that a new energy would be activated in the psyche of those in need of healing. This was perhaps the origin of modern psychodrama. The masks worn, or *personae*, are the root of our contemporary word *person*. So, by assuming the face and adopting the stance of another person or animal, a pathway to healing could emerge (Papadakis, 1988; Mayer, 2004b).

The ability to shape-shift is considered to be an important part of learning how to play the game of life. In esoteric teachings about the game of chess, for example, the pawn symbolizes the ordinary person attempting to cross the board of life as he or she moves through seven grades of initiation (chakras), usually moving only one step at a time, probing straight ahead (unable to reverse course), sometimes attacking its shadow opponent of an opposite color. But when the pawn has triumphed over the world's ordeals, it has moved through the seven rows (chakras), and it reaches the eighth row, it reaches—in musical terms—the higher stage of *the octave*. Here, paradise is regained and the pawn can transform into any piece on the board that the player wishes (Schneider, 1994, p. 291). Anyone who has played chess knows the rush of energy that comes from having their little piece on the chessboard actualize its transformative potentials as it shape-shifts into a more flexible figurine that can reenter the game with more effective, powerful moves. Similarly, the higher octave of any of our lives is rung when we are able to change our psychological state into the form most suited to the occasion ... discovering a self-assertive way of being when we are unduly inhibited, opening our ears to really listen to another when we are feeling defensive, or finding our central equilibrium when we are going to be overreactive.

So, we do not need to think of shape-shifting as some overly esoteric concept, as something relegated to ancient initiation rituals, or only as part of difficult games. In our everyday life, not just our mental state but our whole bodymind shape-shifts as we embody the vast continuum of ways of being in any sphere. In the sphere of self-esteem, for example, as we shape-shift into various different psychological life stances, our chest expands and contracts in various representative ways. Assume the chest position of arrogance, and your chest will push overly outward. Self-assuredness also expands the chest out, but not as much. Being balanced with regard to the fact that you are the most special person in the universe and at the same time just a piece of dust, may bring your chest into a centered position. Self-denigration leading to a deflated stance can puncture the sphere of open-hearted Self-appreciation; and feeling worthless totally collapses the chest. So, even though throughout this book I will be addressing how shape-shifting can be activated by processes from a wide variety of healing traditions, such as symbolic process methods and various Tai Chi and Qigong postures, shape-shifting and changing your life stance is a natural part of everyday life.

Recent modern research into multiple personality disorder adds to our understanding of how the power of changing our life stance and state of consciousness affects health and healing. It was discovered that a multiple personality diabetic had one or more separate personalities that did not suffer from diabetes (Chopra, 1990, p.122). Allergies present in one personality—for example, allergies to orange juice and cats—were often not present in other ego states.

Research by various doctors shows that in different identity states extraordinary bodily changes take place in visual acuity, in brain-wave patterns, and in slowing down the aging process. This supports the belief by researchers that both dissociative and altered states facilitate healing (Braun, 1983).

Not just in multiple personality states but also in other states of consciousness, many health conditions are associated with "state-specific states of consciousness" (Tart, 1968; Rossi, 1986). When shifting our consciousness, health conditions oftentimes disappear. For example, Milton Erickson once cured a woman from her orange juice allergy by age regressing her to the time of the negative association to orange juice (Rossi, 1986, p 65). As the "state dependent memory hypothesis" (Tart, 1968; Rossi, 1986) and psychoneuroimmunological research evolved, it was shown that when we use the powers of the imagination to enter into an altered state, we can create another reality in which disease and general imbalances of body, mind, and spirit can be healed (Ader & Felton, 1991). For example, it is now common knowledge that by activating the relaxation response and imagining we are someone, something, or somewhere else, the immune response is activated and healing oftentimes occurs. For a taste of this experience, try taking a few slow natural breaths, then imagine you are sitting in a beautiful spot in nature with your back against a tree overlooking a river. As you breathe, feel the changes that come to your Self and body.

Found in the Upanishads, one of the clearest statements ever made about the psychology of shape-shifting alludes to this deeper purpose of the use of metaphor. It reads, "By seeing all beings in yourself, and yourself in all beings, enlightenment is found." Not only do the Hindu gods and goddesses shape-shift into animals and other aspects of nature as part of their evolution, so do we in our self-healing process as we become the elements of our wider nature.

Nature not only represents different aspects of the Self, but we are nature. When we are out of balance with those elements of our primordial Selves, images and metaphors from nature restore our connection to the "Way of things."

Metaphors are a particular use of symbol that creates a likeness between our lives and the wider whole of which we are a part. Metaphors from nature have long been used to help facilitate the healing of the psyche, and they have been used in psychotherapy (Asch, 1955; Mayer, 1977; Wallas, 1985) and in clinical hypnosis (Achterberg, 1985). This process is inherent in the deepest layers of our psyches as they manifest in our dreams. Take the example of a modern psychotherapy patient who during a time of a stressful job relocation dreams of his healthy bonsai tree that survived its transplanting into a bigger pot. Realizing the likeness between his life and the bonsai tree, the patient gets a sense of power to cope with the transplantation going on in his life.

Metaphors give wisdom and healing; but in creating a likeness between our narrow Selves and the wilder whole of which we are a part, much more happens. A fundamental part of the suffering of civilized men and women comes from being out of touch with nature, our nature—and as when we are actually out in nature, an experiential journey takes place as we "re-member" our connection with the elements of our wider nature.

Metaphors help to bridge the gap between civilized people and the world of nature, thereby calling on the wider sphere of nature's healing powers to help us. In Chapter Nine on healing addictions and in Chapter Nineteen in the example of a patient with writer's block, you will see the clinical application of how the elements of nature, imagined and experienced in vivo, can be used to facilitate a transformative healing of blocked life energy.

Shape-shifting is one way to harness the power of metaphor in order to make psychotherapy a deeper, more transformative process. In the West, as in the East, it has been known that shape-shifting is a fundamental part of the path to self-knowledge. In Greek mythology, it is said that Proteus, the old man of the sea, changed his form from a lion to a snake and from a leopard to a tree. When Menelaus needed information from Proteus to find his way home, Menelaus disguised himself as a seal and waited with the rest of Proteus's flock until Proteus returned to his true form, and then he got the information he needed.

Similarly, each of us moves through various forms in our everyday lives; sometimes we feel powerful like a lion or grounded like a tree or as if we are slithering around like a snake. After going through our ups and downs and surfing in the waves of our emotional nature, eventually we may find our true form[4] and our way home. In the following chapters, you will see how specifically body movements and postures, as well as metaphors representing nature, can help the lost soul find its way home.

This power that symbolic processes have as tools comes from the fact that symbols, metaphors, and images precede language and therefore exist at a more primordial level of the psyche. For example, in the Jewish Kabbalistic tradition, Hebrew letters symbolize primordial sounds, each of which has its own inherent meaning (Suares, 1973; 1976). Also, an image of an object invokes a deeper primordial healing realm than does the reified term that represents that object. For example, when someone tells you that you are as strong as a tree, you may thank the person and the message may not go very deep. But if you take a moment to shape-shift into the tree to feel and imagine your roots descending into the earth, you may experience how you are rooted in your family relationships and in connection to your own religious/spiritual path. You may come to see that it is from these roots that you draw your strength, thereby deepening the personal meaning and healing power of the tree. A further step on the path to making the imaginal real is found in the Tai Chi Chuan tradition, in which your teacher, or sifu, tests the power of your visualization of the tree and your stance and pushes you see if you are really rooted.

It is in this light that images, like the tree or the river, are used in the bodymind healing methods that follow. When we create a likeness between ourselves and an object in nature, we may shape-shift into that object, imbibing its needed quality for our healing. Next, you will see how the river in the River of Life practice functions as a shape-shifting metaphor for healing the psyche.

The River of Life

The River of Life (ROL) is a key method used to activate both transcending and transmuting dimensions of our psyche's healing journey; and it will be an essential treatment method used in most of the following chapters, which I use with my patients and anyone can use outside of the sanctum of the psychotherapeutic setting. The imagery and breathing methods of the ROL are oriented to activate the transcendent energy of life and induce a felt experience of the glow of our natural being. But the ROL exercise also contains a transmuting dimension as it directs the river of one's life energy to come up against bodymind blockages, then helps a person to focus on those blocks, and finally uses appropriate aspects of the ten-leveled methods of BMHP (explicated next in this chapter) to transmute those blocks. The "river" in this process is not an intellectual symbol, but rather it evokes the essence of "riverness" as an archetypal force, with all of its inherent power to cleanse, take us on a journey, and more. In the ROL practice, we shape-shift into assuming the attributes of various aspects of a river.

As a metaphor, the river provides many psychotherapeutically useful elements, such as the following:

- a metaphor for the soul's journey through life

- a felt experience of Qi down the front, central meridian (Conception Vessel, *Ren* channel, also called the *Jen Mei* or *Jen Mo*)

- a way to activate blocks in the body and psyche and bring them to the surface, where the underlying issues can be brought to light and undergo a process of transmutation

- a tool to dissolve blocks in the bodymind, restore flow to frozen, stagnant, fixated bodymind issues, and bring forth new healing psychological meanings.

Throughout this book and in the case illustrations, you will see each of these different attributes of the river emphasized at different times depending upon the clinical need. For example, in Chapter Eight in the case of a man suffering from the long-lasting effects of unremembered sexual trauma, the ROL helps to bring those hidden memories to the surface and in conjunction with other aspects of BMHP, helps facilitate a process of transmutation. In Chapter Twenty in the Mythic Journey Process, the ability of the ROL to constellate the soulful experience of a person's life journey is emphasized. The metaphor of, and the experience of, the inner river gives us a powerful tool that integrates psychological and energetic healing powers.

In the prior chapter, I outlined Microcosmic Orbit Breathing and the practice of focusing on the energy up the back (Governing Vessel, *Du* channel, also called the *Tu Mei* or *Tu Mo*) and down the front of the body (Conception Vessel, *Ren*). In BMHP, the use of the metaphor of the river adds to the healing effects of Microcosmic Orbit Breathing.

A river is a powerful hypnotherapeutic image that can constellate the river of one's life experience. By combining the image of the river with a breathing method that activates the primordial central energy channel (Conception and Governing Vessels) of the bodymind, the practitioner is further induced into the experience of the river's "psyche/somatic realness." By using the long-breath, discussed in the preceding chapter, we add to the relaxed flow and cleansing ability of the inner river of energized breath. The tradition of BMHP proposes that adding this central channel breathing method (Microcosmic/Macrocosmic Orbit Breathing) to the process of imagining a river helps us to "re-member" further the river within us.[5]

Interestingly, I recently learned from my colleague Hana Matt, who teaches world religions at various universities, that in the mystical Jewish tradition the linking of the long exhalation with saying various divine names was used to produce psychological change. Abraham Abulafia, a famous Kabbalist who lived in Spain (1240–1290), used a method that is somewhat similar to the River of Life practice that I developed. The experiences that Rabbi Abulafia had were so powerful that he thought he could convert the pope to Judaism, and he set off to Rome to prove his point. Idel reported that Abulafia described one of the processes that he taught as follows:

> The human being is tied in knots of world, time and persona . . . and if one unties the knots in oneself, one may cleave to God. . . . This process is accomplished with the help of repeating the Divine Name on the long deep out-breath. One must link and exchange a name of the unwanted behavior with a Divine Name. The extended slow deep breathing renews one and loosens the tied pattern. And then the use of the Divine Name re-ties the loosened state. By this loosening and re-tying you will strip off your binding constraints . . . and dress yourself in a new form.
>
> —Abraham Abulafia
> *Otsar Eden Gamuz* (As cited in Idel, 1988, p. 135)

In another of Abulafia's writings, called *Hayyei Ha-Olam Ha-Ba*, he said that this repetition of the Divine Name with breathing in a slow deep rhythm is a way to attain spiritual energy and help to "Enter the Spiritual Stream." In addition to using the image of the stream, which is central to BMHP's approach, Abulafia's imagery is also striking when he says that as you draw down the Divine Supernal Force with your breath that "your two nostrils are the chariots which force the female aspect of God (*Shekhinah*) to dwell in you . . . and eighteen long-breaths give you vitality of the soul *(Hai)*." In his book *Minyan* Rabbi Rami Shapiro says that this repetition of the Divine Name used by the Kabbalists helps one to get rid of unwanted thoughts and behaviors, as his or her breath slows and deepens. This practice in Kabbalah is called *gurushin*, meaning "dispelling," and in the Bible this method of quieting the mind and stepping back from unwanted patterns is called *hagah* (Shapiro, 1997).

In light of one of the essential themes of this book regarding the importance of tapping into the ancient roots of psychology, it is interesting that "repetition" of eye movements in EMDR while substituting more truthful or constructive cognitions with unwanted thoughts, and repeating tapping movements or sounds in energy psychology, have similarities to these age-old Kabbalistic practices. Likewise, to dispel unwanted psychological patterns in the practices of Bodymind Healing Psychotherapy, we link the image of the River of Life with the long out-breath, while substituting truthful or constructive cognitions, repeating Qigong movements, or adding the use of other Western and Eastern transformative methods.

Whether you use the methods of EMDR, Bodymind Healing Psychotherapy, or various other forms of energy psychology, if you find these practices of exchanging names and repeating movements, sounds, songs, words, or touch to activate altered states to be so empowering and transforming that you want to let the world know about it, take care not to get inflated from your experience. When Rabbi Abulafia went to Pope Nicholas III, the pope ordered him to be burned at the stake. Fortunately for Rabbi Abulafia, he was instead jailed for a short time because the pope succumbed to a stroke (www.en.wikipedia.org/wiki/Abraham_Abulafia).

In the River of Life practice below, and the way the practice is developed in the following chapters, there are some similarities to the above Kabbalistic practices. Yet you will see how in the ten levels of Bodymind Healing Psychotherapy that there are many other principles for, and ways of, "untying the knots," or melting the ice blocks, in order to "... strip off your binding constraints ... and dress yourself in a new form."

Further, if you think that blending breath with healing words or images is just an esoteric method for premodern times, read what Dr. Herbert Benson, professor of medicine, Harvard Medical School and chief of behavioral medicine at New England Deaconess Hospital says:

> Over the course of time your brain develops certain physical conduits that determine how you habitually think, act, and feel. These conduits are your "wiring." Your wiring can become so fixed as to make changing your behavior nearly impossible. When you try to change a deep-seated habit, your best intentions are not enough. Change is not merely a matter of will. Habitual thoughts, feelings and behaviors become hard-wired into your brain, and you cannot change them until you change the wiring. You have to make a physiological change in the brain's old wiring before you can successfully imprint new wiring. Many studies have shown that periods of deep breathing and repeating the Divine Name on the exhale, bring this about. It makes the brain and nervous system more pliable. This is called "neural plasticity." This deep breathing and repeating the Divine Name releases the hold that the old wiring has on your brain and nervous system and allows you to imprint new neural pathways. This enables you to alter the way you think and act, and you create new and additional connections that can, with repetition, come to dominate the old connections, helping to solidify the new thoughts and behaviors. This practice causes the two hemispheres of your brain to begin to exchange information more freely causing them to function in sync with each other. Then your mind tends to operate more creatively, you process information more effectively and you are capable of understanding things in different ways. This is called "cognitive receptivity." Because you are more receptive to new information and new ways of thinking about old situa-

tions, you are open to alternative ways of handling situations. This allows you to make lasting changes in your mind and behavior. It allows for a more successful re-imprinting of the mind. It rewires the brain with the new behaviors that you want.

—Dr. Herbert Benson
The Maximum Mind (as paraphrased by Hana Matt
    from Benson, 1975a, 1975b, 1984)

The River of Life practice that follows contains a blend of guided imagery, hypnotherapy, a Qigong breathing method, and Gendlin's Focusing (1978). As mentioned earlier, this method combines a directive, transcendent imagery practice with a nondirective, transmuting "focusing" process on the crux of a blocked life issue. The transmuting dimension is further enhanced by combining the River of Life exercise with elements of modern psychotherapy, as is explained in the section following this exercise.

The River of Life Practice:
Healing with the Transcending/Transmuting Dialectic
STEP 1: BREATH: MACROCOSMIC ORBIT AND THE RIVER OF YOUR LIFE:

As your breath comes in, imagine it rising up your back. It rises all the way to the sky. Then as you exhale, feel the breath going down the front of your body. Notice how your exhalation gets longer and longer and deeper and deeper the longer you are aware of your breath. Do not try to force your breath deeper. Then imagine that this out-breath is a river that is traveling down the front of your body. The longer and deeper your breath is, the longer and deeper your inner river is. Focus on the pause at the end of your exhalation, as it brings you to an inner peaceful pool slightly below your belly. After that pause by your inner peaceful pool, the river continues to flow down to the ocean beneath your feet. Then the breath rises again for another cycle up your back.

STEP 2: USING THE BREATH TO CONSTELLATE
BODYMIND BLOCKAGES:

Your life has been a journey down a river that came from the mountains; and it will eventually reach the sea. Right now on your life's journey there may be some issue that is constricting or blocking the flow of the river of your life. On the next downward cycle of your breathing, notice where the river does not flow smoothly in your body and allow an image to arise that represents a block in that place on the river of your life energy. Maybe the encumbrance feels like a boulder or an ice block.

STEP 3: TRANSMUTING BODYMIND BLOCKAGES:

As you sense any block in the river of energy, focus (Gendlin, 1978) *on that body sense and allow a word, image, or phrase to emerge from it as you ask yourself, "What is this all about?" Do not try to think of an answer, allow a response to rise to the surface as if something stuck was being shaken loose from the bottom of a riverbed. Then "resonate" that word, image, or phrase back to the body sense to see if it gets the crux of what that block is about. Once you hit the bull's-eye of meaning, you will often notice a felt shift occur . . . perhaps a sighing breath may release the blockage—a sign that you have found what it is "all about."*

These three steps are just the beginning of the process. In many of the following chapters, you will learn how to build upon this practice in different ways to fit different circumstances. Once the patient's issue is constellated, the next transmuting elements of Bodymind Healing Psychotherapy (BMHP) may be applied. Some of these transmuting methods are cognitive-behavioral therapy, various psychodynamic approaches, energy psychology methods, self-soothing, and various transmuting symbolic process approaches to psychotherapy. (The application of many of these methods are illustrated in Chapter Six.) In its broadest scope, BMHP weaves together transcending and transmuting dimensions to create an integral (Walsh and Shapiro, 2006; Wilber, 2000; Mayer, 2009) healing approach for energy psychology.

Toward a Comprehensive Energy Psychology: The Ten Psychoenergetic Holographic Dimensions of Bodymind Healing Psychotherapy

In addition to imaginal and somatic approaches, Bodymind Healing Psychotherapy also contains an integrative psychological approach to heal the psyche, by bringing back into balance the imbalanced elements of the psyche.

In the following chapters, you will see how BMHP includes Western forms of psychotherapy, including psychodynamic psychotherapies, self-psychology, cognitive-behavioral psychotherapy, and energy psychology. BMHP also includes ancient sacred wisdom traditions including Qigong, in the broadest sense of the word. From the perspective of the wider purpose of this book, we can see the limitation in thinking of Qigong as just a physical exercise to create energy in the body. There are other ways to cultivate our life energy; that is, by working on all psychospiritual facets of ourselves. A person's life stance at a given moment, and the energy that expresses that life stance, does not change through the medium of the body alone. Instead, as proposed in BMHP, healing is best done by integrating the following methods and traditions that address the aforementioned facets of ourselves—body, mind, and spirit.

1. Taoist Breathing Techniques and Hypnosis (most often using the River of Life practice)

2. Self-soothing

3. "Focusing" on Felt Meaning

4. Psychodynamics (working with the psychological forces underlying human experience)

5. Cognitive Restructuring (plus using a body-oriented SUDS scale)

6. Energy Psychology Methods, including Eye Movement Desensitization Reprocessing (EMDR)

7. The Belly Massage of Chi Nei Tsang (Chia & Chia, 1990)

8. Acupressure: Phenomenological Approach and Acu-yoga (Gach & Marco, 1981)

9. Practices from Bodymind Healing Qigong[6]

10. Symbolic Process Approaches to Healing

  (These ten methods are specifically illustrated in Chapter Six.)

Bodymind Healing Psychotherapy (BMHP) is "psychoenergetic" in that it combines elements of modern psychotherapy and hypnosis with ancient Taoist energy-healing methods. The dimensions of this method are "holographic" in that each part actually contains the whole. In order for any one dimension to function properly, the others must be present. In practice, the clinician or individual using this approach moves from one part of the hologram to the other, as needed. While one dimension is being focused upon, the other parts of the whole need to be present. For example, even though Taoist breathing techniques and hypnosis enable us to relax, the underlying psychodynamic patterns that create our tension may not be transformed. Thus, we need to have the psychodynamic dimension present.

As another example, if we merely understand how our fear of having our vulnerability exposed is a psychodynamic issue stemming from our family of origin, but we do not feel a felt shift in our body through a body-oriented technique like Gendlin's Focusing, the insight may not develop deep roots and may be short lived.[7] Also, crucial to psychological healing is the need to cognitively restructure our old entrenched thought forms, such as *I can't trust being vulnerable with anyone*, into new thought forms, like *I choose to be in a world where I can be vulnerable with at least some people*. BMHP adds to cognitive therapy a bodily dimension, as do other therapists (Shapiro, 1995), by using a subjective units of distress scale (SUDS) to make sure the cognition is congruent with the "real self." Additionally, having patients check-in with their bodies serves to ground new beliefs. The energetic dimension catalyzes the whole mix.

It should also be noted that many aspects of current energy psychologies are included within the framework of BMHP, which also includes Bodymind Healing Qigong (BMHQ); and there is also some overlap in some current energy psychologies using methods contained within the framework of BMHP. Meridian tapping is part of Qigong and part of BMHQ. However, tapping fits into a larger framework of self-touch methods; because in Qigong, tapping is looked at as a yang method that increases energy, and in psychotherapy, there are times when relaxing yin methods are more appropriate. Therefore, self-touch methods from acupressure, such as the "circle, stop, feel method" are used to open the energy of meridians along with psychotherapeutic methods. Although at certain times, specific acu-points are chosen by the therapist, BMHP favors an orientation where the patient chooses where to touch him or herself, trusting how the natural, primordial expression of movement and self-touch arises from the unconscious (see Chapter Sixteen). Many energy psychologies use cognitive therapies as their underlying tools; and as mentioned in the example above, just as Shapiro's EMDR (1995) uses a body-based SUDS scale to determine the felt effect of a change in belief, so does BMHP. The Emotional Freedom Technique (EFT) has some excellent bodily and verbal healing methods that are used and adapted to BMHP. For example, as a person says *even though I _____, I can still love and accept myself,* BMHP adds touching the heart (Conception Vessel-17) for self-soothing purposes and touching the belly (Tan Tien) to help further ground in the body the new cognition. The verbal "self-soothing" dimension of such new healing beliefs are central to EFT and psychodynamic theories (Kohut, 1977), and BMHP's self-touch methods can easily be integrated with their treatment protocols. However, the hypnotherapeutic idea of *anchoring* is more favored in BMHP than it is in those energy psychologies that emphasize tapping away problems/fixations; in BMHP there is more emphasis on using touch (holding or tapping), breath, imagery, and posture to ground the new state-specific state of consciousness and new belief that has been activated in the felt sense (Gendlin, 1978) of the bodymind so that patients can carry this new body awareness into their everyday lives with a new life stance.

Qigong and Tai Chi: A Soulful Practice for Bodymind Healing

> *You could not find the ends of the soul though you traveled every way, so deep is its Logos.*
>
> —Heraclitus

Finally, although Qigong is usually associated with a transcendent spiritual path, I suggest adding a "soul-oriented" practice of Qigong and Tai Chi to expand the somatic dimensions of psychological healing. Esoteric psychology says that our souls consist of our unique constellation of the elements, such as fire, earth, air, and water (Rudhyar, 1970; Hillman, 1975, p. 127). Qigong and Tai Chi can aid in the cultivation and healing of the elements of our soulful selves by grounding us (earth), activating our energy (fire), helping us to flow with life (water), and helping us to activate our transcendent states (air).

A "soul-oriented" (Hillman, 1975; Moore, 1992) Qigong and Tai Chi can become a center post for energy psychology practice. While we are practicing Tai Chi and Qigong, instead of solely focusing on transcendent, spiritual aspects induced by these practices, we can focus on the memories, emotions, and images that arise, making it into a "soulful practice." For example, when we are practicing Standing Meditation, oftentimes shaking will spontaneously arise in an area of the body that has been blocked, particularly after we have been practicing for a good amount of time. Instead of just appreciating the process of release, we can ask ourselves *which of my life issues am I now releasing?* Then as the body is shaking, we can appreciate the issue that is being released; and we can practice cognitive restructuring, as we say our truthful or constructive new belief. For instance, a perfectionistic person might say while his or her leg is shaking *I'm letting go of my life-long stance of being self-judgmental and fearing rejection.* When the shaking stops, he or she might say *I can feel the solidity of my new stance.*

Another facet of a soul-oriented Tai Chi relates to a proposition put forth in Chapter Three regarding the ancient roots of modern energy psychology. There, I spoke of how a major theme of cross-cultural ancient sacred wisdom traditions is how to shape-shift from one state of consciousness to another with conscious choice. Modern hypnotherapeutic traditions speak of this as an *anchor* that facilitates the movement from one state-specific state of consciousness to another.

Tai Chi is much more than a physical practice, it is an initiatory tradition that has a wide variety of transformative effects. For example, Tai Chi is a practice for learning how to shape-shift smoothly from one state-specific state to another (Mayer, 2004b). A basic theme of Tai Chi training is to shift from a state of oneness with the universe (wuji) to moving into the world of oppo-sites (Tai Chi). In this training the initiate practices alone, and with others (Tai Chi Joining Hands practice), to try to maintain a state of relaxation (wuji) as the oppositional forces of life push on him or her. When under stress different specific body postures and principles become anchors to bring the initiate, back to the state of equilibrium and back into harmony with the universe. Every individual stance, and the transitions between those stances, can be such anchors. Depending upon the particular form of Tai Chi, there are between 24 to 108 stances, more or less. For example, the initiate slowly transitions from White Crane Spreads Wings, symbolizing a transcendent birdlike state, to Brush Knee Forward, one of the most assertive yang movements in the Tai Chi set.[8]

Though usually the initiate is not explicitly told that Tai Chi is a specific training for joining his or her transcendent and assertive selves, this shape-shifting is implicitly embedded in the transition from one posture to the next. With the conscious awareness that the movements involve shape-shifting from one stance to another, a research hypothesis to be explored would be that this awareness may lead to an increased ability to access such chosen psychologi-cal states, that is, that the practice would further generalize to everyday life.[9] As you will see in subsequent chapters, various Tai Chi postures can function to anchor, signal, and evoke desired state-specific states of consciousness (see Chapter Sixteen). Similar to classical conditioning where Pavlov's famous bell was paired with food and eventually the bell alone produced a salivary response; in the Tai Chi tradition, aspects of Tai Chi positions may become associated with activating desired state-specific states.

In Tai Chi practice, there are many types of anchors that become a signal (bell) to change from one state to another. In addition to each specific posture being an anchor for state-specific states, the act of shifting weight can anchor a felt experience of filling or emptying the Self. And rocking back and forth slowly from one posture to another simultaneously signals the bodymind to enter into a relaxed smooth flow and at the same time activates energy. (As noted in Chap-ter Four, the unique attribute of the Tai Chi "alphabet" is that the space between the letters is as important as the letters themselves.) Most important, the breath alone may become a signal to change from one state to another. In Tai Chi training, it is said that eventually just the breath, the intention, or the associated sinking of Qi is enough to re-create the desired state.[10]

From the list of the ten levels of Bodymind Healing Psychotherapy mentioned earlier, we can see that Bodymind Healing Qigong movements are one dimension of this approach and are part of a wider system. In my attempt to make the essence of this tradition accessible to modern psychotherapy, I extracted certain elements of the tradition—such as the use of particular styles of breathing, the awareness of sinking of the Qi on the exhalation, the visualization of animal postures, and the awareness of one's life stance—to make this tradition more accessible to our everyday healing repertoire.

From this wider perspective, we can see that the practice of Qigong methods can be used to constellate, work with, and focus upon the body blockages that reflect the encumbrances to the soul's journey, as you saw outlined in the River of Life practice. In the chapters that follow, you will find many examples of this method and other Qigong methods combined with psychotherapeutic processes used to transmute psychological issues and create "soul." Most specifically, in the chapter on the Mythic Journey Process, you will see not only how the breathing methods of these oriental traditions facilitate the journey into our mythological inner worlds; but you will see how other somatic attributes of the internal martial arts traditions help to anchor the felt shifts created in telling our stories. These methods bring out a soulful dimension to the psychotherapeutic process.

Adding to our psychological processing, the internal martial arts traditions enhance our ability to go through our "underworld journeys."[11] In the following chapters, you will read the stories of those who have met and engaged in the process of transforming their demons. For example, you will hear about a case of a woman who had a passive-aggressive style of withdrawal under stress and how the combination of internal martial arts training, animal forms of Qigong, and the Mythic Journey Process helped her to shape-shift into a healthier way of being (Chapter Twenty). And you will read of man with no internal martial arts training who was cut off from his instinctual self and had lost the ability to banter, and how verbal martial arts and affect modulation skills helped him to be better able to defend himself verbally (Chapter Eighteen). The combination of internal martial arts and psychological processing are an ideal mix to repair and cultivate the vital, primordial Self.

Summary of Applications of Bodymind Healing Methods in Psychotherapy and Behavioral Health Care

The following chapters illustrate the various facets of the energy psychology method that I call Bodymind Healing Psychotherapy (BMHP) in action. In these chapters it will be applied to such issues as anxiety, chronic pain, writer's block, addictions, insomnia, trauma, hypertension, workaholism, and carpal tunnel syndrome. You will read how Qigong (in the broadest sense of the word) can be integrated with psychological inner work and healing of health-related conditions. Though a good portion of these examples came from my psychotherapy office, the transformative dimensions of the practices go beyond the walls of the psychotherapy office. As you are reading these examples, please keep in mind that the clinical examples given in these chapters are not proof of the efficacy of BMHP; instead, they are meant to serve illustrative purposes and to inspire you to carry these pathways opened by my patients into your life. Furthermore, BMHP is not meant to be a stand-alone methodology, but rather its intention is to take its stance and join hands with other healing methods in the vibrant mandala of integrative health care.

Case Illustrations for Common Mental and Physical Health Issues

My philosophy is that psychological issues and bodily disease are divina afflictios (divine afflictions), giving us opportunities for psychospiritual growth, soul making, and finding the source of healing.

—Michael Mayer

CHAPTER SIX

Anxiety and Panic Disorders

Anxiety Disorders: Sociopolitical and Economic Background

Anxiety and panic are some of the most common issues treated by therapists in our culture. The National Institute of Mental Health estimates that anxiety disorders afflict eight percent of the population. Three million Americans are said to suffer from panic disorder or recurrent attacks of anxiety, while eleven million suffer from such variations as phobias, obsessions and compulsions, and chronic levels of apprehension and dread (Breggin, 1991, p. 220).

Many millions of people in our culture use medication for anxiety, creating a multibillion-dollar pharmaceutical industry.[1] A wide variety of questions have been raised as to whether it might be better to make fewer trips to the pharmacy (Altrocchi, 1994).[2] The side effects of antianxiety drugs are many, including severe withdrawal symptoms and "rebound anxiety." The use of the medication can even eventually cause an increase of the very symptoms that the drug is supposed to ameliorate. Some medications may even cause brain damage (Breggin, 1991, pp. 244–253). Also, once a person begins to take these drugs it is difficult, if not impossible, for a therapist or a client to determine whether therapeutic improvements are result of the medication or the other components of the therapy.

Whether or not these drugs are worth the side effects is a complex question that needs to be decided by each individual. There are certainly times when medication seems necessary, for example, when there is an imminent danger to self or others. And many people find antianxiety medications help them function when they feel at a loss to do so. However, natural caution dictates that psychotherapeutic methods should be tried first, before using medication. If these methods fail, then we may choose to move up the hierarchy of responses.

Alternative and Complementary Approaches to Treating Anxiety

In 1991 the Office of Alternative Medicine was mandated by Congress to encourage and support the investigation of alternative medical practices. The ultimate goal was to integrate validated alternative medical practices into health and medical care. The conclusion of the National Institute of Health panel (1996) was that "integrating behavioral and relaxation therapies with conventional medical treatment is imperative. . . ." The panel did not endorse a single technique but said a variety of them worked to lower one's breathing rate, heart rate, and blood pressure."[3]

Various forms of meditation techniques have been shown through reputable studies to affect anxiety and panic attacks. In one study from the University of Massachusetts Medical School's Department of Behavioral Medicine, Doctors Kristeller and Kabat-Zinn researched the effects of Mindfulness Meditation training at their stress clinic and "found that both anxiety and depression dropped markedly in virtually every person in the study" (Kabat-Zinn, 1990, p. 336).

What Qigong Offers to Anxiety Treatment

Having practiced and taught Qigong for more than twenty years, I began to wonder whether elements of Qigong could help psychotherapy patients suffering from anxiety disorders. As a traditionally trained psychologist, I was suspicious of claims that any single type of physical intervention could be a panacea for anxiety.

Our anxieties have deep roots in our character structures, our internalized family of origin messages, our beliefs, and in the very condition of being human. The roots of our problems cannot be superficially remedied by a drug, by the activation of chemicals in the brain that are stimulated by Western forms of exercise, or even by meditative techniques, such as Qigong.

In this sense, anxiety is not, in its deepest essence, a demon to be slain or defeated. Since the time of the cavemen and cavewomen, anxiety has operated as a signal to warn of danger. Homo sapiens would not have survived without acting on their anxieties about a noise the saber-toothed tiger made in the woods at night. Likewise today, anxiety signals the fight, flight, or freeze response in the modern individual who faces the dangers of modern society; and it alerts us of emotional threats, and it lets us know when we have strayed from our life's purpose. To attempt to slay anxiety is to attempt to destroy the barometer of our souls.

However, despite our intellectual understanding that anxiety has purpose, anyone who suffers from an anxiety disorder knows how vital it is to find a moment of relief from its debilitating effects. Relaxation tools can provide these moments of relief, thereby serving as anchors in the sometimes chaotic or overwhelming sea of life. Once relaxed, we can get in touch with our observing selves in order to reflect upon our issues. Qigong, with its breathing methods and internal martial arts techniques, has evolved over many thousands of years to help us hone the awareness and ability to meet fearful situations by cultivating "a neurophysiology of harmony" (Diepersloot, 1995, p. xvi).

Combining the wisdom of psychotherapy, hypnotherapy, and Qigong provides us with the ability to integrate two different modes of healing—transcending and transmuting. Qigong and hypnosis give us the ability to relax, center, and transcend our ego's limitations by tapping into a wider source of energy—the energy of life, called *Universal Qi*. We thereby can get distance from the "demons of life" and meet them from a place of connecting with the powerful energy of our transpersonal Selves.[4] On the other hand, Western psychology provides the skills to go into, understand, work through, and transmute our underlying psychological patterns—including debilitating forms of anxiety.

Bodymind Healing Psychotherapy's Ten Psychoenergetic Holographic Dimensions Applied to Anxiety/Panic Disorder

Bodymind Healing Psychotherapy is a psychoenergetic approach that integrates Western psychotherapy and Qigong. Its ten psychoenergetic holographic dimensions can be applied to anxiety and panic disorders in psychotherapy and in our everyday lives. Though these ten dimensions often progress in order, they can also emerge organically—in their own time and way—in psychotherapy or in your own inner processing. As you extract these methods from this therapeutic process and work with the methods on your own, you may omit one or more levels as needed. The ten dimensions may eventually be seen as a hologram, each part containing the others. These psychoenergetic methods provide the basis for the comprehensive energy psychology tool kit introduced in this chapter and throughout the rest of this book:

1. Taoist Breathing Techniques and Hypnosis (most often using the River of Life practice)

2. Self-soothing

3. "Focusing" on Felt Meaning

4. Psychodynamics (working with the psychological forces underlying human experience)

5. Cognitive Restructuring (plus using a body-oriented SUDS scale)

6. Energy Psychology Methods, including Eye Movement Desensitization Reprocessing (EMDR)

7. The Belly Massage of Chi Nei Tsang (Chia & Chia, 1990)

8. Acupressure: Phenomenological Approach and Acu-yoga (Gach & Marco, 1981)

9. Practices from Bodymind Healing Qigong[5]

10. Symbolic Process Approaches to Healing

The following case example of a woman with severe anxiety manifesting as a panic disorder illustrates many of these BMHP methods, as they combine Taoist healing techniques with traditional forms of Western psychotherapy.[6] As you listen to her story, reflect upon how her inner work paves the way for you to work on your own anxiety alone or with a health professional.

Case Illustration: Panic Disorder

The story of a young woman, whom I will call Shelly, is one of those turning-point cases that helped to create Bodymind Healing Psychotherapy (BMHP).

Working with her on her panic disorder helped me to see the limitations of my approach to psychotherapy, because certain elements of my approach that had worked with so many other patients, did not work with Shelly. Therapists grow, and the field of psychotherapy grows, as we meet the limitations of our methods. I owe Shelly a debt of gratitude for showing me how each of the ten components of BMHP was necessary for her healing. But in addition, through our work together, she helped to forge a pathway that has led me to help many subsequent patients over the years.

Shelly was a twenty-three-year-old woman who had just landed her first job as a graphic artist for a big company. When she first came into my office, she was very stiff and her face was frozen, showing almost no emotion. She told me: "Whenever too many jobs back up, I have to leave my cubicle. I tell my fellow employees that I have to go to the bathroom—but in reality, I'm sweating, heart palpitations and dizziness come over me like an unwanted plague. Sitting on the toilet seat in the bathroom with the door closed, I hope no one will discover what's going on with me. Finally the panic lessens."

Shelly was literally petrified that her boyfriend and friends would find out about her attacks and reject her. Before our therapy Shelly suffered from adverse side effects from medications used to alleviate her anxiety, so she wanted to find an approach that did not require medication. She told me that she had been to a psychiatrist, who according to Shelly, "tried to push on me the idea that my issues related to the fact that I had been adopted when very young." She left treatment with the psychiatrist because she felt that her anxiety could not have anything to do with her early life because she had such a loving relationship with her adopted parents.

After establishing rapport with Shelly, and sending her to a doctor who ruled out medical complications, I first wanted to help Shelly gain control over her symptoms.

Taoist Breathing Techniques and Hypnosis

One popular behavioral psychology method for treating anxiety, phobia, and panic attack is systematic desensitization. In this method, a patient's fear is desensitized by combining a state of relaxation with imagining moving closer to the feared object—in Shelly's case, her fear was of being overwhelmed by the multitasking required of her at work. Shelly's anxiety was so strong that she had a difficult time finding a sense of relaxation with traditional therapeutic methods, such as Jacobsen's technique of tensing and relaxing each part of the body.

Elevator Breathing

After establishing Shelly's openness to experimenting with alternative treatments, I taught her how to activate a deep state of relaxation by using Elevator Breathing, a variation of the Microcosmic Orbit Breathing method illustrated in preceding chapters.[7]

Notice your out-breath, the pause after the out-breath down in your belly, and the in-breath that comes from there. As you inhale, imagine your energy rising up from the basement below your navel, and up to the crown of your head connecting to the heavens above. As your breath goes out, imagine an elevator descending down to a point just below the belly (Tan Tien). With each succeeding exhalation, you will sink down a little deeper into yourself. Notice how many floors you go down on each breath. How low and how high does your elevator travel? Allow your breath to take your elevator to the level to which it wants to go, without trying or forcing.

The length of the breath that is associated with the development of Qi is called long-breath. To find it, imagine that your exhalation is like a tire that has a slow leak in it and that someone is sitting on the tire. This can be differentiated from short-breath that is like a blowout in a tire. Long-breath builds Qi and provides a grounded feeling.

Do not try to force the breath in and out; just notice your natural breathing. As your rate of breathing slows down naturally, the length of time of each part of the process will take longer to complete. For example, if at the beginning you count to four for each in-breath, pause, and out-breath, after doing a few cycles, the count for each phase of the cycle may increase to seven.

Using a water metaphor may further induce the feeling of the descending of the breath and thereby the sinking of the Qi. Imagine that your fingertips and bottoms of your feet are like hoses with the central faucet being just below the belly button. As you breathe out, the water flows down to the sea, carrying out stress and toxins and relaxing you. On the inhalation, new fresh "water" (or energy) comes in from the universe around you and the ground under you. Just like water eventually wears away rough spots on a riverbank, so will the energy you are contacting wash over your tension and naturally wear it away as it travels down to the sea.

The Taoists believe—and virtually anyone can experience as did Shelly—that breathing out, with focus on this central meridian line, does indeed give the feeling of sinking the energy (Qi) as this many-thousand-year-old tradition reports.[8] For virtually every patient with whom I have tried this method, it was of major significance in reducing his or her panic attacks. But for Shelly, it only provided minor relief. I discovered later that this was because of how critical she was of herself and that she feared I would judge or abandon her if she did it wrong.

Chi Nei Tsang—Belly Massage

In addition to the Elevator Breathing technique, another Taoist technique can be helpful for treating our anxiety, as this one proved to be for Shelly. The following is an adaptation of this technique called Chi Nei Tsang:[9]

1. *As you are lying down, place your hands on your belly. Just feel your inhalations and exhalations; notice the way you normally breathe, and whether your hands rise or fall as you breathe in.* (The Taoists say that in natural breathing, called *diaphragmatic breathing*, as the breath comes in, the stomach should inflate and the hands should rise.) *As you breathe out, your stomach should deflate and your hands should follow the falling of the stomach.*

2. *Follow the breath out, and using your hands, press firmly yet sensitively into whatever tension you feel there. Gradually increase the pressure on the succeeding out-breaths. On the inhalation, let the hands slightly rise and follow the stomach back up. When you feel a spot that is painful, imagine that you have the healing hands of a spiritual Being (your Self) who is sending loving energy to your belly. You will know when you have spent long enough on a spot by the release you feel.*

3. *Imagine a clockwise spiraling circle around your navel. Imagine that the top of this circle extends out as far as your rib cage, and the bottom extends to your pelvic floor. Picture this circle to be like a clock. On each point on the clock—the 12, 3, 6, 9, or all the points in-between—make little circling movements, pressing in with your hands until you reach the point of greatest depth in your body at the end of your exhalation. Then stop and feel.*

Shelly found this process to be helpful. For the first time, she was able to feel a sense of having some control over the anxiety in her body without psychiatric medication. Though she was very happy to have found some momentary symptom relief from her feelings of anxiety, the symptoms returned between sessions. And though she gradually learned to use these methods herself outside of our sessions, the work was far from complete. In the realm of psychological/spiritual interface, it is often the case that if the psychological complex behind a life issue is not worked through, the spiritual altered state accessed may not be long lasting. In such instances the transcendent state merely serves as a temporary anchoring—similar to the effects of a drug. This is the land where spiritual traditions can benefit from psychological knowledge regarding how to transmute the underlying issues.

Psychological knowledge helps us come to terms with our panic in a variety of ways by helping us to understand how it developed; develop new coping skills; activate new cognitive methods, including modulating catastrophic thinking; transmute dysfunction messages; and foster a compassionate relationship toward our issue. In this way anxiety becomes the dragon's claw that grips us, taking us on a journey of emotional evolution, sometimes against our will.

Reframing the Meaning of a Symptom

Though BMHP most often uses cognitive restructuring as its preferred cognitive method, with Shelly, I first started with another cognitive therapy method called *reframing*. Psychotherapy research teaches that a panic attack is often based on fear of fear, and that reframing fear as a normal part of the human condition can help to reduce the escalation of anxiety into panic. Reframing a symptom with a metaphor from nature or the outside world helps to de-pathologize a quality of being and to begin a healing process with it. For example, I pointed to the electric outlet in my office to reframe Shelly's fear. I told her, "A wall socket can handle just a certain amount of voltage. Just as the fuse box and circuit breaker in the house shuts off the power to give the current running through the line a rest, so do our bodies signal us when we go into overload. Sweating, dizziness, and tightness are 'friends' reminding us that we need to find a way to relax."

Shelly felt a sense of relief after hearing this metaphor, as if she could accept that maybe her symptom of overwhelm had a purpose of reminding her to relax. We will see how another purpose of this symptom was to initiate her into a transformative inward journey to heal long-standing life issues.

"Focusing" on the Felt Meaning of Anxiety

Shelly felt incompetent and troubled that she did not know what her feelings of panic were about. Once again, this is where psychological knowledge and Western psychotherapeutic methods help us to discover the specific unique meanings of our individual feelings. One such method is Gendlin's Focusing (Gendlin, 1978).[10] I like to think of Focusing as a psychological method of deep-sea diving for hidden treasure; or perhaps better put, it is a way of sitting by a river and reflecting, as answers to your life issues arise from the depths of the water and emerge onto the surface of the water (your awareness). The process, as I have adapted it to combine with BMHP, consists of the following six steps:

1. You learn to "clear a space" from painful feelings and the "subpersonality" (Assagioli, 1965) that is associated with those feelings. As mentioned earlier I added to the Focusing technique the idea of imagining a river traveling down the "macrocosmic orbit"[11] on the exhalation in order to facilitate further clearing a space from these distressing feelings.[12] Through this integration of Qigong and Focusing, a temporary, healing dissociation from your issue can be created. In this combined method, on the exhalation you imagine negative feelings releasing down the river of breath and coalescing into an image of that subpersonality at a distance from you. This honors Focusing's emphasis on finding the right amount of "breathing room" from your

issues—not too close and not too far. It is from this "right distance" that you can get a "felt sense" of what this issue is "all about."

2. You find a "felt sense" of the issue, which can be distinguished from a feeling by the fact that it is unclear, is experienced as more holistic, and it combines meaning with a body sense. The unclear sense in the body is a place where the meaning feels like it is "on the tip of your tongue." The difference between a feeling and a felt sense is like the difference between being immersed or drowning in the water of a feeling and sitting next to the river of your experience and noticing words or images arise that capture the essence of what that feeling state is all about. This involves not thinking about the issue, but directly referring to the body in this state-specific meditative state and allowing meanings to arise. (This is a key component of the transmuting dimension of the River of Life practice.)

3. You find a "handle word or image" that opens the door to the description of that sense.

4. You "resonate" the emerging thoughts or images back with the body sense to see if you are hitting the center of the target and get a "bull's eye."

5. You "ask questions" of the felt sense, such as *what's the worst thing about this issue* or *what's so _____ about this whole issue* or *what's the crux of this issue?* You wait until one of the images, words, or sounds gives you the sense that you have discovered the "felt meaning" of the issue and a "felt shift" occurs.

6. You "receive" the information you get from your bodymind with appreciation and explore where the information leads you in terms of life changes.

As Shelly embarked on the journey of focusing on the tension that blocked her inner river, she discovered a "held back" feeling in her jaw and heart. When she resonated the words *holding back* with the felt sense of all this, she realized, "No, it's more like I feel *ashamed* that I don't have it together." Though this was an important step at getting closer to the crux of what Shelly's panic was all about, identifying this feeling of shame still did not produce a felt shift. Still another level of descent into "the underworld" was needed for Shelly to transmute this issue at a deeper level.

Psychodynamics: The Family of Origin Roots of Your Energy Blocks

Psychodynamics relate to the psychological forces underlying our life issues. The question of *what feels so scary about not having it together* enabled Shelly to find the bull's-eye of felt meaning, and it led her to the psychodynamic roots of her current issue. As she continued to focus on the unclear felt sense of "what this whole thing was all about," an image came to her mind. The image of an infant being given away brought tears to Shelly's eyes; and at first, she said, "No, it couldn't be about this."

But as the tears turned into sobs, she realized that the deepest, earliest root of this issue was her feeling of being rejected by her birth parents. Though her past psychiatrist had been correct in his assessment, I believe that because he told her his interpretation, rather than allowing it to come from her own body-mind, the interpretation did not take hold, and produced a defensive reaction instead. Shelly knew she had hit the target of felt meaning, because she felt it arise from the depth of her own guts. For the first time, she was able to cry about this abandonment. She realized that her current fear of being rejected by her friends felt similar to her fears that her adopted parents would reject her if she did not meet their standards. We then worked on developing the reparenting tools needed to soothe herself.

Though Shelly had this deeply cathartic experience, and for a while the panic attacks subsided at work, her panic soon returned and scared her. This led to a next layer of her process and a next level of the development of Bodymind Healing Psychotherapy.

Self-Soothing Using Acupressure Points: The Tao of Reparenting

The Tao of reparenting uses the felt sense in the body and imagery to facilitate the reparenting of vulnerable emotions. First, we try to find an image and felt sense of our actual parents soothing us; but if blocks exist, archetypal imagery can be used to find an energetic connection with a universal mother or father figure.

In the beginning Shelly held a pillow and tried to imagine her mother soothing her by being compassionate and nonjudgmental about her problems getting enough things done at work. Since her natural parents had rejected her,
and though there was much love with her adopted parents, Shelly realized she
did not fully trust the unconditional love of her adopted parents. Because she
had a hard time finding a self-soothing figure in her personal life, she searched
for an archetypal image that could accept her the way she was. Mother Teresa
came to her mind, and Shelly's anxiety level fell from a 7 to a 4 on a 10-point
SUDS scale.[13]

Chinese medicine, with its knowledge of the acupuncture and acupressure
points, positively complements this imagery work. Along with using archetypal
or personal healing imagery, the therapist can suggest that the patient self-
touches an acupressure point on his or her heart with the right hand and a point
just below the navel with the left hand. These points can provide an anchor, so
that any time an unwanted feeling arises in the patient's life, these points can
be touched, outside of the session. Similar to when the master hypnotherapist
Milton Erickson (Rosen, 1982) said, "My voice will go with you," here the tool
of self-touch goes with the patient and serves as an anchor in difficult circumstances, even outside of the therapeutic encounter. One anchoring point that
often proves useful is Conception Vessel-17, located at the center of the heart
chakra according to Taoist theory; and according to Chinese medicine, this
point functions to "unbind the chest" (Deadman, Al-Khafami, & Baker, 1998, p.
518). This point, also called the Sea of Tranquility (Gach, 1990), is on the center-line of the breastbone, four fingers' width up from the base of the breastbone,
in an indentation there. To contact your heart's energy, you touch this point
with the middle finger of the right hand or the whole hand, make small circles,
stop, breathe, and feel the energy.[14]

Shelly practiced this method; and with the middle finger of the left hand,
she also touched her Tan Tien acu-point, beneath the navel, which the Taoists
believe is the power center of the body. Shelly was the first patient whom I tried
this physical method of self-soothing with, suggesting it to her as an experiment. She later described this self-soothing as one of the most beneficial tools
of her therapy.

Self-soothing is deemed by psychoanalytic psychotherapists to be important to repairing the Self (Kohut, 1971, p. 64; Pearlman & McCann, 1992), particularly when soothing was not provided by a person's early primary caretakers (Schore, 2003, p. 171). Bodymind Healing Psychotherapy proposes that physical self-touch of the body, in general, and on particular acupressure points on the heart (CV-17, also called *Du*-17) and the belly (*Ren*-6, Tan Tien), adds a key dimension to self-soothing. I have had many patients tell me that this is one of the things they most remembered about our therapy.

After my work with Shelly, I was feeling that sense of accomplishment and personal satisfaction that comes from having discovered a new addition to the realm of psychotherapeutic healing. I presented this at a few major conferences to spread the word and see if it worked as well for my colleagues' patients as it had for mine.[15] Then one day while I was doing some anthropological research I saw the picture at right:

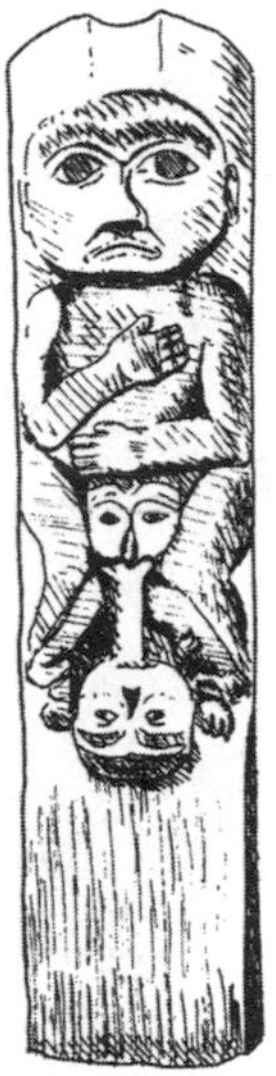

Figure 3. Chiltan Spirit Posture

I was amazed when I saw this picture of the Chiltan Spirit Posture, which shows standing figures that have one hand on the heart and the other on their belly (Goodman, 1990). It was exactly what I was doing with my patients. I discovered that the image of this posture was found in Alaska, Arizona, and Tennessee; on along the Northwest coast of America; among the Olmecs in Central America, in Bolivia; as well as in Asia in the valleys of Uzbekistan (Gore, 1995, pp. 60–61). At first I felt deflated that the contribution I thought I had made to the field of psychology was known so many years ago. But, then I felt a sense of deeper satisfaction because I was aligned with my psychological colleagues from ancient times who took the time to carve in wood this healing totem, rich with potential healing meanings. Rediscovering this self-soothing gesture was another step on my path of traveling into the earlier roots of psychotherapeutic healing "before modern psychology 'began' in the laboratory of Wilhelm Wundt."

Though we cannot be sure of what meanings these totem carvers intended, it can prove enlightening to follow the tradition of psychological archaeology that was developed by Dr. Felicitas Goodman (1990) and her colleagues, and to explore holding postures and repeating hand gestures used by indigenous traditions. From doing so, I felt a renewed sense of connection with the importance of a primordially based energy psychology.

Drawing from psychology's age-old indigenous origins provides a deeper root system that helps all the branches of modern psychotherapy. Touching the heart and belly have cross-cultural healing significance from the chakras of Hinduism to the energy centers of Taoism and are also represented in Native America. Chinese medicine gives us more than just these two points to help alleviate anxiety. For example, Kidney-1 (located on the ball of the foot, in the middle, slightly in front of center, toward the toes) is particularly helpful for public speaking phobias. This point is also helpful to ground energy, bringing it down from the head, at times when the ego experiences fragmentation under stress. The Kidney meridian in Chinese medicine is used to deal with the polarity of fear and vitality/strength.

Cognitive Restructuring

Cognitive restructuring could be defined as a type of spiritual transformation of the mind—a spiritual exercise.

—L. Rebecca Propst (1981)

In the process of touching acupressure energy points or doing various movement-based interventions, it is helpful to do "cognitive restructuring" (Beck, 1979). And it was also an important key for Shelly's healing. Recently, cognitive therapy techniques have been combined with somatic interventions. For example, in Dr. Shapiro's Eye Movement Desensitization Reprocessing (1995), the patient is instructed in using particular movements of the eyes along with restructuring their beliefs; that is, instead of an abused person being fixated on a negative cognition, such as *the world is an unsafe place,* they might instead verbalize a truthful or constructive new cognition, like *it's over; I'm safe now.* In Thought Field Therapy (Callahan, 2001) and the Emotional Freedom Technique (Craig & Fowlie, 1995), a patient taps on various locations on the body while saying constructive new beliefs, such as *even though I am not a great public speaker, I can love and accept myself the way I am.*

This restructuring of statements creates a positive transcendence by allowing the mind to access our compassionate observing self, who is then able to put the symptom that we are identified with into proper perspective. When the statement is truthful or constructive, it also allows a transmuting of a dysfunctional false belief. Before and after treatment, a measurement is often taken on a Subjective Units of Distress Scale (SUDS). For example, a patient may say *I can feel okay about myself even though I still feel a little_____* and then check his or her SUDS level to determine how much he or she was actually soothed by the cognition.

Bodymind Healing Psychotherapy (BMHP) adds to cognitive approaches the power of self-touch of key acupressure points, in order to allow us to dip into and activate the well-known primordial healing streams of the ancient sacred wisdom traditions of our ancestors. For example, as you read previously, touching the Sea of Tranquility (CV-17) in the center of the chest may lead to a felt sense of a relationship with our transcendental compassionate Self. When we also touch the belly (Tan Tien), we may access the psychoenergetic dimensions of love and power, which may aid us in transforming our relationship with our symptom by providing somatic anchors for the new belief. Finding the specific thought forms that express a person's old and new beliefs is an important key.

In Shelly's case she began with the catastrophic negative belief that if anyone knew how messed up she was, she would be rejected. In the field of psychology, it is well known that catastrophic thinking is one component of panic attacks. BMHP proposes that adding a somatic component to cognitive therapy helps to develop a more grounded, compassionate way of thinking. Through this work, Shelly developed a new, grounded, more-constructive cognition: *I deserve to be loved for the way I am, vulnerable and all. I'm willing to take the risk to put out who I really am and have people in my life who won't abandon me for who I am.* Shelly anchored this new cognition by touching the two acupressure points on her heart and belly, using this BMHP self-soothing method. Her face and breath relaxed. Her SUDS level reduced to 0 when she focused on her fear in session, and she said that using the self-touch methods outside of session helped her to maintain the connection to our work and reduced her SUDS level there as well.

Shelly eventually became more comfortable discussing her anxieties and panic attacks with her boyfriend. Another step forward on her path came after telling her boyfriend her deep dark secret about her panic attacks, after which he shared a secret with her regarding abuse in his childhood. This led to increased intimacy between them. Another sign of Shelly's growth was that she was better able to handle the job stressors of being a graphic artist.

A dream she had at this time provided Shelly with more validation of her inner work. Early on in our therapy sessions, Shelly had dreamed that she had a beautifully colored flower tattoo that turned into a gray, lifeless flower. During our termination process, she had another dream that the flower's color returned and was even more vivid than it had ever been before. She interpreted this to mean that trying to hide her fears and invalidating her vulnerabilities took the color out of her Self—now her colorful Self was returning.

Similar to the tradition in the Aesclepian temple that a healing dream signaled it was time to leave the temple; Shelly and I saw this dream as a signal to begin the termination phase of her treatment. We were able to discuss how all the elements that we had been working with—the breathing, belly massage, self-touch, new beliefs and their connection with her wound from the past—were coming together for her. This was a first step for me in confirming the holographic dimensions of the model that was to become Bodymind Healing Psychotherapy. Breathing and self-touch without the cognitive and psychodynamic levels are less complete; and similarly, the cognitive and psychodynamic levels less complete without breath and self-touch. It seems to be best when each level is contained within the other; for example, when breath and self-soothing is in the cognition, and the cognitions are in the breath and self-soothing. As discussed in Chapter Two on energy psychology, the research on self-touch and cognitive therapy showed that cognitive therapy alone was not as successful or as long lasting as when the two methods were used together (Andrade & Feinstein, 2004).

In our termination session, after about six months of therapy, Shelly said: "It's not that feelings of anxiety don't arise anymore; but they haven't turned into panic for a long time because I'm able to soothe myself when they arise. I look at life's difficulties as an opportunity to practice 'sinking my Qi.'"

Standing like a Tree Qigong—Finding Your Stance

Other Qigong methods may help with your anxiety as they have helped patients of mine who suffer from anxiety disorders. For example, Standing Meditation Qigong (Standing like a Tree or Zhan Zhuang Qigong)[16] is a method of psychoenergetic healing whereby a practitioner learns to find a relaxed stance in life.[17]

In Chapter Fifteen you will read about one of my patients with severe anxiety that stemmed in part from his brother's physical abuse coupled with the brother's message of *I'm better than you at everything*. I believe combining psychotherapy with Standing Meditation practice led to a pivotal moment in his therapy, when he found his stance and was able to say to his brother, "You're not better than me at everything, you're not better at being a kind brother." This new belief coupled with his new stance became *I deserve to be treated with kindness.*

Internalized messages from our childhood often contribute to the scattering of our Qi, or in psychoanalytic terminology *fragmentation*. For this reason, everyone can benefit from a practice that uses breath and stance to constellate our observing Selves. From this place of compassion and equanimity, as we watch abusive thoughts arise, we can find a way to return to our ground in kindness and appropriate self-assertiveness. By integrating Western psychological methods with the body-mind-spirit healing methods of Qigong, the modern person may benefit from the joining hands of Eastern and Western traditions.

CHAPTER SEVEN

Qigong and Behavioral Medicine: An Integrated Approach to Chronic Pain

Perhaps everything terrible is, in its deepest being, something helpless that needs our love.

—Rainer Maria Rilke

Case Illustration: Qigong with a Disabled Car-Accident Victim

Because my patient "Terry" was a nurse at a local hospital, she had the best hospital care money could buy when a terrible car accident crippled her and required her to use a crutch. Her lawyer referred her to me as part of a lawsuit against the person who crashed into her car, pinning her in so badly that the "jaws of life" had to be used to free her crushed foot from the automobile. For six months Terry suffered with a bad limp, and any time she tried to reduce her pain medication, she found herself in excruciating pain. The doctor who prescribed the pain medication told her she would probably need it for the rest of her life. By the time she came to me, Terry was developing an addiction to the medication. I advised her to reduce the pain medication under the advice and care of her doctor, so that she would be able to determine to what extent the methods we used in psychotherapy were helping her.

Pain and Economics

Surveys indicate that eleven to twelve percent of the adult population in the United States report difficulties related to chronic pain (Sternbach, 1986). According to *The Pain and Absenteeism Report* (1996), employee benefit managers believe that twenty percent of their employees suffer from various types of pain conditions; and employees think that more than two-thirds of all full-time employees—the equivalent of more than eighty million people—suffer from pain-related conditions.[1] It is hard to fathom that estimates for the direct and indirect costs of pain-related syndromes in the United States each year range from $90 to 100 billion, and that 20 million tons of aspirin are consumed annually (Taylor, 1991).[2]

Research on Complementary Treatment of Pain

A wide variety of well-documented research studies, and the National Institute of Health's (1996) report in the *Journal of the American Medical Association,* show that strong evidence exists for the ability of various techniques of behavioral medicine to alleviate chronic pain, including techniques in relaxation, hypnosis, and meditation.[3] Additionally, moderate evidence exists for results in reduction of pain using cognitive behavioral therapy and biofeedback (NIH, 1996, p. 313). The data of meta-analysis consistently showed positive effects of these behavioral and relaxation programs, although evidence was insufficient to show that one technique was more effective than another in reducing chronic pain. "For any given individual patient . . . one approach may indeed be more appropriate than another" (NIH, 1996, p. 315). According to the report, the successful techniques all shared some basic components: repetitive focus on a word, sound, phrase, body sensation, or muscular activity; the adoption of a passive attitude toward intruding thoughts; and a return to the object of repetitive focus (NIH, 1996, p. 314). Even though Qigong was not mentioned specifically in this report, the above criteria are the very essence of Qigong practice.

In spite of the beneficial results of relaxation methods in general—and Qigong and Tai Chi in particular—for pain relief, we hear less about these natural, no-side-effect alternatives for those suffering from the severe debilitating effects of pain than we do about medication. Fueled by drug company advertising and our culture's propensity for instant gratification, mass marketing has programmed us to search for miracle cures in a pill the moment we feel pain.

Certainly, many people suffering from extreme pain have good reason to be thankful for modern pharmacological and medical advances.[4] The decision between when to use these or other pain-reducing drugs and when to try to find a more natural choice is a complex one that needs to be decided by each individual.[5] There are certainly times when the advances of modern medicine can be useful, but it seems that caution dictates that natural methods should be tried first before treatment with medication. If these methods fail, then a person may choose to move up the hierarchy of responses.[6]

Modern neuroscience has demonstrated that many chemicals of the outer world are produced in our brains, like the "natural morphine" found in endorphins. An interesting fact is that thirty to sixty percent of patients will experience pain relief by being given a placebo, that is, an inert pill.[7] This shows that the mind has the ability to activate inner pain medication if we can learn how to turn the key. The questions become how and to what extent can we increase our abilities to unlock our natural powers?

In a culture like ours, so oriented to the outer world, we oftentimes forget our inner healing resources, just as we forget the old traditions that existed long before the advent of Western medicine that once held knowledge of how to use these abilities to effect healing.

Research on Qigong and the Treatment of Pain

Qigong is one age-old tradition of relaxation and healing that can help sufferers of chronic pain. There are peer-reviewed (Morris, 2000; Wu et al., 1999) and non-peer-reviewed (Jin, 1944; Anderson, 2000) articles showing the benefits of Qigong and Tai Chi for the treatment of pain.[8]

It is interesting that in one of these peer-reviewed studies (Wu et al., 1999), the researchers chose the most severe patients with complex regional pain syndromes; and this group of researchers, which included two medical doctors, concluded that Qigong practice resulted in reducing pain and long-term anxiety. However, the study emphasized that the Qigong result for pain reduction was transient and did not last after the patients stopped practicing. This illustrates one of the problems with scientific research—the wrong question can be asked. The important question to be answered is whether Qigong can continue to reduce pain with continued practice.

Qigong and Tai Chi come from a "practice model" of healing—meaning one needs to continue the practice to achieve results. Just as we do not expect pain-reducing pharmaceuticals to be taken one time and produce results for difficult pain syndromes, it is unreasonable for us to expect that the benefits of short-term, time-limited Qigong practice will last without continued commitment. Still, this was a very well-designed study that is important in showing Qigong's beneficial effects even with patients with severe pain.

Methods of Qigong and Visualization: Partners in Pain Relief

The work that Terry and I did together helps illustrate how Bodymind Healing Psychotherapy applies the methods of Qigong in a psychotherapeutic or behavioral health setting. As a psychotherapist, my goal is to speak to my patients in common language, using methods that would not be perceived as "selling Qigong" or advocating an Eastern method that might seem strange to some of my traditionally oriented Western patients. To those of my patients familiar with hypnotherapy, I present Qigong methods under the umbrella of the well-researched field of clinical hypnosis in that Qigong adds another method of *trance induction*.

A next step for researchers will be to study how Qigong compares to other hypnosis methods regarding how it facilitates a relaxation and healing response. For everyday use outside of a therapist's office, the following methods that I taught Terry can be used by anyone as a first line approach to deal with pain (within the parameters previously mentioned about due caution needed to properly diagnose the cause of the pain).

Microcosmic Orbit Breathing

When Terry came into my office, I asked her to give me a current rating of her pain on a SUDS scale—10 being the greatest it had ever been, and 0 being pain free. She said it was an 8 because she had reduced her medication, as I had asked her to do with consultation with her physician. She wanted to "see what this hypnosis stuff could do" for her.

After taking a case history, I introduced Terry to an approach that integrates Qigong and hypnosis without mentioning a word about Qigong. When presenting the methods to patients, this background can be revealed or not, depending upon the given patient's background and the clinical relationship.

The first step in helping to relieve Terry's pain was to teach her how to activate her Qi by noticing her inhalation coming up the "microcosmic orbit." Classical Taoist literature claims that Microcosmic Orbit Breathing, when done properly, can help induce a healing state. As discussed more fully in Chapter Four, this breathing method consists of inhaling and allowing the breath to rise up the back, and on the exhalation, imagining the breath going down to the belly (Tan Tien), thus creating a circular circuit of breath.

Macrocosmic Orbit Breathing

After Terry moved into a state of relaxation with Microcosmic Orbit Breathing, I introduced Macrocosmic Orbit Breathing (Huang, 1974), which is an extension of the above method whereby the person enlarges the circle of breath, imagining it coming up from the ground over the head on the inhalation, and then down the front of the body on the exhalation (see Chapter Four).

As discussed with the River of Life breathing exercise in Chapter Five, the use of imagery adds to the healing effects of Qigong.[9] On Terry's exhalation, I had her imagine a waterfall coming down over the top of her head that became a river flowing down through the front of her body and out her damaged foot.

Terry told me that another health practitioner told her to imagine putting healing energy into the pain in her right leg, but that just seemed to make it more swollen. This illustrates the Taoist notion that when there is an excess of yang, we want to decrease the energy there not increase it, which may happen when we concentrate too much on a point that is already suffering from excess. I told Terry to experiment with focusing, not on the spot that hurt, but on the river above and below that spot. Because she described the pain as having a hot, stuck quality to it, the following image was constellated to use along with her Macrocosmic Orbit Breathing:

> *Where you feel the energy blocked, you might imagine it as stuck leaves in a river, or anything else that you picture the block to be; and without forcing it, notice how many breaths it takes for the cool waters to flow through the dammed-up place.*

Visualization is a hypnotherapeutic tool often used with chronic pain patients (Hilgard & Hilgard, 1983). The Taoistic parallel and addition to this idea is to use the thousand-year-old understanding of the meridian lines and vital points of the body to activate the vital energy of the body (Qi) to aid this process. Terry visualized the Bubbling Well point (Kidney-1) at the bottom of her foot with water being drawn into her body from there, then spiraling up her leg and up the back of her body over the top of her head, to the Baihui point.[10] Then Terry visualized it coming down the front of her body and exiting at the foot through the Bubbling Well point. The Taoists, and practitioners of Chinese medicine, believe this point is one key place where energy can be drawn into the body, as well as being a point where the waters of life can wash out toxins from the body.

In the first session, Terry's pain decreased to a SUDS level of 2. She was amazed because this was the most pain-free she had been without medication since her accident six months before. During subsequent sessions Terry learned these and other methods to use with her pain. She was able for the first time, in our second meeting, to experience a SUDS level of 0. With the consent of her doctor, she started to use medication on a less-frequent basis. In our third and subsequent meetings, we focused our efforts on Terry learning how to achieve this state outside of our sessions.

Yin-Yang Balancing Method

One other method I taught Terry to ease her pain was the Yin-Yang Balancing Method. I derived this method from a hypnotherapeutic technique called *pain transferal* (Hilgard & Hilgard, 1983, p. 65; Crasilneck & Hall, 1985, p. 105), which involves a person imagining the transferal of his or her pain from one to another part of the body.

By adding to this the idea of yin and yang in Taoist theory, we have the benefit of adding a ancient understanding of the pathways of energy in the body, thereby allowing the person to transfer the pain, or energy, by coming into alignment with a ready-made stream. Whether we want to believe that this stream is "real" when we visualize it and imagine that it is real, our mind activates our healing powers.[11]

In the Yin-Yang Balancing Method, a person imagines more energy flowing through the *yin* (cold, weakened) part of the body and less energy going through the *yang* (hot, strong, acutely injured) part of the body. Terry learned to imagine and experience her breath turning into warm water flowing through her uninjured left leg and cooling gentle waters flowing through her injured leg.

She learned to play with the sensations and to control and trick her body. Never mentioning a Chinese word or the term *Qigong*, I introduced Terry to an idea from the tradition of *Yi Chuan* (the mind or intention behind the various systems of Chuan) that energy (Qi) follows intention (Yi). While she was in a relaxed trance state, I gave her the hypnotic suggestion that her left leg was the one that was hurt in the accident instead of the actually injured right leg. She did indeed experience that this left ankle felt very painful. Then I brought her out of trance and she was able to see how powerful her mind was in creating pain. When I presented this case at one conference, I was criticized for using hypnotherapeutic methods to create pain. However, this temporary "creation of pain" serves the higher purpose of helping a patient to discover the role of his or her mind in creating, controlling, and healing pain. After seeing how Terry's mind alone could create pain in her left leg, I taught her how to release this pain by imagining a river of breath coming all the way down to the bottom of the foot (Kidney-1). As a further way of working with left-right imbalances and one-sided pains common in many cases of chronic and acute pain, I introduced her to the following method, which I call the Energy Hula Hoop:

Imagine a vertical hula hoop with water flowing through it, circling through the points on both ankles and going up to the hips. Between the two feet there is a break in the hula hoop, where the water can be released to the earth, when desired. Breathe in and up through the left leg around the hips and on the out-breath, down and out the right leg and foot.

Each time the sensations of pain arose in her right or left ankle, I asked Terry to imagine what it felt like. At first the hula hoop was blocked like stuck leaves where her injury was; but gradually, as she imagined the water flowing through the leaves, she felt the blockage clear. While she was playing with her mind-body connection, Terry forgot which leg was the one in the accident.

Finding the Healing Ball of Qi with Your Hands

The use of various postures is another Taoist contribution to alleviating pain. One posture involves experiencing the magnetic force between the *Lao Gong* points in outstretched palms to enhance the healing ability and cultivate the Qi (vital energy) in our hands.[12] A world apart and a thousand years later, directing a patient to imagine that there is a force that attracts outstretched hands together is well known in hypnotherapy. In the Stanford Hypnotic Clinical Scale, one of the methods used to assess a patient's ability to enter into trance is by having them practice this method.[13]

Another hypnotherapist who uses the outstretched hands to create trance is Dr. Ernest Rossi. He uses it for the purpose of ideomotor (ideodynamic) signaling to measure the patient's responsiveness to the inner work that is occurring. According to Rossi and Cheek (1988), "If your creative (healing) unconscious is ready to begin therapeutic work, you will experience those hands moving together all by themselves to signal yes; but, if there is another issue that you need to explore first, you will feel those hands being pushed apart" (p. 39).

In Qigong practice, a similar posture is held, though the methodology is more intricate (having developed over thousands of years) and the intention is broader. The two traditions could benefit much from learning from each other. The hypnotherapist focuses on using the outstretched hands to create a trance and to facilitate the reorganization of the psyche. For the practitioner of Qigong, the energy in the outstretched hands is developed for the purpose of self-defense, personal empowerment, as well as healing acute and chronic disease. In addition, a long Taoist lineage promotes the practice of meditation in these postures in order to find keys to open the energy gates to the spiritual healing energy of the body and the cosmos.[14] Cultivating the energy in-between the hands is viewed as a way to affect the universe of energy that the practitioner holds, qualitatively and quantitatively.

For example, the Yi Chuan Qigong tradition is oriented to cultivating a "ball of Qi," which can then be used for whatever purpose the practitioner chooses.[15] *Yi* translates as "intention," and *Chuan* literally translates as "fist." But the esoteric meaning of holding the five fingers into a fist is to grasp, or bring into a whole, the healing energies of the five elements: fire, earth, metal, water, and wood. Depending upon the practitioner's intention, the Yi Chuan postures can be used for self-defense, healing, personal empowerment, or transforming Qi into *shen* (spirit). The outstretched hands in the position used in the Stanford scale and by Rossi is virtually identical to position number six of the eight postures used in the Yi Chuan.

In this tradition a period of sitting or standing in stillness is advised as a first step before raising the two hands into a fixed posture. These meditation positions are very specific and are oriented to developing the body's energy in a multiplicity of ways.

There are many postural elements to be aware of while practicing Sitting or Standing Meditation. For example, while sitting, place yourself on the edge of the chair, the spine is straight, chin is slightly tucked, hands are facedown on the knees, and your feet are straight forward and under the knees. For Standing Meditation, the hands are by the sides, the feet are straight forward, knees are slightly bent, chin is slightly tucked, and the pelvis is slightly tucked so that the Ming Men (located behind the Tan Tien, in the center of the lower back) is filled out.[16]

The spine is naturally stretched by these methods so that the Qi sinks and the spirit is raised. Once in position the practitioner may be instructed to practice Microcosmic Orbit Breathing for a few minutes, to focus on the natural breath, or to focus the intention on the Tan Tien.[17] Then the teacher may tell the practitioner to allow the hands to rise, as if in water, until they are in front of the heart. In this movement the palms are facing each other as if they are holding a helium balloon and the elbows are slightly away from the body and are not locked. The practitioner continues the breathing techniques mentioned above with the hands in this position, and then the practitioner is instructed to see if he or she can experience a "stickiness" as the hands are gently pulled apart, away from the ball of energy. Likewise, the person is instructed to try to squeeze the ball of energy and see if he or she can experience its substance (see Chapter Twenty-one, Ocean Wave Breathing).

In more advanced practice, a student of the tradition learns to direct the Qi of the meridians with his or her intention. One method is to focus the intention on one hand and note any sensations or energy that follow the movement of awareness (as in the similar practice in Chapter Four). Small, circular hand movements are sometimes used to enhance this direction of healing energy into the *Lao Gong* points in the center of the palms or fingertips.[18] For example, in the Tai Chi Ruler Qigong tradition (Tai Chi Chih), wooden balls are held between the palms and circular movements are practiced to open the *Lao Gong* points.[19] The practitioner is also taught how to cultivate Qi by moving the hands in small circles without the ball there.

It would be heuristic to explore further how the combination of hypnotherapeutic visualization techniques with Qigong postures enhances entering into a trance state, and healing. In my private practice, for example, I may ask a client to imagine the following:

The ball that you feel in your hands can be filled with whatever you desire, and its energy can be directed to wherever you choose. First, you might imagine that the love in your heart enters into the balloon. Then, just as when earlier you felt energy enter into one hand through the direction of intention there, so can you feel its energy spread throughout the body wherever you want to direct it. By letting go on your exhalation and imagining the compassion of your heart melting any ice blocks in the rivers of your Qi, you can gradually let go of tension in your body and direct that liberated healing energy to wherever it is needed.

Acupressure Points and Pain

In various Qigong traditions (such as acupressure), touch is used to focus the Qi. By teaching psychotherapy clients to touch their own acupressure points, rather than a practitioner touching them, various ethical and clinical problems can be avoided (Kilburg, 1988, pp. 487–491; Goodman, 1988, pp. 492–500).

After Terry learned to hold her hands apart to activate the experience of the ball of Qi in her hands, we moved on to practice how she might direct that energy for her own self-healing. I showed Terry how to use the Yin-Yang Balancing Method combined with touch. When the inside of her inflamed ankle hurt, she learned to touch and direct healing energy to points on the outside of the ankle more strongly, to shift the energy there. To respect the need for a yin relationship to the inside point that hurt, she did not touch it at all, but instead directed her healing intention to that point with the other hand from a few inches away.

When Terry touched a point in the little hollow anterior to the outside ankle-bone (Gall Bladder-40) known to be beneficial to ankle pain, she reported a release of the pain down to a SUDS level of 0 within 10 exhalations, accompanied by a perception of green light filling the room. (Terry had never had an experience of seeing light like this before.) If the outside of the ankle hurt, we would have similarly had her experiment with touching a point next to the inside of the anklebone (such as Kidney-4). Also, Terry learned to press acupressure points more strongly on the ankle opposite to the one that was hurt, and to touch points on her hurt ankle more softly or not at all. This helped her to learn to balance the energy in both legs. In the very first session that she tried this, she had the experience of creating that balance.

Terry began to see her homework as a spiritual practice to learn to work with her pain and let it teach her. She imagined opening her heart to send love to the hula hoop of her pain. She also reported an experience of the water in the hula hoop dissolving into water vapor and leaving her body—as the boundaries between herself and the world dissolved into a pleasant feeling of lightness and heaviness combined. If an old Taoist was listening to modern Terry, he or she might describe the boundless feeling she experienced as *wuji*, described in ancient texts as the void, emptiness or healing reservoir from which Qi derives.[20]

After five sessions Terry felt like she no longer needed to see me because she was able to achieve a SUDS pain level of 0 every time she did the above practices. In addition, she noted improvement in her ability to walk during this time (although from a scientific standpoint, we cannot know whether this improvement in her ability to walk was a function of time and would have occurred without treatment).[21]

An important final note of caution: Not all people will find relief from these methods as quickly as Terry did. From the perspective of Qigong, the path to spiritual growth involves more than just eliminating pain, it involves letting go of *trying* to get rid of pain. "Trying" constricts the river of Qi; whereas, "letting go" of our process allows the river to expand and find its natural course. There may be moments when we hit rocks in the downward currents of the river of our pain; these moments can serve as reminders to breathe in and out of our pain in order to find our center as we ride the rapids of physical and emotional agony. At other moments our breath leads us to merge with wuji, and we are held in the warm embrace of the ocean of energy that is the mother of all life.

With any technique we need to be careful that we do not produce a personal attribution of shame when a "cure" does not come as quickly as we might like. Hence, the distinction between *cure*—the absence of symptoms—and *healing*—an attitude that whatever life presents us is an opportunity for psychospiritual growth in the midst of suffering. Many patients who have described more-severe and long-lasting pain than Terry report being thankful that they have Qigong as a partner that gives them breathing room and helps them to find a compassionate relationship to being with pain.

Dealing with Various Types of Pain: The Medicine Wheel of Possibilities

Each different type of pain leads us on a journey to different methods from the wide variety of healing traditions. Native Americans would say that each place on the "medicine wheel" has its value (Storm, 1972). For example, sometimes the pain due to a subluxated vertebrae may be best helped by a chiropractic adjustment. At times when through our own Qigong practice we are unable to remove a given energy block, an acupuncture treatment may help. When a person is too debilitated to practice Standing or Sitting Meditation, perhaps doing yoga postures while lying down will be the best way to breathe and work with the pain. Sometimes prayer may help (Dossey, 1993).

It is in these various ways that pain leads us on a journey to rediscover the natural healing elements of the world around us. The most basic elements of the yin and yang of life, such as hot and cold, may become the medicine we need. We might experiment with using ice packs during the early phases of an acute injury and using warm compresses during the later stages; or in the case of some chronic blockages, we might find that going back and forth between warm and cold packs may do the trick. An herbalist may have information to remind us that the world of nature is our ally (Heinerman, 1988). Homeopathic remedies (Edinger, 1985) are based on the notion that "like cures like": They use the minutest amounts of a substance to create a healing response in our immune system—for example, using a highly diluted amount of nettles to heal pain. Homeopathic treatment opens our minds to wonder about the healing potentials of the things around us that we take for granted.

Western doctors and medications may help us to appreciate being part of an evolving civilization, because the pain-killing medications used by modern pharmacology often derive from the biological intelligence that has been developing for eons in the natural world. For example, a new pain-relieving drug, SNX-111, is a synthetic copy of a natural neurotoxin isolated from the venom of sea-going snails.[22]

Qigong energetic practices can be viewed as a center point in the medicine-wheel approach to pain; they can be combined with any other approach, including pharmacological. For example, in a research study in China, 127 patients with advanced cancer were divided into two groups: a Qigong practicing group and a control group that did not practice Qigong. Both groups took medication. The Qigong group improved significantly in strength, appetite, diarrhea free, weight gain, and in the phagocyte rate of their immune systems compared to the control group. In addition, the Qigong practices helped to ameliorate the effects of the medications (Sancier, 1996b).[23]

Each different type of pain initiates us into the lessons of its own particular pathway. At times, finding ways to distance ourselves from the pain is helpful. We use our breath to find a calm place inside where we know we have pain, but we are not identified with that pain. We may thereby learn to cultivate concentration and equanimity in the midst of our suffering. At other times we may choose to go into the pain. Buddhist Mindfulness Meditation practice can be very helpful at such times—to be with the sensation of pain instead of distancing from it.[24] As we explore its various qualities, such as temperature and tightness; metaphors may arise of pinpricks, knife stabbing, or demons grabbing our stomachs while we shape-shift into yogis, internal martial artists, or any subpersonality that can explore and handle the elements of pain. Something about us may indeed transform in the "being with it"—a self-sufficient, isolated person may reach out for others or a critical, judgmental person may finally find compassion for his or her pain instead of fighting against it.

"Focusing" on the Meaning of Pain

Our complexes are not only wounds that hurt and mouths that tell our myths but also eyes that see what the normal and healthy parts cannot envision.... Afflictions point to gods, gods reach us through afflictions.

—James Hillman

Every pain contains a message that has its own unique meaning and its own voice. If we listen to its message, we are led to appropriate action. Sometimes our stomach pain says that a certain food is disagreeable to us, other times that pain may mean that a psychological issue needs to be faced. Learning to read the deeper messages behind our feelings is the missing ingredient in "symptom relief" schools of thought on pain.

Western psychotherapy has many tools to discover the meaning of pain; for example: psychoanalysis uses free association; phenomenological methods allow a person to explore his or her own unique experience; hypnotherapeutic traditions have contributed imagery and relaxation methods; and cognitive-behavioral psychology has contributed techniques involving shifts in attitude, distraction, and imagery. Gendlin's Focusing (1978), as outlined in Chapter Six, involves a six-step process for finding the felt meaning of any psychological issue, including pain.

For example, using the Focusing method, one man in his early forties focused on the thoughts that arose while breathing into, and out from, his chronic lower-back pain. He remembered his mother repeatedly beating him with a wire coat hanger when he was a child. He was able to begin a process of working through his feelings about this, and releasing the held emotions that had been stored there for years. Also, in the case of a placating, continuously smiling teacher who focused on her recurring headaches, she realized that they often occurred when her husband did not help with the housework and meal preparation. By being conscious of the meaning of her pain, she was able to work through a long-standing message from her matrilineal lineage that women are supposed to grin and bear it. When she expressed her feelings, including anger, she noticed that her headaches disappeared.

Generally speaking, in cases of internally generated pain—such as with headaches, muscular aches, and energy blockages—stress begins at the level of mind, signaling us that inner emotional reprogramming needs to take place. These symptoms, or off-centered patterns, first manifest on the level of Qi; then they are translated into the musculature; and finally, they may manifest as spinal subluxation. By using psychotherapy in conjunction with Qigong practices, we can work on realigning ourselves and finding our center in the midst of the cross-currents of our emotional terrain. The Yi Chuan Standing Meditation Qigong practices discussed earlier can be particularly helpful in experiencing and realigning structural deficits that derive from our genetic and characterological makeup.

CHAPTER EIGHT

Trauma and Post-Traumatic Stress

Trauma often disconnects a person from her or his center or self—the
essence of positive emotional wisdom and guidance that is best equipped
to guide us.

—Asha Clinton (2002)

The New Biology and Somatic Approaches to Healing Trauma

Since both Qigong and Tai Chi have self-defense and empowerment methods at their core, it is natural to look at what they and other body-oriented, mind-body methods might contribute to those suffering from post-traumatic stress. First, I will review the growing field of stress research, in which recent research helps us understand more about the role of brain and biochemical reactions in the creation of and healing of stress.

In his book *Why Zebras Don't Get Ulcers*, Robert Sapolsky (1988) shows that when our bodies face stressors perceived as life endangering, our arteries constrict—like a hose maximizing its powerful force—in order to maximize our power. However, if prolonged, this adaptive stress response creates excess glucocorticoids, which lead to certain physiological dysfunctions. When primordial survival mechanisms are activated in modern high-stress situations for which they were not designed, the mechanisms are no longer adaptive. Thus, a big key to transforming locked-in stress responses is to use various bodymind healing methods that unlock such nonadaptive patterns.

The field of "new biology" has also contributed to this understanding. Dr. Bruce Lipton (2005), one of the foremost thinkers in the field of the new biology, says that there is a primordial, psychobiological ground to the stress response. As we approach danger, we activate the hypothalamus, pituitary, adrenal, (HPA) axis; this stops our ability to fight disease as we focus on survival. When our "survival-self" hears the sound of a lion, our bodies halt the fight against infection in favor of mobilizing energy for flight and fight. The HPA axis interferes with our ability to think clearly. The forebrain center of logic is significantly slower than the reflex activity controlled by the hindbrain. Stress hormones constrict the blood vessel in the forebrain, thus reducing its ability to function (Lipton, 2005, p. 150). This sheds some light on why, when we are fixated in a state of overstimulated sympathetic nervous system overarousal, we develop various chronic diseases and lose our ability to think clearly. Many of my patients, and I am sure other therapists' patients, feel a sense of profound appreciation when hearing about this research. One patient cupped his hand to his head in a gesture of relief and said, "Now I understand why I've always felt like I was stupid when I was in a major conflict."

In the arena of post-traumatic stress, there have been many contributions to understanding why the role of the body is significant to healing. Dr. van der Kolk (2002), the prolific author of one hundred articles in the field, says that "the basic assumption that finding words to express the facts and feelings associated with traumatic experiences can reliably lead to a resolution turns out to be wrong" (p. 62). His research in brain functioning shows that when trauma occurs, the trauma is held in the right brain where it is inaccessible to verbal therapies. He posits, and much research is now confirming, that for many conditions, psychotherapies that incorporate the body are more successful than traditional therapies (Shapiro, 1995; Andrade & Feinstein, 2004; Wells et al., 2003).

Dr. van der Kolk and others have therefore reoriented their research direction due to understanding the importance of the body in healing. For example, infants have demonstrated the ability to heal from trauma and stress from being touched, making sounds, and through movements—such as rocking (van der Kolk & Fisler, 1995). Also, Dr. Levine (1997), author of *Waking the Tiger: Healing Trauma,* draws from animal sources showing the way that animals, such as impalas, heal from trauma. He explains that when the impala is chased, it will often play dead once its fight, flight, or freeze response is activated; once the impala stops moving, its predator—the cheetah—takes its awareness off the impala, and the impala is able to escape. The impala then heals through shaking, and by replaying the trauma by reenacting with fellow impalas the drama of the cheetah attack. This has formed part of Dr. Levine's method of *Somatic Re-experiencing*, that is, using the body to heal from trauma.

In realizing the importance of the body in healing, Dr. van der Kolk became interested in new methods of therapy, such as Eye Movement Desensitization Reprocessing (EMDR). In EMDR (Shapiro, 1995) traditional cognitive restructuring[1] is combined with a body-oriented approach of moving the eyes back and forth across the center-line. This method has shown promising results with post-traumatic stress, though it is still unclear as to exactly why. Some posit that it breaks up fixations in the brain where "dead spots" stop normal cognitive functioning from operating (Ruden, 2005). The key to a person's healing from trauma is to be able to be in the present, rather than react with the inflexible responses based upon the past trauma. Drawing from theories in physics, many therapists are now pursuing a *bottom-up*, meaning "from the body to the mind," approach.[2]

Researchers like Dr. van der Kolk put forth experimental evidence from brain scans about the effectiveness of various types of body-based psychotherapy approaches in healing trauma (van der Kolk et al., 1996; van der Kolk, 2002; Rauch, van der Kolk, & Fisler, et al., 1996). One of the keys to healing post-traumatic stress is the stimulation of the meaning reorganization centers of the brain, such as the amygdala (LeDoux, 1986; 1992), where new metaphors and new contexts emerge. After such body-based therapies as EMDR, brain scans do show a reactivation of these and other important areas of brain functioning (van der Kolk et al., 1996; van der Kolk, 2002; Shapiro, 1995).

You read about the importance of the role of the body in healing in the introduction and in Chapter Five on Bodymind Healing Psychotherapy's approach energy psychology. In Chapter Three you learned how preliminary research in the field of energy psychology, substantiated by brain-wave imaging and independent raters assessments, shows that meridian-based tapping plus cognitive therapy is more effective than cognitive therapies alone in dealing with anxiety (Andrade & Feinstein, 2004). Some postulate that one of the key elements of body-oriented energy psychology, such as tapping on acu-points on the body, may have a neurobiological basis behind its ability to work (Ruden, 2005).

In this era of bringing body-oriented approaches into psychotherapy, Qigong and Tai Chi have much to offer to help reverse sympathetic nervous system overload that comes from the fight, flight, or freeze response. As internal cultivation (*neigong*) traditions (Cohen, 1997; Kohn, 1989), Qigong and Tai Chi have developed over many centuries to help reverse the fight, flight, or freeze response for purposes of health and self-defense.

So, it is no wonder that a psychiatrist, such as Dr. van der Kolk, is experimenting with using Qigong in his trainings of trauma therapists. From the catalogue at his workshop on *Frontiers of Trauma Treatment* given at Esalen Institute (February 2005), he says, "Recovery needs to incorporate physical experiences that contradict feelings associated with helplessness and disconnection. The goal of treatment is to help bring the traumatic experience to an end, in every aspect of the human organism. This includes experiencing physical mastery to initiate new ways of perceiving reality and promoting new behavior patterns." In his workshops, toward this end, Dr. van der Kolk incorporates yoga, EMDR, Mindfulness Meditation, theater, breathing, touch, and Qigong.

I feel very honored that he is using my *Bodymind Healing Qigong DVD* in his trainings of trauma therapists. In addition to their long history of helping practitioners move from sympathetic nervous system overactivation to parasympathetic nervous system relaxation, Qigong and Tai Chi have other benefits. For example, the various movements of Qigong and Tai Chi activate *fongsung*, defined as "relaxed awakeness;" so these traditions both relax and re-empower—a valuable contribution to those suffering from trauma. A wide variety of Tai Chi and Qigong movements can also be useful for establishing new state-specific states of consciousness that "contradict feelings associated with helplessness and disconnection," as is shown in the case illustrations throughout this book.

One of the unfortunate outcomes of early childhood trauma is the development of "reactive instead of stable attachment styles" (Schore, 2003). This is one of the most common problems standing in the way of making relationships work for those who have suffered from childhood trauma. In cases of early childhood trauma, of general experiences when the stability of the self was not nurtured, or of neglect or ongoing maltreatment (Briere, 1997), Tai Chi and Qigong have the potential to be ideal complementary practices to psychotherapy. Those with reactive attachment disorders oftentimes respond to life stressors with retriggered fear and the activation of emotionally labile qualities rather than with modulated coping strategies. Tai Chi and Qigong can help to develop a cohesive center when the everyday issues of life assault or impinge upon a person's sensibilities; and they both can provide a bodily base for developing affect modulation and affect tolerance.

Using Qigong to Modulate the Sympathetic Nervous System Stress Response

Tai Chi Ruler (for an illustration see Chapter Twenty-one) is one such exercise that helps to reverse the fear response in the body by the action of simultaneously lifting the hands while sinking the body's energy to the center of the body in the belly and lower back (the Tan Tien and Ming Men). As an example, I recall a perfectionistic manager of a local company who was preparing to be a witness in a court case involving the murder of a family member. As part of his psychotherapy, we practiced Tai Chi Ruler; and he found the body movements and the sinking of the Qi helped to ground him in a state that countered his introjected paternal critic and the resultant obsessive need to get everything right. Then during the trial, he reported success when he touched his belly (Tan Tien) as a cue to remind him of the sinking of the Qi that he had experienced with the Tai Chi Ruler practice in his psychotherapy sessions to anchor this centered subpersonality. This is similar to the common behavioral treatment method of "systematic desensitization" when the relaxation response is used to reciprocally inhibit an unwanted behavior (Wolpe, 1958). Instead, here we are using Tai Chi and Qigong movements to decondition and reciprocally inhibit an unwanted response.

It may be impractical or incongruent with modern psychotherapy to ask a patient to stand up and practice Tai Chi Ruler in a session; however, psychotherapists can extract the essence of the internal martial arts tradition to help patients in a variety of ways. For example, patients can be introduced to the Elevator

Breathing method (see Chapter Six) as a way to sink their Qi without doing a Qigong movement. In everyday life any person can use Elevator Breathing and other Qigong methods to help reduce stress and find our central equilibrium in the midst of the emotional crosscurrents of life. In the following chapters, you will find various examples of how patients can significantly increase their relaxation response, producing useful effects for psychotherapy, behavioral health care, and our everyday lives.

Dr. van der Kolk et al. (1996) say that the first task of treatment is for patients to regain a sense of safety in their bodies: "Assault victims often benefit from 'model-mugging' programs, and physical challenges such as Outward Bound programs. Many women whose bodies have been violated report having been able to regain a sense of physical safety with the help of therapeutic massages" (p. 18).

One of the deepest injuries of severe trauma is that it "disconnects a person from her or his center or self—the essence of positive emotional wisdom and guidance that is best equipped to guide us" (Clinton, 2002, p. 101). Multimodal treatment approaches are a key element of many psychotherapeutic approaches that attempt to help restore patients' connection with the core of themselves. Finding a new ground of safety in one's body is a key to healing inside and outside of a therapist's office. As this ground in safety is found, emotional work can begin and overreactivity can begin to be modulated. For example, Krysal (1978), Pennebaker (1993), and Nemiah (1991) have all discussed the critical importance of learning to identify and utilize emotions as signals rather than as precipitants for fight, flight, or freeze reactions.

Bodymind Healing Psychotherapy (BMHP) proposes that many elements of the internal martial arts tradition, such as learning to sink Qi in response to an imagined or actual aggressor, can be beneficial in finding a new ground in safety in the body of those who have suffered from trauma. Once this ground is reestablished, this person can begin the inner work required to heal from his or her trauma.

Helpful Methods from Qigong and Tai Chi

In general, the practice of Tai Chi and Qigong have long been used to reprogram the body and the nervous system to reestablish a neurophysiology of harmony. Not only in the East, but in the West as well, enactments of physical movements have been a part of the healing process. For example, I mentioned earlier one of the rituals of the first holistic healing temple in the Western world, the temple of Aesclepius. As part of the healing process, people were sent to the Dionysian theater to act out a part in a play, which would be helpful to their healing.

With respect to healing trauma, I have suggested, when appropriate, to my trauma patients that they practice various Animal Qigong movements or other aspects of the Bodymind Healing Qigong tradition. Tiger movements from Yi Chuan Qigong and from Hua Tau's animal frolics (Mayer 2004b, p.135–137; Feng, 2003) are one type of practice that has particularly helped quite a few of my patients in reestablishing power in the re-empowering phase of treatment. A rape victim still carrying the trauma ten years later reported having benefited from the courage to practice Tai Chi Push Hands; she reported that these practices taught her how to feel in her body the ability to use her gentleness and a yielding movement to turn back an aggressive force of an attacker. Certainly due caution needs to be exercised to not be overconfident of our abilities to fend off an aggressor; here, I am addressing the re-empowerment that is part of the recovery phase in trauma care.[3]

Depth Psychotherapy and Trauma

Healing of trauma involves much more than just finding safety and groundedness in the body. What depth psychology teaches is that oftentimes the psychological results of trauma "develop not in response to the trauma per se, but in reaction to the fantasies through which it gets an attributed meaning" (Kalsched, 1996, p. 95). Thus, a fundamental aspect of psychotherapeutic healing is to help patients come to terms with the meaning of the trauma. It is common for those who have been a subject of abuse to develop patterns—such as withdrawing from conflict, being a victim, or being an unconscious perpetrator—because "when innocence has been deprived of its entitlement it becomes a diabolical spirit" (Grotstein, 1984).

In Dr. Kalsched's (1996) profound book *The Inner World of Trauma*, he says that one aspect of the depth psychological answer to healing such patterns is through *lumen* (light) and *numen* (meaning). This type of "light" that heals trauma in the Western mystery tradition has been called *lumen naturae* (the light of nature), or *soma pneumatikon* (spirit body), which is related to the body's animating spirit. Dr. Jung, drawing from an old alchemical text, put it this way, "There is in the human body a certain aethereal substance . . . of heavenly nature, known to a very few, which needeth no medicament, being itself the incorrupt medicament" (Jung, 1955, para., 114n).

The parallels between the Western notions of this healing lumen and the Qigong practices that have remained intact in the East are striking. I propose that these lumen-generating practices can be incorporated to help heal trauma. Likewise, regarding the healing tool of numen, after going though the descent into the felt darkness of the traumatized complex, a key moment in healing often comes when the patient finds a new meaning, such as *this abuse led me to be a healer, or it helped me to be more sensitive to the suffering of others.* You will later see how finding a new meaningful life stance is a key element in the Mythic Journey Process, and in various other aspects of the Bodymind Healing Qigong tradition.

Healing Trauma with Bodymind Healing Psychotherapy

In many of the following chapters, case illustrations of patients are presented who would easily have fit in this chapter, but instead I used their cases to illustrate other important themes of Bodymind Healing Psychotherapy. For example, in Chapter Sixteen on incorporating patients' gestures, you will read about a case of a female victim of sexual abuse who naturally came up with a posture like the Tai Chi movement called Fist under Elbow, which helped to give her a sense of safety and groundedness in her body. This helped her to have the confidence to deflect the assaultive energy she felt coming from aggressive men. She reported that the sense of groundedness that developed from her Standing Meditation and Tai Chi helped to give her a safety zone, where she was better able to differentiate men's intentions and better able to modulate her responses to men.

In Chapter Fifteen about changing your life stance, you will read about a young man who was the victim of his brother's physical abuse and how Standing Meditation Qigong helped him find his stance of power with his brother.

In Chapter Twenty on the Mythic Journey Process, you will review an example of a woman who was a rape victim and had passive-aggressive tendencies that were endangering her marriage. A combination of psychotherapy, learning the animal movements of Qigong, and a Mythic Journey Process helped her to realize she was being "an ostrich rather than an openhearted crane." She reported that all of the above traditions, including doing the Crane movement from the animal forms of Qigong, helped her to transform her withdrawing pattern and develop a more open, modulated, and expressive communication style with her husband.

It is important to remember the advice in Chapter Four from Master Hon and his Ping-Pong Ball analogy in which he said that that isolated movements may go along with the technique-oriented Western mind; yet the real key to healing involves filling the dented Ping-Pong ball of our lives with the "warm tea" of our life energy. This is analogous to the wisdom of the Western mystery tradition that we just discussed regarding finding the *lumen naturae.* The wide range of psychotherapeutic and Qigong methods are part of the process of finding our inner heat and recovering our inner illumination. Specific movements like Tai Chi Ruler, Standing Meditation Qigong, and Tiger or Crane movements can be an integral part of reconnecting to a life stance that shapeshifts a trauma victim back into being grounded in his or her primordial Self. Also, the Mythic Journey Process can be part of the process of transmutation of our self-identifications.

Case Illustration: Treating the Long-Term, Retriggered Effects of Past Physical Trauma

The following case shows how—even without doing Qigong or Tai Chi or a Mythic Journey Process—Bodymind Healing Psychotherapy (BMHP) methods can facilitate the healing of trauma. By extracting certain aspects of the essence of these traditions, we can use the River of Life practices and shapeshift into new stances grounded in new meanings.

To exemplify how BMHP functions in the case of a past trauma affecting a patient's physical health, I will refer to a patient called "Gerry," a single father in his early forties, who was referred by an orthopedic doctor to our integrative medical clinic. While Gerry was taking out the garbage one day, his back went into spasm. For three months he was unable to walk up the stairs to the second floor of his house and switched bedrooms with one of his children downstairs. One surgeon had already recommended surgery, and our orthopedic back specialist wanted to see what a noninvasive approach could accomplish before he concurred with the first doctor's opinion.

In our second session, after some rapport had been built, Gerry was lying on the couch in my office in pain. Because he could not sit up comfortably in my office, I suggested he take an acu-yoga posture—sometimes called the child's pose while touching Bladder meridian acu-points in the inside corner of the eyes (Gach & Marco, 1981, p. 150). While Gerry was in that posture, I introduced him to the combination of breathing and guided visualization used in the River of Life practice (see Chapter Five), in which Gerry sensed a river of energy traveling down his body along with his breath. He described a sensation in his back like a block of ice stopping the flow of the river. I asked Gerry not to try to change this, but just to imagine the sun shining on the block of ice, gradually melting it. I then asked him while focusing on the body block to report any images or words that arose from the block while it was melting. After a few minutes, his subdued crying turned into deep sobbing. Gerry exclaimed, "It couldn't be this, it couldn't be this . . ."

Gerry then proceeded to tell me how when he was sixteen years old he was hitchhiking and he got into a car with two men. They sexually assaulted him, stabbed him in the back, and left him in a ditch. He made his way back to his parent's house but never told them about this until after our session. When he was a teenager, his parents had forbidden him to hitchhike. Gerry did not want to admit to his parents that they were right about hitchhiking, and so he suffered his shame in silence.

Over the next sessions, we worked with healing the trauma of this repressed incident. Gerry released his shame and feelings of victimization by experiencing his anger toward his perpetrators, and he forgave himself for not sharing this story with his parents for all of these years. Most important, he was able to see that his current pattern of not sharing with others and standing up for his truth was related to this past trauma. He realized that this had been a major factor contributing to his divorce. Gerry saw that "developing spine" in his interpersonal relationships was an important part of his life's meaning and not "holding back" his truth. Gerry had found his numen.

Because I am not a therapist who generally believes in miracle cures but instead one who knows that transformation often takes long hard work, I was surprised to hear Gerry's report on his progress. Within a few weeks of this session, he was back to his old jogging schedule of running up mountains and was able to move back to his upstairs bedroom. Not only was there a healing on a physical level, but Gerry also took the metaphor of "the pain held in his back" as a numinous symbol of his life's journey—to work on not holding back his truth and to work on developing his spine in relationship with others.

Whenever I tell this story of Gerry's transformation, I am careful to point out that I cannot be certain that his dramatic change was due to our therapy. Gerry had also been seeing the chiropractor and an acupuncturist at our clinic. However, I must say that I believe and hope that the type of integrative treatment for patients with certain somatic complaints will be the standard approach to medicine sometime soon in our twenty-first century—using the least intrusive and most cost-effective methods first before moving to costly, more invasive methods.

CHAPTER NINE

Addictions

Bodymind Healing Psychotherapy for Addictions

Carl Jung once said that only "a radical rearrangement of consciousness" could have any lasting effect on individuals suffering from chronic addictions (Sparks, 1993). Using the etymological definition of the word *radical* as meaning "returning to the roots," from the perspective of Bodymind Healing Psychotherapy, one aspect of addiction involves returning to the roots of the "ego-Self axis." This requires not only dealing with the ego's dysfunctional coping strategies that first led to the addiction and replacing them with more healthy coping strategies, but also it requires helping patients' higher Selves find a pathway to link to the wider whole of which we are a part.

The following method can serve as an adjunct to either a broader psychotherapy or a Twelve Step approach to healing addictions. It is useful for those who suffer from addictions, as well as for the helping professionals who serve them. It is a way to help overcome addictive patterns and return to the roots of the primordial Self who basks in the natural ways to feel "high." A basic instinct fundamental to being human is the ability to enter into altered states naturally; for example, through breathing, rocking, moving, imagining, and so forth. It has been hypothesized that one of the roots of addictive processes is our culture's lack of adequate initiation rites where the individual learns to find natural ways to link with the higher power that is the source of our life's energy—by whatever name we call it, and through whatever means we access it.

The resources we need in order to cope with a difficult world are within us, if we could just take the time to tap these inner wells. Our body's biochemistry activates endorphins when we are in need of pain relief; our breath can put us into a pleasurable altered state as we activate our parasympathetic nervous system and the well-documented relaxation response occurs; and our imagination creates images that have neurobiological correlates so that we can not only imagine a river, but also experience its healing effects.

Next, I will outline the Bodymind Healing Psychotherapy (BMHP) method for addictions, using cigarette smoking as an example. Those who suffer from addictions can do this method in one or more sessions with a health professional or as a self-practice method. The process can be done in its entirety, as it exists below in its five parts, or it can be trimmed to suit individual needs. While describing the method, I incorporate the case of a married woman, named Mary here, who was working in the mail sorting room at a local corporation and who was smoking about a pack a day. She came to me after hearing from our clinic that I did hypnosis for smoking addictions. She said that a close friend of hers had just died from emphysema; this finally motivated her to try to stop.

The BMHP Process for Smoking Addictions

Preliminary Questionnaire for Smoking and Other Addictions

- **Take a History:** When did smoking begin? What were the psychological reasons for beginning? What feelings were associated with these times, such as feeling insecure and trying to fit in with peers, not feeling cool like someone who you admired who was following this addictive pattern, and shame over not living up to some standard. Do you realize that your smoking, or following another addictive pattern, was because you did not know another way of coping with this feeling? Was it your way of medicating this feeling? What was that feeling?

- **Past History of Attempts to Stop:** What methods were tried? What happened?

- **Reasons to Stop:** What are the reasons you want to stop smoking now? What kind of negative effects has this addiction had in your life?

- **Triggers:** What are the current places that trigger you—that are your most chosen locations where you self-medicate rather than using alternative methods of coping? What are the feelings associated with those trigger times? Where do you feel these triggering stresses in your body? Does some image express what that feels like? For example, maybe it is at work when you are overwhelmed by all that you have to do.

This was the case for Mary as she worked in the mail sorting room. When overwhelmed, she felt like electrical wires shooting out electricity in all directions with no ground.

- **Identifying a Favorite Object:** What is your favorite flower, animal, and place in nature? What is your favorite houseplant? (This will be used later as a sacrificial object.)

Part I: River of Life Preparatory Induction

Breathing: *Check abdominal breathing by putting one hand on your belly. As you inhale, does your stomach go out? This is correct abdominal breathing. Then use Microcosmic Orbit Breath: Naturally inhale and feel the breath rising up the back, on your exhalation feel the breath coming down the front of your body. Notice how long the out-breath lasts, and be aware of the pause after the exhalation. As you are noticing the out-breath going down your body, your eyes will naturally feel like dropping or closing.*

Imagine a River: *Picture the most beautiful river you have ever seen, or the most beautiful one you can imagine. What kind of trees and flowers are growing next to it? How fast is it flowing? Perhaps you can hear it rushing or dribbling over rocks or smell some element of nature around the river. As you breathe out, imagine that river flowing down the front of your body: The longer your exhalation, the deeper the stream. Do not try to let go of tension but just imagine the river flowing over that tension, as if water was flowing over leaves or encumbrances and gradually freeing up the blockages so that they get washed down stream. At the end of your out-breath, the river comes to a still pool where you are seated with a nice tree against your back. What is your favorite tree? Feel its strength supporting you. This is the river of your life. Get a sense of how it came from the rain of the heavens, flowed down through the mountains, and formed your life-stream. Maybe you will see some images about those places where the river became constricted or blocked as you felt _____ (fill in your feeling here that you medicated through using your substance of choice).*

Identifying Your Triggers: *Picture the time in your life right now that you find your-self getting most triggered. What time of day is it? Where are you? Can you picture something, a color or an object, that is in those surroundings? Can you feel how your body gets some certain feeling, perhaps a blockage, when that situation exists? Imagine that blockage as a block of ice (or choose your own image) in the river.*

Coalescing Your Blockage into a Belief: *Focus on that felt sense of your body block and what it is about. Can you get a sense of a belief, phrase, or image that gets the worst of it? For example, Mary's sense of overwhelm was associated with her belief of* I'm a failure for not being able to get done as much as other employees. *Assign your-self a number for how strong you feel this belief, phrase, or image on a SUDS scale (10 being the most you have ever felt stress and 0 being totally relaxed). Mary was a 9 on this scale. Imagine writing this belief on the block of ice and feel how the issue blocks the river of your breath.*

Restructuring Your Belief: *What is a more constructive or truthful belief (not nec-essarily a more positive belief)? Mary first came up with a belief of* I'm acceptable the way I am with all my limitations. *This brought her SUDS level down to a 6. I asked Mary how much she believed this statement on a 10-point scale (10 being the most) and she said, "not that much." I asked her what would be a more truthful or constructive belief? She said, "Even though I am slower than others, I deserve to be loved the way I am." This brought her down from her original 6 to a 3.*

Self-Soothing: *Put one hand on your heart and one hand on your belly. As you say your constructive belief, imagine that you have in your hands the love that you have given to another at a time when they were in difficulty. Or imagine the person who has most loved you and imagine his or her hands on your heart. How many breaths does it take to let that love in?*

Identifying Underlying Psychodynamics: *For some people more rounds may be necessary to get to the crux of what is creating the block. Both Mary's mother and father had had high expectations of her and were always comparing her to other children and to her brother. She remembers being hit on a few occasions when she brought home a "bad" grade (C) in school. She was criticized rather than coached. So, not living up to other's expectations activated a sympathetic nervous system fight, flight, or freeze response.*

Melting Your Blockage with Compassion: *Go back to your breathing and see the old ice block with the negative belief written on it. Imagine as you are touching your heart that the compassionate light of the sun is shining on the ice. The sun shines on everything on the earth regardless of how light or dark, good or bad it is. Gradually the sun melts the ice. (Do not try to do anything, just let the sun's love gradually melt your ice.) Sometimes this takes a short time, sometimes it takes a day, and sometimes it takes longer. Allow the love of the sun to turn the ice into water. As you let go with your exhalation, can you feel the water flow all the way down to the still pool within you?*

Part 2: The River of Life Practice Targeted to Smoking and Other Addictions

Imagine you are sitting with your back against a tree by the side of this river. In front of you is a fork in the river. Recognize that you are at a turning point in your life—a fork in the river. Imagine walking alongside one of the two rivers. In and along this river are cigarette butts, and the river is an ugly yellow color. You continue to walk down the river where there are dead flowers and dying trees along its banks. Be aware of your own sensitivity to these life forms as if you could hear them crying out in pain from dying from the tobacco-laced river. Eventually you have walked past many crying life forms: fish lying belly-up, deer lying dead from drinking from the river, and so forth. Finally you reach the stagnant, putrid pond at the river's end, where cigarettes butts have accumulated over many years. Can you smell it?

Allow an image to arise of the many people who thought they could beat the odds and are lying here with emphysema or other diseases—maybe an image will come of one of those people lying in the hospital, attached by a tube in his or her throat to a machine that is breathing for him or her. Here on the river, your favorite animal is lying down, making sounds of pain as it takes its last few breaths after being poisoned by the river. You apologize to the animal for your lack of strength to not pollute the river; you make excuses to the animal (all the excuses you usually make about why you cannot stop smoking). Your favorite animal looks at you pleadingly; but when it tries to utter something, it just emits a hacking cough. You stop and pause and let in the message of this suffering animal, and you think about how this is like the pleading of others in your life who care about you and look pleadingly at you. (Notice how your breath is right now and how your body feels. Do you recognize that this polluted river is one of your choices?)

Next, imagine that you are again by the tree at the fork in the river. Feel its strength against your back. Notice your exhalation going to its strong roots. Be aware of the beautiful, clear river that flows right in front of you and down the other river fork, and begin walking down that fork of the river. Notice the beautiful flowers, trees, and foliage along the banks. You can even see fish swimming through the clean, clear waters. Be aware of other images that might arise to represent the path that would emerge in your life if you followed this river. What is the posture that you hold as you are walking with a sense of accomplishment, pride, and strength of character on this path? Notice the admiration from those whom you care about, admiring that you have had the strength to choose this path. At times there may be difficulties with this path—your cravings for your old habit of walking down the other stream may produce irritability and headache; but the beauty, power, and flowing vitality of the river you are now walking along strengthens the conviction that you are following the path meant for you. Follow the river down to the ocean. As you feel the sand under your feet, you look out at the sea of healthy new life possibilities that await you. What feelings are associated with your sense of accomplishment? And what postural stance do you now embody? Touch or tap on the part of your body that you associate with this new stance to awaken further its energy.

Part 3: Anchoring the Process

Imagine those habitual places where you smoke in your everyday life. Just as you are located where you are seated now and imagining you are in those habitual smoking spots, when you are located where you smoke, you can imagine you are in the location where you are now—or back in your sanctuary by your inner river. Your breath and the body part that you just touched will be your anchors. This River of Life practice will become your practice one day, one hour, one minute at a time—to choose to travel down the path of the river of increased health.

If you want to smoke, put your fingers (of the opposite hand from the one you use to smoke) up to your lips without a cigarette in them. Say to yourself smok-

ing is a natural desire; but I have distorted the desire to smoke fresh air and replaced it with a toxic mimic (smoking). I will now smoke fresh air. Take a few puffs of fresh air through your fingers, and feel the fresh air taking you back to the healthy river of your inner sanctuary.

You have the choice of which river you want to travel—the one of disease, and shortened life or the one of _____ (fill in the reasons you listed in the Preliminary Questionnaire for wanting to stop smoking). The healthy river is one where you will achieve your goal(s) of _____ (repeat the reasons for wanting to stop smoking).

In the next days or weeks, you will continue to make choices between which river you want to travel down. Feel the place in your body where your commitment to walk down the river of your health and to follow your desire to fulfill the goals (reasons for wanting to stop smoking). Touch or tap on that part of your body to anchor that commitment.

Part 4: Post-Session Options

Outside of your Bodymind Healing Psychotherapy session, you have two choices.

1. Throw away all of your cigarettes today and stop smoking today. Then when you feel the desire to smoke, try one (or all) of the above practices that worked best for you. If you still cannot resist smoking, do the *sacrificial object* method below.

2. With the advice of your medical doctor, smoke more cigarettes than you ever have at one time, until you get sick. By overloading with an excessive, distasteful amount of cigarettes, this can create an extremely negative association to cigarettes. However, if you still have a desire to smoke at some point, try the *sacrificial object* method below.

Part 5: The Sacrificial Object Method

Save all of your cigarette butts and put them into a big glass of water. Pour the water into your favorite flowerpot or houseplant. Make sure that this plant is in a place that you walk by regularly, or is in a place where you regularly smoke.

Create a ritual where you ask for forgiveness from the plant for needing to sac-rifice it to find your path. Promise the plant that its sacrifice will not be in vain: tell the plant that you will use its sacrifice not only to follow a healthy life path but also to give, in some way, to loved ones or the planet that will make this plant's sacrifice more worthwhile. Tell the plant that any time you see another plant of the same species, you will pay it special attention, water it, and/or send it loving wishes.

Overview of the Process

This method of smoking cessation provides a means to stop not only smoking but also other addictions. These are the basic components of the protocol:

- Establish an altered state of consciousness by Microcosmic Orbit Breathing and guided visualization of the River of Life practice.

- Imagine sitting at a fork in the river with your back against a tree. Then take a walk alongside one fork of the river imagining the negative outcomes of this addictive path. Walk down the other riverbank imagining the positive out-comes from breaking the addiction.

- Create a ritual during which you acknowledge that you have a choice to stop your addictive pattern or you will transfer harm to some element of nature that is significant to you. This sacrifice should not be taken lightly, and it is done to induce a commitment to use this sacrifice for the world's, and your life's, higher good.

Additional Helpful Methods

Sometimes our psychological patterns are so entrenched that even the previ-ous ritual will not be enough to handle our inner demons. In this case the other elements of Bodymind Healing Psychotherapy can be of assistance.

- **Psychodynamic dimension:** Explore the underlying patterns that lead to self-destructive behaviors. What created these patterns in our family of ori-gins? What costs do we pay? What secondary gains come from not changing? And what benefits would accrue from a new path?

- **Cognitive Restructuring and Focusing Dimensions:** What beliefs stand in the way of changing? And what would be more truthful or constructive new beliefs? Focusing on what is behind these patterns and beliefs that are stuck in the body can lead to finding the crux of what keeps them entrenched and can create felt shifts, new meanings, and new pathways.

- **Symbolic Process Dimension:** Try doing a Mythic Journey Process (see Chapter Twenty) to activate the archetypal layer of the psyche and thereby find a new healing path.

Various other elements from the healing mandala of life are useful, such as changing diet; increasing liquid intake; and drinking herbal or green teas, aloe vera juice, and so forth. Just as Twelve Step programs have taught us that social support is an important part of recovery, you need to assess whom you can call when you are tempted to go back to your substance of choice. Check with your doctor and/or other health professionals for the most current treatment methods. Chinese medicine and herbs and acupuncture have some significant research pointing to their benefits as an adjunct. Find a Qigong movement that helps to remove the stuck energy that comes from detoxifying. In particular, Tiger Qigong (see Volume 1 on the Yi Chuan Tiger) can help to release irritability and strengthen the Lung meridian (Mayer, 2004, p 135).

During our follow-up session three months later, Mary announced she had totally stopped smoking because she did not want to "hurt something living (her favorite plant)." She realized that her lungs and her life were also something living. In the process of stopping smoking, Mary realized that she had started smoking again when her mentally ill father had committed suicide, and she had felt responsible. Mary made a choice to embark on a course of depth psychotherapy to heal her patterns of taking on other's issues and feeling bad if she did not meet other's expectations. She realized that these patterns were affecting her relationship with her husband and made this conscious decision, "Now that smoking is out of the way, it's time to look at other problem areas of my life." Mary's subsequent therapy regarding these deeper issues is beyond the scope of the current chapter.

Case Illustration: Binge Eating

The process outlined above can be adapted to use for any addiction. For example, a patient, whom I will call Amy, was binge eating at night. As she focused on the feeling she experienced right before eating, she first said it was a sense of being bored. But then a deep feeling of sadness emerged as Amy realized she had been avoiding dealing with the loss of her oldest brother, who she described as being like a father and her companion. She felt alone and abandoned. Even though Amy was married, she felt abandoned when her husband went off to work on his computer at night. This paralleled her past, similar feeling of emotional abandonment by her parents.

Amy had been in talk therapy for many years and complained about it not working; and now, in addition, she was taking Prozac to treat her depression. Amy reported that her psychiatrist had told her that she should be over her grief, which added to Amy's guilt. The self-soothing practice of one hand on the heart and one hand on the belly was helpful in getting Amy out of her intellectual mode of dealing with her loss. Also using the Emotional Freedom Technique method, she said, "Even though I have pain, I can accept and have compassion for my feelings of grief and abandonment." This statement brought solace and lowered her SUDS level significantly. Her favorite place was the ocean, so it fit in well with the BMHP River of Life breathing method. Amy jokingly said that her inner sanctuary of the river merging with the ocean provided her with an "interesting inner movie to watch," and that it helped as a substitute to self-medicating with food.

Sacrifice: A Key Tool in Addictions and in Therapy in General

Sacrifice of something in the real world is an important part of ancient rituals. Our ancient psychological colleagues knew that when they sacrificed a goat or an animal this could lead to a transformative effect on the human psyche. Though we can take pride in that as modern people, we have evolved to a point where we do not need to sacrifice a young maiden to create transformation in ourselves or in our tribe; nonetheless, there is still something useful that can be extracted from such rituals. Sacrifice, when done with mindful awareness, can add psychic energy to produce healing effects. In a primordially based psychotherapy, it is one more tool given by the powers of the universe and nature for our healing.

For Mary, the anticipated sacrifice of a plant helped her to save her lungs. It is important to realize that the object to be sacrificed needs to be one that is very significant to the particular patient. In my experience the anticipated sacrifice of a living thing from nature, or a meaningful object, can be a motivator for many people to stop an addiction.

The Case of the Batterer and the Baby Grand Piano

I remember a situation in which the sacrifice of a meaningful object was a transformative agent in a case of couple's therapy. A man, whom I will refer to as George, had impulse control problems and had battered his girlfriend on a few occasions. She said she would give their relationship one last try. After they came to see me and a few sessions of teaching them nonviolent communication, George's partner "Alice," in the midst of tears, said she still did not trust George. She said she could not think of anything that would make her believe he would not batter her again—regardless of the progress that he seemed to make in therapy. I asked George what his most valuable possession was. He replied that his grandfather's grand piano was what his life was about; and after a long day at the office, the opportunity to play a tune on this family heirloom was what he lived for. (He qualified the statement with a wink at Alice, clarifying that she was his grand, grand piano and also what he lived for.) I then challenged George about how much Alice really meant to him: I asked if he would be willing to put a contract in her safety deposit box, stating that if he ever hit her again, he would sacrifice his grand piano. He paused for a brief moment and then said, "Yup, I'd be willing to sign."

In the sessions that followed, this agreement helped Alice regain her trust, along with the work that they continued to do on their relationship. It worked. After termination, I heard from Alice and George about a year later to thank me for the work we had done and to let me know that there were no further incidents of violence and that they had just been married.

Twelve-Step Programs

A twelve-step program is a useful complementary tool that works well in conjunction with psychotherapy for addictions. Specifically, for alcoholism, sex and love addictions, and various major drug addictions many people achieve beneficial results from the philosophy, camaraderie, support, and the spiritual path based on connecting with "a higher power" involved in these programs.

I have had the experience of doing psychotherapy with quite a few people who are simultaneously in such programs. Other patients, who do not appreciate aspects of twelve-step programs for a variety of reasons, will chose only to do psychotherapy. Depending upon the person, and the severity of his or her addiction, this may or may not be successful. I have known patients who wanted to avoid twelve-step programs; and at times I have agreed to work with patients without their entering into a twelve-step program on the condition that they are honest with me and will agree to go to a twelve-step program if they slip back into old addictive patterns. Appropriate assessment of the severity of an addiction regarding a person's ability to gain control over his or her addictive patterns without the support of a twelve-step program is a key element of treatment.

Case Illustration: Working with Codependence— A Kabbalistic/Qigong Perspective

When a loved one is suffering with addiction, it tests our own limits and boundaries. Such was the case for a man, called Mark here, who had been in depth psychotherapy with me for about six months, working on his "reactive attachment style," among other things. This had caused him problems in many of his relationships, including his son, over the years. Mark's twenty-five-year-old son had recovered from alcoholism due to a twelve-step program; and he had not had a drink for four years. Yet Mark's son had begun smoking again.

Mark's mother had died of lung cancer, and during the son's teenage years before he moved out of the house, Mark had many arguments with his son trying to convince the young man to stop smoking and drinking—to no avail.

As part of Mark's therapy during those years, he worked on his codependence; that is, looking at the sense of self-righteousness that he felt from being the all-knowing father. But Mark noticed that he still had a hard time catching himself from falling into this old, codependent pattern. It was particularly difficult when Mark saw his son for the first time in about a year and saw him smoking. Mark reported that by remembering his breathing, this helped him to sink his Qi and not be reactive. In addition, Mark told me about how he applied a principle he had heard from me many months earlier: when he wanted to tell his new girlfriend how weak she was regarding her overeating problem. At that point we discussed the principle of *tsimtsum*, from the Kabbalah, meaning "a withdrawal or retreat" (Scholem, 1969, pp. 258–264). In the creation myth of the Kabbalah, it is said that God created the world by stepping back; and from the space created, the world came into being.

Mark found meaning in acting out the creation myth of the Kabbalah with his girlfriend and with others, by withdrawing and stepping back from his judgments, thereby following the path of *tsimtsum*. And when Mark saw his son the next time, we were in the process of exploring his affect modulation skills regarding how to balance right assertiveness versus withdrawing and making space. Mark proudly reported to me that although when he saw his son smoking, he felt like strangling him with words, he first exhaled and then remembered the stepping back of the Kabbalah. During the week that his son stayed in town, Mark did not confront him as he had done in the past. At the end of the visit, the son told Mark how much he appreciated that his father was not getting on his case about his smoking. Mark replied, "Why should I get on your case? You are an adult now; and I know you have the strength to stop when you decide to, as you did with alcohol and with cigarettes in the past."

Mark's son expressed deep appreciation for his father's nonconfrontational attitude; and in a few months, the son quit smoking on his own. When Mark expressed appreciation for his new changed attitude in one of our sessions, he commented on how the Tai Chi Push Hands practice that he was learning (from another instructor) was teaching him how to avoid force when interacting with others. Mark said, "This nonforce stuff is really beginning to take root in my body."

CHAPTER TEN

Insomnia

Research

A record 43 million sleeping pill prescriptions were filled the United States in 2005, fueled by almost $300 million in drug companies' advertising, which resulted in more than $2 billion in sales. Consider these statistics for a moment: More than 70 million people in the United States may be affected by sleep troubles, according the National Institute of Health. The National Commission on Sleep Disorders Research estimates that 40 million Americans suffer from chronic sleep problems, and as many as 30 million more have occasional difficulty sleeping. The use of sleeping pills by adults, ages twenty to forty-four, doubled between 2000 and 2004; and according to IMS Health, a market researcher, the 43 million prescriptions issued by doctors last year represent a thirteen percent increase from 2004. Sleep deprivation and related disorders cost the nation $16 billion in annual health-care expenses and approximately $50 billion in lost productivity, according to the U.S. surgeon general (Laszarus, 2005).

According to Dennis McGinty, a professor of psychology at University of California, Los Angeles who specializes in sleep disorders, insomnia can result from a wide variety of factors: some physiological, some psychological, and some behavioral. But McGinty says, "one cause that hasn't yet been closely studied by experts is the impact on sleep of American's increasingly stressful lives . . . and that's something you can change through your attitude . . . by getting more exercise, or by just looking up at the sky from time to time" (as cited in Laszarus, 2005). Rachel Manber, director of the insomnia program at the Stanford Sleep Disorder Clinic (in California) says, "the biggest concern is that people are getting swayed by the drug companies' marketing campaign and are accepting that little if any risk is attached to frequent use of so-called hypnotics to catch some shut-eye. This means that people are taking a shortcut to circumvent insomnia, rather than addressing whatever the root causes may be. Sleep problems relay to us a message that something is wrong. Taking medication is the same as killing the messenger" (as cited in Laszarus, 2005).

Solid research shows mind-body interventions to be effective in helping with insomnia. For example, a randomized trial found that cognitive-behavioral therapy (alone and in combination with pharmacologic therapy) effectively reduced the amount of time it took elderly patients to fall asleep after going to bed. Only those subjects treated with the behavioral approach maintained treatment gains at follow-up: While pharmacological treatments produce somewhat faster sleep improvements in the short-term; behavioral approaches show comparable effects in the intermediate-term (four to eight weeks); and in the long-term (six to twenty-four months) behavioral approaches show more favorable outcomes than drug therapies (Morin, Culbert, & Schwartz, 1999; Morin, Mimeault, & Gagne, 1999).

Regarding Qigong in particular, Dr. Pelletier (2000) reports, "Qigong exercises helped patients with insomnia, according to a 1996 review of the literature by Dr. Kenneth Sancier, president of the Qigong Institute in Menlo Park, California" (p. 360). Specifically with seniors in a randomized controlled study (which used a well-respected self-report measurement called the Pittsburgh Sleep Quality Index [PSQI]), Tai Chi showed greater benefit compared to stretching exercises on sleep-quality outcomes (Li et al., 2001). In another randomized controlled study, Tai Chi Ruler, or Tai Chi Chih, was shown to improve sleep quality in adults with moderate sleep complaints. The participants, ranging from fifty-one to eighty-six years old, showed these results after sixteen weeks of practice—three times a week for forty minutes each session. A research design was used which randomly assigned 112 participants from the surrounding community to a Health Education class (HE) or to a TCC group without telling them the purpose of the study. This helped to eliminate the problem of long-term, enthusiastic Tai Chi advocates potentially (consciously or unconsciously) biasing the outcome measures. Nearly two-thirds of the TCC group, as reported on the PSQI, showed improvements in sleep quality as compared to one-third of the HE control group. These gains held for nine weeks after completion of the training (Irwin et al., 2008, p.1006). These results are particularly significant for seniors, because although aerobic exercise can help people sleep better, vigorous workouts are not an option for many seniors. (The Tai Chi Ruler practice is illustrated in Chapter 21 of this book and can also be seen as a You Tube link from the front page my Web site www.bodymindhealing.com.)

In the rest of this chapter, I will discuss how Bodymind Healing Psychotherapy integrates some aspects of Qigong with other BMHP methods for the benefit of those who suffer with insomnia. Of course, for severe sleep disorders, such as those involving sleep-disordered breathing, it is helpful to attend a sleep clinic and draw from the whole range of integrative medicine—which includes the latest measures, such as polysomnography. However, for most sleep-related problems, combining the known benefits of exercise and Qigong with the deep emotional healing abilities of Western bodymind healing approaches creates a viable, powerful alternative to pharmacological medications.

Pharmacological treatments have several disadvantages compared to bodymind healing methods. Pharmaceuticals oftentimes produce "rebound insomnia"; when the patient stops taking the medication, they have side effects. And pharmaceuticals disempower the person regarding having confidence in his or her own inner resources. According to a recent report by CNN, taking the most common sleeping medication, Ambien, may be related to sleep walking and "sleep driving" in some patients.[1] For this reason it seems that the intelligent consumer would try to use the best mind-body approaches before using medications, at least as a first line of defense. Pharmacological treatments fit well with the prevailing corporate worldview that pushes "outside fixes" and hypnotizes the public through advertising hype to de-emphasize the need to do inner work to find healing. Certainly there is a place for using "outer world"-oriented solutions for insomnia. Awareness of the effects of caffeinated drinks and appropriate exercise are keys; and use of medications and herbal remedies, such as Valerian can be important adjuncts to treatment (Pelletier, 2000, p. 171). Be aware of your body's unique reactions to Valerian to see if it has any unwanted side effects. Check with your medical doctor regarding such remedies as Melatonin, which helps some people, but stimulates others, causing nightmares or hangovers, and it may harm the reproductive system (Pelletier, 2000, p. 111).

However, since symptoms are often symbolic messages from the deep recesses of the unconscious mind, it is important to listen to these messages as learning opportunities. As we move into a horizontal position and go to sleep, we leave the world of everyday life and we get a chance to lie horizontally at one with the truth of our spirit. If issues are in the way of our spirit being at rest, we have a chance to be at peace with these issues before gaining entry into the deeper recesses of the sacred world of sleep.

To address these wider, deeper dimensions of insomnia, Bodymind Healing Psychotherapy uses the following eight-leveled holographic approach, which can be used by any of us whether or not we are in psychotherapy.

Bodymind Healing Psychotherapy Treatment Protocol for Insomnia

I. Nonattachment to Falling Asleep

One major reason why people suffer from various natural autonomic nervous system disorders is that they are trying to force something that is natural. For example, many who are suffering from sexual impotency issues try to force sexuality when the body is trying to express a message. As sexual potency naturally declines in our later years, rather than accommodating these natural changes— fueled by a culture that worships youth and a drug industry that profits from selling us unnatural fantasies—we buy into an unrealistic vision. I am not speaking against taking an occasional Viagra pill but rather about the excessive use of medication in a compensatory manner that damages our health in the short- and/or long-term (Pomeranz & Bhavsar, 2005). Likewise with anxiety, fighting against it can contribute to panic attacks. So, the first step in treatment of autonomic nervous system disorders is to try not to fight something that is natural in many cases, and to say the following when having difficulty sleeping:

This is an opportunity to catch up on my relaxation/self-healing meditation practice. If I was in a monastery now, I would have to get up to the sound of a bell; and though I would have an opportunity to appreciate this hour of the morning and the silence around me, I would have to sit up and be in a cold uncomfortable room. Instead now, at this hour of the morning in my comfortable bed, I can be aware, enjoy my surroundings, and notice my breath. Going into a deep state of trance or relaxation will be as healing for me as going to sleep.

2. Microcosmic/Macrocosmic Orbit Breathing and the River of Life Practice

Notice your inhalation as the energy rises along with it up the back, and on the exhalation notice your energy sink down to your belly. Continue the oval breathing circle from the perineum to the top of your head. Then extend your breathing all the way down to your feet using the River of Life practice (see Chapter Four, where both the Microcosmic and Macrocosmic Breathing methods are explained in greater detail).

3. Self-Soothing: One Hand on the Heart, One on the Belly

For more details, refer to Chapter Six.

4. Acu-point Self-Touch

CHI NEI TSANG (CHIA & CHIA, 1990)

Making your way around your belly clock, press in gently on the exhalation (see Chapter Six for more on this method).

ACUPRESSURE POINTS

It is best to go to an acupuncturist to find which meridian imbalances relate to your ideographic condition, and then to use those acupressure self-touch points on your own. I usually favor the circle, stop, breathe, and feel method described in Chapter Three. Here are some general self-touch points often used for insomnia (Deadman et al., 1998; Gach, 1990):

- For relaxing the central nervous system: try touching the third-eye point (GV-24.5).

- For calming the spirit, agitation of the heart, palpitations, overexcitement: try touching the point at the inner wrist crease in line with the little finger (H-7).

- For fright, agitation, sadness and worry with diminished Qi, and fear of people: try touching the point where the bent pinky finger hits the crease on the inside of your palm, in line with the little finger (H-8).

- For relieving nervousness, blocked Qi in the chest/heart, and anxiety: try touching the acu-point on the center of the breastbone three thumbs' width up from the base of the sternum bone (CV-17).

- For mania, fear, palpitations, nausea, disorders of the chest, and distention in the stomach: try touching the point two thumbs' width above the center of the inner wrist crease (P-6).

- For fear and back pain that make it difficult to sleep: with your hand or foot, try touching an acu-point in the first indentation directly below the outer anklebone (Bl-62).

- For hypertension, nightmares, and deficiency conditions in the elderly: try touching the acu-point directly below the inside of the anklebone in the slight indentation (K-6).

When touching all the above points, use the River of Life practice, your own imagery, and your heart's love, to relax and melt into the calm lake of life's energy. In BMHP as we touch these points, when needed, we also integrate the methods below to maximize the healing potential of integrating East and West, transcending and transmuting traditions.

5. "Focusing" on the Felt Meaning of What's Keeping You Awake

For the six-step Focusing process combined with BMHP's River of Life imagery process, see Chapter Six (Gendlin, 1978).

6. Cognitive Restructuring

What are the thoughts and beliefs that are keeping you awake? Take your negative thought/belief that is keeping you awake and give it a SUDS level. What is a more truthful/constructive thought? Now what is the SUDS level? In addition to this cognitive method, you may want to try one of these practices:

- Practice thought stoppage and thought substitution.

- Serenity prayer: Recite aloud or say silently with a hand on your heart, "God grant me the serenity to accept the things I cannot change, the courage to change the things I can change, and the wisdom to know the difference." How will worrying about the issues you are preoccupied with, help?; versus, can you let yourself deal with it tomorrow? Imagine the situation that is creating your upsetting feeling (worry, anxiety, fear); and on your exhalation, imagine letting go of the associated feeling, watching it float like a dead log downstream.

7. Psychodynamic/Object Relations Issues

To illustrate the importance of this dimension, read the case about "Carl" beginning below.

8. Bodymind Healing Qigong Exercises

Some of the BMHQ practices that have been reported as useful for those with insomnia are Yi Chuan Holding the Golden Ball of the Heart, Tai Chi Ruler, Cloud Hands, Buddha Opens the Heart to the Heavens, using the sound *ha* and Raising Qi to Heavens and Returning It to Earth (Mayer, 2004b.) Trust your body regarding which movements or static postures are best for you. For some people, activating *fongsung* (relaxed awakeness) with a Tai Chi movement helps. While doing Qigong movements, try focusing on one of the acu-points mentioned above. For other people, static Qigong postures serve presleep purposes better. For some people, doing Qigong before going to sleep gives a nice balance of relaxation and fuel for the night's journey into sleep; for others, it is too stimulating. Listen to your bodymind.

Case Illustration: The Unresolved Issues That Invade Your Sleep

"Carl" was a forty-five-year-old married man who came to me suffering from insomnia. His past psychiatrist had prescribed sleep medication, but it did not seem to work. Carl still awoke from nightmares with a sense of being invaded.

When he came to see me, we began BMHP's integrated treatment approach. Because Carl wanted to get off his sleep medication, we worked with his psychiatrist to taper his sleep medication as we began to unravel the deeper meanings of his symptoms.

We discovered that the sense of being invaded in his nightmares was correlated to the fact that his father physically abused Carl during his childhood. His father would barge into Carl's room when he was resting, or even when he was asleep, and hit him for "being bad." In addition to the physical abuse, Carl had internalized messages about not being good enough, resulting from his father's blaming messages when Carl did not meet his idealistic expectations. When Carl was not functioning well in his work, he felt his boss was judging him, and then Carl hid his feelings of ineptitude behind a cloak of placating behavior—similar to the way he had responded to his father's abuse and demands. Although Carl's boss was different from his father, Carl's emotional body and the hypervigilance of his childhood were triggered as he projected on his boss the physical abuse by his father. From not feeling safe to express himself with his father, Carl developed a stance in life that was overly accommodating to others. Adding to his fear of expressing his feelings was the fact that his father had a heart condition. Though Carl had held anger toward his father, Carl was afraid that if he really expressed himself he would cause his father to have a heart attack. This learned holding-back survival strategy was the same style Carl used with his boss. But as Carl continued to hold in his feelings, somatic symptoms began to flare up, including neck and back pains. From not expressing and honoring his limits at work, he developed repetitive stress syndrome in his right arm; and from the tension he carried from the accumulation of unexpressed feelings during the day, his sleep was invaded by nightmares related to these unworked-through issues.

After doing some good inner work on the above issue with Bodymind Healing Psychotherapy, the pain from Carl's repetitive stress and his other somatic symptoms gradually disappeared. He attributed this healing to expressing feelings by setting boundaries at work regarding the time he needed to finish projects and to the various Bodymind Healing Qigong movements that he practiced.[2] The reversal of somatization disorders (Gatchel & Blanchard 1993) is a miracle to behold when a person opens a blocked pathway for expressing what has been internalized and finds the source of healing.

Through role play during therapy, Carl practiced how to express his anger to his father constructively. Then, after not speaking to his father for many years, Carl finally called him. This conversation led to his father apologizing for hitting Carl during his childhood, and a new relationship developed between them. After this phone call, Carl's insomnia disappeared for a while.

Often in depth psychotherapy, layers of the underlying pattern lie beneath the surface as a psycho-archeological dig takes place. The next layer for Carl was the layer of his current feelings about his mother. After his parents had divorced, due to his father's physical abuse of both him and his mother, Carl lived with his mother. During one session while focusing on the feeling he had in his body when he woke up, Carl realized that another layer of his insomnia was because of his guilt feelings for not taking care of his mother, who lived in a third-world country. As the oldest son, Carl had been shouldering most of the responsibility for sending money to her. Through the course of therapy, he realized that he had been holding back his anger toward his other siblings about their not shouldering their fair share of the financial responsibility for taking care of their mother. As he had just learned to do with his father, Carl was able to express this feeling to his two siblings constructively. This helped him to let go of some of the burden he had been carrying. He also spoke up to his mother to renegotiate the amount of money that he was sending to her. This led to his mother assuming responsibility to reactivate her sewing business to help support herself and decrease some of her dependence on Carl and his siblings.

Carl worked on his beliefs with cognitive and energy psychology methods. He no longer believed *I'm no good, and I need to do all I can to get other's love, even if it means not having rest myself* (SUDS level of 9). Instead, his new truthful and constructive belief was *even though I have my limits in terms of what I choose to give, I deserve to have people in my life that take responsibility for their own lives, and I will help them to the extent that it doesn't endanger my own health and economic well-being* (SUDS level of 1).

Many of the other elements of BMHP also helped Carl to maintain an anchor in the state-specific state of letting go of his tension and accepting his chosen limits. Using Microcosmic Orbit Breathing and visualizing the river washing away the old patterns were keys to his healing, as was practicing Tai Chi Ruler at times during the day to let go of tension. When the pattern reoccurred in his bed at night, Carl repeated his new constructive belief along with his River of Life practice. While doing these practices, he also found it helpful to press the acupressure point on the inside of the wrist crease in alignment with the little finger (called Spirit Gate [H-7]), a point often used for insomnia (Deadman et al., 1998). During one session while holding this acu-point, Carl said with tears in his eyes, "It's sad that my mom doesn't have more money." However, he realized that his codependent way of trying to fix everything for everyone was putting a financial burden on his relationship with his wife. Carl expressed his newfound realization "It's better to mourn my mom's limits than it was to be in that state of continuous guilt that was stopping my spirit from resting."

By the end of our therapy, Carl's repetitive stress injury had disappeared, and he was speaking up more in his significant relationships. The insomnia that he had had every night had significantly decreased, but it did reoccur when triggers activated him. He told me that when it did reoccur, on somewhat rare occasions, he was able to use our bodymind healing methods to go to back to sleep much more quickly than he had before treatment. Carl had totally stopped all medication.

Carl's case exemplifies that those who jump on the bandwagon of medication to alleviate symptoms (and risk "rebound insomnia" when they get off medication) are missing the growth potential involved in unearthing the deeper meanings behind their patterns. Also, such inner work enables people to discover self-healing methods as they learn to deal with the underlying issues. It is also important to realize how medication affects our access to dreams. Like physical symptoms, our dreams are messages waiting to be deciphered. By prematurely shutting off the "messenger" with medication, we risk not hearing the message. By using a combination of psychotherapeutic and other bodymind healing methods, the encumbrances in the river of our life energy can be removed and our spirit can find its way to its natural state of rest.

Alternative Visualization Methods

Though the breathing methods of the River of Life practice have been effective with most people whom I have worked with over the years, there are a few people who are "meditative-breath resistant." For example, sometimes a person has had a traumatic experience learning to meditate or breathe when inner feelings emerge that he or she cannot handle. Sometimes that trauma is still linked to meditation or breathing. With other people the difficulty may be linked to a perfectionistic critic who compares himself or herself to others who "can meditate." Sometimes it helps to apply energy psychology methods like saying *even though I can't relax, meditate, and breathe as well as others, I can still love and accept myself* (Craig & Fowlie, 1995). In BMHP this is done while one hand is on the heart, practicing self-soothing.

Though the preceding BMHP methods (cognitive restructuring of the negative beliefs, self-soothing, and so forth) can be useful to heal these traumas, other methods are occasionally useful as well. For instance, there are times when attending a sleep clinic where differentially diagnosing for sleep apnea and other disorders can be helpful. Likewise, changing the form of imagery from a river to a specific place that has been relaxing to the patient can be beneficial. Then the patient is instructed to use the eight-item protocol protocol (at the beginning of this chapter) and to imagine being in that place with or without the use of focus on the breath.

Pleasant dreams....

CHAPTER ELEVEN

Hypertension

Research

Hypertension affects twenty percent or more of the adult population in Western societies, and it is a significant risk factor for stroke, myocardial infraction, and congestive heart failure. These together account for more than fifty percent of deaths in the United States (Wollam & Hall, 1988). It is estimated that about fifty million Americans have elevated blood pressure (BP), which is defined as systolic BP of 140 mm Hg or greater or diastolic BP of 90 mm Hg or greater (Joint National Committee on Detection, Evaluation and Treatment of High Blood Pressure [JNC-V], 1993).

The problem with conventional treatments that use medication is that patients suffer from high costs and side effects. For example, research points to hypotensive drugs negatively affecting carbohydrate and lipid metabolism (Pollare, Lithell, Selinus, & Berne, 1989; Medical Research Council Working Party, 1985) mood state, cognitive functioning, and sexual performance (Kostis et al., 1990). Therefore, a growing body of research in the West has focused upon lifestyle modification as an alternative to anti-hypertensive drugs. According to the Joint National Committee report (JNC-V, 1993), lifestyle modification can provide "multiple benefits at little cost and minimal risk" and may be used as a first step therapy for individuals within a high range of normal or who have Stage 1 hypertension. Lifestyle modifications can also be used for reducing the number and doses of anti-hypertensive medications required (Little, Girling, Hasler, & Trafford, 1991).

It is now well known that hypertension is a disease with a psychosomatic component, and that mind-body interventions are an important part of the new paradigm of treating hypertension (Mann, 2000). Qigong and energy psychology are some of the leading-edge components of an integrated approach that will give self-healing power to people to affect their hypertension.

Qigong Research

In my earlier two peer-reviewed research articles (Mayer, 1999, 2003), I reviewed thirty-three studies representing approximately 5,545 people who used Qigong to treat hypertension. Almost all of the studies suggest that Qigong lowers blood pressure (BP) to various degrees over various time periods.

The most in-depth of these studies is the Kuang study (Kuang et al., 1991, updated by Wang et al., 1995), which took place over twenty years. The basic design involved 204 patients with hypertension who were randomly assigned to Qigong practice and control groups. The ages of the subjects were not mentioned. Both groups were given anti-hypertensive drugs. The Qigong group of 104 patients reportedly practiced, for twenty years, twice per day for thirty minutes. During the first two months, the blood pressure of all patients dropped in response to the hypotensive drug. Subsequently, and consistently over the period of twenty years, the blood pressure of the group practicing Qigong stabilized, while the blood pressure of the control group increased ($P < 0.01$). Due to the stabilized blood pressure, forty-eight percent in the Qigong practice group reduced the hypotensive dosage; and for thirty percent in this group, the BP medication was eliminated. In contrast, thirty-one percent in the control group increased the hypotensive dosage (Kuang et al., 1991). Kuang reports, in his twenty-year study, less cardiovascular lesions ($P < 0.05$), decreased blood viscosity, improved platelet aggregation, decreased triglycerides, and increased high-density lipoprotein cholesterol (HDL-C, good cholesterol) in the groups practicing Qigong. Beneficial changes were reported in the Qigong group in total peripheral vascular resistance, plasma cholesterol, and in two messenger cyclic nucleotides (cAMP and cGMP) compared to the control group (Kuang et al., 1991).

Most important, in an update of the research of Kuang by Wang et al., (1995), significant differences were reported in subjects who reportedly practiced Qigong for thirty years, twice a day for thirty minutes. The accumulated mortality rate was 25.41 percent in the Qigong group and 40.8 percent in the control group. The incidence of strokes was also significantly different in the Qigong practice groups at 20.5 percent as compared to the control group at 40.7 percent. The death rate due to strokes was 15.6 percent in the Qigong practice groups and 32.5 percent in the control group (P < 0.01) (Wang, 1993, as cited in Sancier, 1996a and b).

I concluded my peer-reviewed research by saying that the weight of evidence of these studies, representing approximately 5,545 subjects, suggests that practicing Qigong has a positive effect on hypertension in the following areas: blood pressure; blood circulation; other cardiovascular measures; and other health-related measures, including strokes, deaths due to strokes, and overall mortality. In another study it was found that two months of Qigong practice helped to significantly reduce hypertension compared to a control group using medication alone (Li, Pi, Zing, et al., 1994). Updated meta-analytic research (Lee, et. al., 2007) confirmed the findings of my review and reported that Qigong has positive results in some relevant outcome measures, such as lowering systolic blood pressure.

However, my review of the literature and Lee's (2007) meta-analysis both found that due to inadequate addressing of methodology issues it was difficult to determine just how effective Qigong is, and what other factors may contribute to the positive effects reported in the studies reviewed. In an update on the research on Qigong and hypertension, Guo's (2008) meta-analysis showed the following: (1) Qigong is better than no treatment controls in decreasing blood pressure, (2) Qigong combined with drugs has a better effect than drug treatment alone, and (3) Qigong helps not just in improving hypertension but also in adding to improving quality of life. For those interested in research methodology issues, refer to Palmer's scholarly text on general problems with research in China (2007), my articles (Mayer 1999; 2003), and Guo's (2008) article. Guo et al. updates my examination of various research studies and reports on the results of Chinese studies, which I could not read. I said in my final abstract that whether Qigong alone can affect hypertension is not necessarily the most important question. I called for further research to assess and understand better the effect of adding Qigong into an integrated, multifaceted program that selectively incorporates diet, moderate aerobic exercise, relaxation training, and social and psychological dimensions.

Guo (2008) answered my call (Mayer, 1999; 2003) to include an exercise group as a control group in future research; and he could not find in his meta-analysis of studies he overviewed that Qigong was superior to control participants who did other active forms of exercise. However, the type of Qigong used in the comparisons was not oriented to treat hypertension, and the Qigong practitioners may not have had enough time to learn to do the practice effectively (Lv, Yu, Liu, et al., 1987; Cheung, 2005; Lee, 2007). An interesting study comparing Qigong to standard muscle relaxation therapy with hypertensive patients concluded that Qigong was more effective in improving well-being, sleep, and relaxation during the intervention as well as later on (Ritter & Aldridge, 2001).

My opinion is that a problem many researchers have in looking at Qigong as a treatment alone is similar to the problem of those who use a mental/psychological approach alone to healing hypertension. A more expansive vision is needed. In this book, and in the discussion that follows, you will begin to understand why I advocate for an integrative approach to treat this major disease.

Qigong and the River of Life: A Quick Fix for Hypertension?

When I was at the Health Medicine Institute, Medical Director Dr. Len Saputo, whom I cofounded the clinic with, asked me to work with one of his patients, who was suffering from hypertension, in a public forum. The Health Medicine Forum (HMF) is a leading-edge group of multidisciplinary health professionals trying to combine the best of modern traditional and age-old methods of healing. HMF is part of the movement to bring forth integrative medicine as the norm in the twenty-first century.

During the forum, in front of an audience of approximately 200 interested people, each doctor or health professional on the panel described how he or she would work with this patient. I always learn so much from hearing the dialogs between ayurvedic doctors, acupuncturists, medical doctors, psychologists, and bodyworkers. At this event, Dr. Saputo asked me to work with the aforementioned patient, who was a man in his late sixties, and to take a risk and do something experiential in front of the assembled group. One of the chief medical researchers from a local hospital was there with a blood pressure monitor. He measured the systolic blood pressure rate of the patient at 168. I then did the River of Life hypnosis method (see Chapter Five) with this patient in front of the group. Within about five minutes, the patient's systolic blood pressure had gone down to 128 (Mayer, 1997b). Many in the audience were impressed, as was I—because I am naturally shy, and I wondered what my blood pressure would be in front of such a large group if someone took it.

There are many reasons why blood pressure reduction on a single occasion is not something that should overly impress us; but in particular, we need to consider some of these research methodology issues. First, we know that the relaxation response is capable of creating significant positive changes in blood pressure (Jacob, Chesney, Williams, Ding, & Shapiro, 1991; Linden & Chambers, 1994; Schneider et al., 1995). More important than any brief reduction in blood pressure, by whatever means, we would want to know how long such reduction lasts, and whether the hypertensive person can call on this method at times when his or her blood pressure rises. This would be one of the behavioral health-care tests to determine whether a deeper, longer-lasting healing has taken place.

Case Illustration: The Hypertensive Executive— What Lies Beneath the Surface?

In accordance with the viewpoint of Bodymind Healing Psychotherapy (BMHP), a person needs to work through his or her deeper psychodynamics, cognitions, and beliefs before deep, long-lasting healing can take place. I recall a patient, named Richard here, who was a very wealthy married man and an executive in a local company. Richard's marriage was about to fall apart due to what his wife said was "his inconsiderateness," exemplified by his going out and buying expensive motorcycles without asking her first. An equally important factor in his upcoming divorce was that Richard's wife described him as a workaholic, sleeping only about four hours a night, who did not pay enough attention to his young children.

Richard was suffering from severe hypertension, and he came to me after hearing about my articles and research on hypertension. Being very busy, he was interested in the quick fixes that he hoped would be part of this "Qigong/hypnosis thing." He was more than a little upset when after our first session, I suggested that a combination of marital as well as individual therapy might be important to consider. He reluctantly agreed. Later, after a few sessions of both individual and couples therapy, I asked him to do our River of Life breathing method and focus on what came up as he followed his exhalation down the river of breath through his body. As Richard focused on his body sense, he became aware of a high energy, yet disconnected quality to his energy state. As he stayed with the felt sense of this a bit longer, he described the feeling as being like a disconnected live wire, after which a sense of anger arose in him. I asked him to stay with the sense of anger and to ask the feeling, "What is this all about?" When Richard did this, another image arose.

Richard remembered a childhood scene from his dinner table when he came home with a D on his report card. He vividly recalled his father saying to him in a demeaning tone, "You'll never amount to anything, you dummy." All of his brothers joined in the shaming process. Laughing, mocking, and pointing at Richard, they said, "Don't worry, when you grow up, you can always work on one of Uncle Jimmy's garbage trucks and pick up the garbage from our mansions." At that moment Richard promised himself, "I'll never rest until I make twice as much money as all of them combined."

Indeed, Richard kept that promise and more than fulfilled this goal—but he had forgotten the promise he had a made to himself. He did not realize how this unconscious motivation was driving him in his current life, and just how literally he was following through on his childhood promise when he had said, "I'll never rest."

This insight began the process of Richard changing his behavior. He became aware of the advantages and disadvantages of this compulsion, which had made him successful but had endangered his health and family. His wife marked this session as the beginning of Richard's change in behavior, which saved their marriage and led to the opportunity to reduce and eventually eliminate his hypertension medication.

There are many interesting clinical points that can be learned from Richard's story. His case illustrates how the "quick fixes" of relaxation modalities may not get to the deeper underlying psychodynamic issues that need to be addressed. Richard shows the power of using an integrative psychotherapy; and because one in twenty Americans suffer from hypertension, and fifty percent of Americans may die from its effects (Wollam & Hall, 1988), Richard's case has bearing on the importance of a bodymind approach to solving a portion of this health crisis.

Chinese Medical Approaches to Hypertension

Regarding a Chinese medical perspective on Qigong and hypertension, we need to be aware that Qigong practices are not so easily oriented toward Western notions of prescribing a single pill or movement. Western, nomothetic (general) categories may provide ease of scientific measurement, but they do not fit into holistic Chinese medical philosophy with its more ideographic (unique) ways of looking at various disorders. For example, the diagnostic category of Western hypertension as perceived in Chinese medicine may be due to a wide variety of energetic imbalances, such as "an imbalance of the Yin and Yang functional aspects of Deficient Kidney Yin and Excess Liver Yang, and/or an overabundance of phlegm and dampness within the body" (Johnson, 2000). In Chinese medicine, two different persons with the same Western diagnosis of hypertension may be treated differently depending upon specific diagnostic considerations that come from such general categories and tongue and pulse analysis. Ideographic factors related to the unique patient and the background of the particular Qigong healer/Chinese doctor are also part of the decision about what treatment, or combination of treatments, is chosen. Unique combinations of herbs, acupuncture, and a wide variety of Qigong movements are prescribed, based upon what is suited to the individual whole person.

Despite this caveat, and the insights discussed in Chapter Four in Chinese Qigong Master Hon's Ping-Pong ball story, I would like to suggest some general Qigong movements that may prove beneficial to those suffering from hypertension.

Breathing

One key element that may be a factor in hypertension occurs when a person's stomach goes in as he or she inhales, which is called *reverse breathing* in Qigong language. In a comprehensive clinical text on Qigong, Johnson (2000) states, "scientific studies confirm that 90 percent of hypertensive patients practice *Reverse Breathing* chronically (p. 352)." Though no reference citation is given for the research behind this claim, many of us in the health-care field have found that changing habitual reversed breathing is one factor to be considered in restoring parasympathetic relaxation to a person suffering from hypertension.

Standing Meditation Qigong

The key to any form of Qigong is first to balance our energy state with a Standing Meditation practice, according to Master Hon, the Chinese Qigong master who told the Ping-Pong ball analogy in Chapter Four and Master Ha, my teacher. Standing Meditation Qigong is a method to develop *fongsung,* or relaxed awakeness, which you can experience if you follow the illustrations and instructions in Chapter Twenty-one. My clinical experience shows that Standing Meditation can be particularly beneficial for hypertensive patients. This may partially be due simply to getting a person to slow down enough to do the practice, like any form of meditation. But the specifics of Standing Meditation, and imagining that we are standing like a tree rooted in the earth, helps to ground the energy of those hypertensive patients who have a high degree of pressure from the various pressures of life that lead to pent up energy or resentment (excess liver yang). There is some research support for the beneficial elements of Standing Meditation to create balance in life and in the brain.[1]

Qigong Movements: Lowering the Qi with Heavenly Palms

To treat hypertension, Johnson (2000) suggests patients move their hands with palms downward along the front and side of the body in order to purge and guide the imbalanced Qi so that it descends down the liver and Gall Bladder channels, or down the torso to the hips. This is similar to the practice I call,

Lowering the Qi with Heavenly Palms (Mayer, 2004b, pp. 81–88). Specific acupressure points, such as acupuncture point GB-30, are also prescribed by Johnson (2000). Additionally, Deadman et al. (1998, p. 652) uses a variety of points, like Lu-7, LI-4, Lv-3, and K-1. BMHP uses the River of Life practice and the circle, touch, and feel method while the patient touches these acu-points.

Just as Chinese doctors use acupuncture needles to treat different points for different people based upon their diagnosis of the tongue and pulses, I choose different points—either by borrowing the points used in the patient's last acupuncture treatment, points suggested in consultation with an acupuncturist, or based my own assessment of the patient and his or her unique issues. When I suggest acu-points, I hope that I compensate for not being a Chinese doctor and not having sophisticated pulse and tongue diagnosis methods in my tool kit by helping patients evoke their life energy through various BMHQ methods. Some of these BMHQ methods include breathing methods that focus on the exhalation and sinking the Qi to the belly (Tan Tien), and visualizations such as imagining warm water flowing in down the front central meridian (*Ren*) as in the River of Life practice. Sometimes I, as well as other Qigong healers (Johnson, 2000), use specific sounds to help patients relax and release pent up energy. In BMHQ, I use various nonforced sounds accompanying the exhalation, such as: *s-s-s-s* to release excess liver Qi; *ha* to let go in the heart; *whooh* or *chir-ee* to help the vitalizing functions of the kidneys; and *huh* for spleen stagnation. But I prefer a phenomenological approach (see Chapter Five) to all of the above, trusting each patient's own unconscious process to come up with sounds, images, visualizations, and movements that feel right to him or her. Though there is a treasure-house of knowledge in the specific series of points chosen by experienced Chinese doctors, the perspective outlined here is a way to respect the essence of their tradition as Western clinicians. Though limited in our understanding of their breadth of knowledge, Western bodymind health professionals can perhaps add an equally significant knowledge base to the multilayered bodymind methods needed for healing hypertension.

Case Illustration: Is Qigong Palatable to Fundamentalist Christians?

In conclusion as a cautionary tale, I would like to mention a case to remind us of problems that can occur when integrating practices from traditions that may be unfamiliar to people in our culture. I tell this story in my trainings so that my students will not make the same error that I once did.

A doctor in our clinic referred a patient, called Paul here, to me who was suffering from hypertension. After our first session, his SUDS level of 8 went down to a 3, and Paul asked if there was anything he could do in-between sessions for homework. I suggested that he continue to practice the exercises we had done in the first session: Microcosmic Orbit Breathing, the River of Life visualization, and the Lowering the Qi with Heavenly Palms Qigong movement. I also offered Paul a booklet that illustrated these and other Qigong movements, which he took home.

At the next session, he came in and told me that he was a Fundamentalist Christian, and he asked me, "Why are these practices not the work of the Devil?" He indicated that he had seen the exercise called Buddha Opens the Heart to the Heavens in my booklet and that he believed, "Jesus is the only son of God. It is only through Jesus that a person can find his way to heaven, and that any others were destined to go to hell."

After taking a breath, I complimented Paul for coming back to this session, and I told him that it showed he was a true Christian by wanting to discover the truth of things (*gnosis*). I went on to indicate that many people misunderstand the idea of the Buddha—that Buddha is not a God, as many believe Jesus is. The Buddha, I explained, is a state of mind that involves compassionate and enlightened awareness, and that any deity may be used in discovering this state of mind. I told him about Tibetan Buddhism when you do certain practices (*Phowa, Tonglin*) of opening your heart to the compassion and light of the heavens, any deity—for example, Jesus—can be imagined to be raining its light of love on you (Rinpoche, 1993, p. 218).

When I asked Paul if he would like to try these practices, he said yes. I instructed him to open his hands to the side and after they were raised over his head, to imagine Jesus in the sky. With a slow exhalation, I told Paul to lower his hands in synchronization with his out-breath and to imagine bringing the love of Jesus down through his body. He reported that his SUDS level went down significantly more as he imagined Jesus's love coming down from the heavens.

Paul thanked me for our work together and said it had really helped his hypertension. He then asked me for a referral to a therapist who specialized in a Christian approach to psychotherapy, which I gave him.

This case illustrates, among other things, how important it is to be aware of an individual's cultural and religious beliefs when doing Qigong or any form of therapy.

CHAPTER TWELVE

Depression

Research: Medication versus Behavioral Health

Almost 19 million Americans are thought to suffer from depressive disorders; however, only twenty-three percent of individuals with clinical depression seek treatment, and only ten percent of these people receive adequate care (Dunn, 2005). The purpose in addressing this pervasive malady here is not to give an exhaustive review of treatment, but to give a sense of how Qigong and BMHP can add to current treatment options.

The literature on the treatment of depression is substantial (Yapko, 1997; Morrison, 1999), showing that cognitive-behavioral approaches can be effective (Beck, 1979). Moreover, there is much research showing that medications can be of help (Morrison, 1999). There are patients and studies that report medication as being a useful, and even necessary, tool in treating cases of severe depression, bipolar disorder, and general inability to function. However, because there is so much conflicting information about the efficacy and side effects of medication for depression, the aware consumer should—in conjunction with consultation with a trusted health professional—read the research on contrasting views regarding the benefits versus side effects of medication (Kramer, 1997; Breggin, 2001). The overall effectiveness of antidepressants has recently been called into question by a meta-analysis of many studies conducted by the National Institute for Health and Clinical Excellence on the most popular SSRI (Selective Seratonin Reuptake Inhibitors) antidepressants and found the positive effects were so small that they were deemed unlikely to be clinically important (Moncrieff & Kirsch, 2005).

The most serious concern is that there are numerous reports discussing the detrimental side effects of antidepressant medication (Breggin, 2001). Unfortunately, it seems that during recent years that the U.S. Food and Drug Administration (FDA) cannot be trusted to be guardians of our health due to political lobbying by drug companies and the FDA's political and economic ties with these lobbyists. One eye-opening overview of this literature can be found at http://www.mercola.com.[1] The *British Medical Journal* reported increased suicide rates in adults and children taking serotonin reuptake inhibitors, the most popular form of antidepressants (Moncrieff & Kirsch, 2005). Concerns have also been raised that some of the violent homicides and suicides have been correlated with or caused by certain antidepressant medications (Bingham, 2000; O'Meara, 2002). A study reported in *Blood* magazine, reported cases of lowered immune function when taking common antidepressants that target 5 HT uptake and release (O'Connell et al., 2006). Also, a study from the Northwestern University Medical School says that SSRI antidepressants can cause internal bleeding (http://msnbc.msn.com/id/7876902).[2]

Exercise

With so many potentially negative consequences involved in taking these medications, it seems prudent to start with less potentially deleterious methods when medications are not absolutely necessary. Dr. Pelletier (2000) facetiously describes exercise as a widely accessible, mainstream-friendly new drug that promises no medication side effects (p. 34). Though obviously not a cure-all for all kinds of depression, it is a well-known fact that exercise is an important treatment component of depression. In a study that involved eight adults, twenty to forty-five years of age, who were diagnosed with mild to moderate depression, when Dunn et al. (2005) looked at exercise alone to treat the condition, they found the following:

> Depressive symptoms were cut almost in half in those individuals who participated in 30-minute aerobic exercise sessions, three to five times a week after twelve weeks. Those who exercised with low-intensity for three and five days a week showed a 30 percent reduction in symptoms. Participants who did stretching flexibility exercises for 15 to 20 minutes, three days a week, averaged a 29 percent decline.

In everyday standard of care, therapists often prescribe exercise to activate energy in depressed patients. So why not consider using Qigong, one of the oldest exercise systems in the world, for depressed patients? Recent research in the *International Journal of Geriatric Psychiatry* adds credence to the intuition that Qigong would be beneficial for depressed patients. In a randomized control trial eighty-two participants with a diagnosis of depression and chronic physical illness were recruited and randomly assigned to a Qigong group or a newspaper reading group. After sixteen weeks the members of the Qigong group were significantly improved in mood, self-efficacy, personal well-being, and physical and social domains of self-concept compared to the controls (Tsang, Cheung, & Lak, 2002).

Qigong: An Exercise That Is More Than Exercise

BMHP proposes that in addition to the cardiovascular and energizing attributes of traditional exercise, and along with the known benefit of stretching exercises, Qigong and Tai Chi should be considered as recommended adjunctive treatments of choice for depression. Not only do these age-old practices complement other methods of exercise; but they also enhance psychological treatment in the unique ways mentioned throughout this book.

One beneficial, yet unrecognized, attribute of Qigong and Tai Chi is that they are easy to use as hypnotic anchors at moments when one is not physically exercising. For example, the combined breathing methods and meridian visualizations in the River of Life practice—as well as the practices of experiencing the "energy ball" between your hands—can be activated at moments when negative cognitions overwhelm the ego. Likewise, the empowerment postures in the animal forms of Qigong, such as the Tiger or the Bear, provide state-specific anchors, which can reactivate these state-specific states of consciousness (Rossi, 1986).

The deeper dimensions of Qigong practice involve the very thing that is needed in the sedentary settings of the modern office and modern life—the ability to activate an empowered, energized state when one is not in the act of exercising. For example, in the Bear practice (Feng, 2003; Mayer, 2004b, pp.126–129), you start by imagining you are a bear, practice Bear Breathing, and then do various movements to activate the Liver meridian, which in Chinese medicine is associated with anger and depression. Afterward, see if you can bring back the energy of the "bear-specific" state of consciousness just by doing Bear Breathing. These multiple access channels provide ways to identify with and shape-shift into activating the soft, grounded power of the Bear.

The Integrated Approach of Bodymind Healing Psychotherapy

Following an integrative treatment approach, BMHP incorporates many of the common standards of care for depression, such as cognitive-behavioral therapy. Qigong has the potential to be an important adjunct to psychotherapeutic treatment by its ability to activate the energy of a patient's vital, primordial Self, regardless of which type of Qigong is integrated into a therapist's practice.

Case Illustration: "I Never Had a Happy Moment."

A young woman, named Gloria here, reported early on that she was unable to remember ever having had a happy moment. She was in a relationship with a man who continually made denigrating comments to her, adding to her long-standing feelings of worthlessness. Our therapy involved some deep psychodynamic work, which uncovered how, according to Gloria, "both my mother and father hated me." Her internalization of these self-deprecating messages led to her sense of worthlessness. From many undeserved beatings, and from being fearful of communicating her feelings to her abusive father, "learned helplessness" developed and Gloria found herself often in a victim stance in life. At her job as an executive assistant, she reported being "walked over" by her office mates; and she complained to me about being "totally incapable of asserting myself to my boyfriend and other people—due to freezing up whenever I am criticized."

The methods of BMHP were helpful in her long-term therapy. As Gloria revisited her early childhood memories, she recalled that she came to her parents as a third child just when her parents were having financial difficulties and did not want another child. From this, Gloria realized that when her parents had deprived her of many of the things that her siblings had received, it was not personal, but circumstantial. She saw the parallels between her relationship with her father, and how she projected and reenacted this old abuse in her current work situation and her relationship with her boyfriend. As she cognitively restructured her belief about being worthless, Gloria realized *I have worth and deserve to be treated with respect.* Even though this cognition, along with energy psychology tapping methods, was helpful to some degree, the anchoring was not long lasting or accessible at key moments due to Gloria's severe wounding at an early developmental age.

Our therapy is too extensive to outline here, but one more aspect worth noting came from my suggestion that Gloria ask her mother for a good picture of her from her childhood. To Gloria's surprise, she found one in which she was smiling. This became a useful anchor for those times when Gloria felt worthless and incapable of smiling about anything. She also found it helpful when I suggested that she try pretending that she was getting $100,000 to act the part of a genuinely happy person in a play. When she acted "as if" she was happy, she was able to shape-shift into the long-buried, happy part of herself. After these interventions and for the first time, I saw Gloria smile, and we built on this in subsequent sessions. She learned to focus less on the abuses in her life, and more on how she responded to these things. She began to find things in life that she was grateful for; and she realized that she could find pleasure in taking a self-assertive stance—even if the person did not respond exactly the way she wanted.

Another anchor we used was the Bear Breathing exercise that she had noticed in *Secrets to Living Younger Longer* (Mayer, 2004b, p. 126). Gloria said, "Since my Teddy Bear was my only friend in my childhood, I thought I'd check out that Bear exercise." In addition to her childhood picture, Bear Breathing became another anchor to help empower Gloria at moments when she regressed to her "worthless" self. Bear Breathing consists of raising the hands (claws) palm up to the heart on the inhalation, and turning of the palms (claws) downward on the exhalation down to the belly. I believe that the role of the Bear Qigong, along with the broader dimensions of BMHP, helped reverse Gloria's learned helplessness and helped her develop a "cohesiveness of self" (Horner, 1990, p. 30).

Toward the end of our therapy, Gloria reported that she was now better able to take her stance of power with her coworkers. Eventually after trying to work things out with her boyfriend and asserting herself with appropriate affect modulation skills to no avail, Gloria left him. In our termination session after about year of therapy, she joked about the Bear being her "medicine animal" (Storm, 1972); and she said that the things that used to bother her bounced off more easily now that she had this new stance in life. Last I heard, Gloria was in a new relationship with a man who treated her better.

The specific anchors chosen must be suited to the particular person. As you learned in Chapter Four, auditory anchors in the form of songs have either transcendent or transmuting attributes. These songs can play an important part in the context of a wider psychotherapy process. To review, I discussed an orthodox Jewish man who was suffering from severe negative thinking and resultant depression. Among other aspects of our depth psychotherapy over a one-year period, he found that singing the song "This Too Is for the Good" (*Gam Zeh Tovah*) was helpful in countering negative cognitions when they arose. When he did this, it created a felt shift from a negative, constricted feeling into a bodily felt sense of openheartedness.

In addition, I mentioned the principle of not just singing a happy song, but singing one that is in tune with the pain felt, that is, like songs from the blues. Along these lines, I recall the female patient suffering from situational depression from having just lost a long-term relationship, and she did not know how she could ever put her life back together again. She found herself singing "I'm Free Falling" in the shower; and along with our longer-term therapy, she used this song to identify with everything in the universe that falls, survives, and is freed up to create new realities. This became her anchor when she was in the midst of her deepest pain, which helped to remind her, coupled with her ongoing psychotherapy, that life goes on.

Cultivating the energy of life comes not just through Chinese Qigong practices, but through finding the songs of your heart. (And it doesn't hurt to add a little Qigong rocking or bodily expression of the song while you are singing.)

CHAPTER THIRTEEN

Additional Syndromes Alleviated by Qigong and Bodymind Healing Psychotherapy

In earlier chapters I addressed a variety of syndromes for which Qigong and Bodymind Healing Psychotherapy (BMHP) can play an ameliorative role. In this chapter I will touch upon some of the prevalent syndromes that are affecting a large number of people, and how a combination of Qigong and BMHP may be of benefit. However, I will not delve as deeply into how BMHP applies to these conditions as I have in previous chapters due to space limitations. I hope that you will draw from the earlier chapters and apply the previously outlined BMHP principles and methods to the health issues included in this chapter. It is not my purpose in these clinical chapters to be exhaustive in addressing all possible clinical syndromes, but rather to lay a groundwork upon which others may build regarding how BMHP and BMHQ may contribute to an integrative energy psychology approach to our current health crisis.

More resources are becoming available on the Bodymind Healing Psychotherapy approach to other health-related issues. Audiotapes on chronic diseases and cancer are available; and a DVD on death and dying is in process.[1]

Arthritis, Joint Problems, and Musculoskeletal Disorders

Arthritis and Tai Chi

A number of peer-reviewed research articles from reputable journals show the efficacy of movement therapy (Van Deusen & Harlowe, 1987) and Tai Chi for a variety of arthritic conditions, including rheumatoid arthritis (Kirsteins, Dietz, & Hwang, 1991) and osteoarthritis (Hartman et al., 2000).

Rheumatoid arthritis (RA) is a chronic progressive disease that consists of joint and generalized pain, swelling, stiffness, fatigue, sleep disturbance, weakness, decreased range of motion, and limb deformities. It affects approximately one percent of the general population, with women almost three times more likely to be affected. This disease's onset occurs most commonly between ages of twenty and fifty, with prevalence increasing with age (Young, 1993).

There is increasing evidence that RA is an autoimmune disease (Young, 1993; Sapolsky, 1998, p. 138), and there are many psychological interpretations for why the body activates such a course of action. It may be that the body is expressing its limits by attacking what is hurting it—itself. Some have theorized that when the body mistakes itself as an invader and attacks itself, it may be related to psychophysiological issues. For example, a person may be severely overdoing things and not listening to his or her body's limits, or the body may be expressing itself metaphorically. For a more extended discussion, refer to Gatchel & Blanchard (1993), Sapolsky (1998), and Wickramasekera (1998). From the perspective of BMHP, it is important for each individual to focus on the felt meaning behind his or her unique symptoms (Gendlin, 1978). It has been shown that autoimmune disorders are highly correlated to stress; yet it is not the stress itself, but a faulty response to stress that may provide an important clue to healing.

Increasing research points to how the consideration of psychological causes and related treatments are an important component of an integrated treatment approach. For example, RA has been associated with learned helplessness (Garber & Seligman, 1980; Stein, Wallston, et al., 1986), and a study showed that arthritis helplessness significantly predicted impairment twelve months later, independent of disease activity (Lorish, Abraham, et al., 1991). Among other relevant psychological variables are self-efficacy (Lorig, Chastain, et al., 1989) and disease-related cognitive distortions (Smith et al., 1988). An article in the *Annals of Behavioral Medicine* concluded that patients who rely on passive, avoidant, or emotion-focused strategies—such as self-blame or catastrophization—for coping with RA, typically report lower self-esteem, poorer adjustment, and greater negative affect. The converse is true for those patients who engage in active, problem-solving coping styles (Zautra & Manne, 1992).

Traditional Western research has shown that appropriate exercise can be beneficial for RA patients to increase aerobic capacity, endurance, strength, and flexibility, and to significantly decrease depression, anxiety, and pain (Minor, 1991). An article in the *American Journal of Physical Medicine and Rehabilitation* says that Tai Chi is safe for RA patients and has the potential advantage of stimulating bone growth and strengthening connective tissue (Kirsterns et al., 1991). But studies like this merely begin to demonstrate what Tai Chi is capable of doing. A next step in research would be to do comparison studies between Western forms of exercise and Tai Chi to see which help which groups the most and which symptoms of RA are best alleviated by each tradition or combination of traditions.

In my limited experience with RA patients at the Health Medicine Institute, I discovered that they usually preferred relaxed Tai Chi movements compared to more vigorous or forceful Western exercise, due to the unique ability of Tai Chi to relax and strengthen simultaneously and not overstimulate an already taxed immune and nervous system. Patients who found vigorous forms of Western exercise too much to handle often experienced Tai Chi easier to practice. For example, when one RA patient, named Mary here, was in her most painful state, she told me that physical exercise was out of the question and Tai Chi was even too much. However, static forms of Qigong that included slight rocking (like the Circle That Arises from Stillness exercise) and just a minimal amount of Tai Chi Ruler were both soothing helped her to feel more in control of her pain.

Osteoarthritis (OA) is a degenerative joint disease characterized by degeneration of joint cartilage and adjacent bone that can cause joint pain and stiffness. It is the most common joint disorder equally affecting men and women. The differences between the treatment of RA and OA are beyond the scope of this discussion. For example, injections of various antioxidants (such as superoxide dismutase) to protect cells against damage from free radicals have been used successfully to treat osteoarthritis, but results with RA have been disappointing (Pelletier, 2000, p. 105).

The world press has reported on the favorable outcomes of Tai Chi in reducing pain for osteoarthritis sufferers. Dr. Rhayun Song (2005), of Soonchunhyang University in Korea, presented his research findings recently in San Francisco at the annual meeting of the American College of Rheumatology. He found that twelve weeks in a Tai Chi program eased women's pain and made their daily activities more manageable. Dr. Song stated that previous research has suggested that the art, which focuses on improving strength, balance, and flexibility through gentle movements, can help treat arthritis and lower blood pressure. He cited the following results of his randomized designed trials: Forty-three women were randomly assigned to one of two groups. Twenty-two subjects performed Tai Chi exercise for twelve weeks, while the rest received standard treatment only. After twelve weeks, there were significant differences between the groups. Song reported, "Women in the Tai Chi group reported less pain, less difficulties with daily activities, improved balance, and greater abdominal muscle strength."[2]

Meditation and mind-body interventions have proved to be very helpful for sufferers of various forms of arthritis (http://nccam.nih.gov/health/meditation). Dr. Kate Lorig (1984, 1993), of California's Stanford University School of Medicine, and her colleagues conducted two studies in which arthritis patients who participated in a behavioral pain management program experienced an increase in self-efficacy, an average twenty percent decline in pain, and a forty percent reduction in visits to their doctors (Lorig, Laurin, & Gines, 1984; Lorig et al., 1993). It is promising to hear that this Stanford National Council for Complementary and Alternative Medicine funded program will extend their research to arthritis patients learning Mindfulness Meditation (Pelletier, 2000). Since there are many similarities and differences between Qigong/Tai Chi and other meditative and mind-body approaches, it would be interesting to explore for whom which treatments work best.

Through my experience, I know that Qigong can be beneficial for many types of arthritic conditions and joint problems. The general axiom is that those who suffer from such conditions need to listen to their own bodies when doing any exercise. In Bodymind Healing Qigong, I advise participants to first build up a sufficient amount of Qi by spending time in static Qigong postures. After building up Qi, then they may flow back and forth from stillness to movement, and back to stillness. Wuji Standing Meditation (see Chapter Twenty-one) is ideal for this, if standing is not too difficult for one's condition. If standing is difficult, then Qigong is practiced while sitting or lying down. An additional aspect of the Taoist notion of going from stillness to movement, and back to stillness, is to first make circles and then go back to stillness. As you do these practices in Chapter Twenty-one, you may grow to understand the wisdom stemming from Wang Xiangzhai, the grandmaster of the Yi Chuan Qigong tradition, who said, "Big circles are very good, small circles are even better, no circles are best." The idea here is that whether one is sitting, lying down, or standing such practices promote healing.

As you will see in Chapter Twenty-one, in BMHQ after Qi is built up into one's "bank account" and the Circle That Arises from Stillness is practiced, we add another practice that involves spirals. The three-sequence practice—Moving a Snake through the Joints, Dipping Your Hands into the Waters of Life, and Opening Your Heart to the Heavens—is another practice that may be useful, as long as the practitioner listens to his or her own body. To make this practice most beneficial, move back and forth from spiraling to no spiraling movements, finding the stillness in spiraling and the spiraling in stillness.

What integrative medicine adds to the treatment of arthritis sufferers is a multidisciplinary approach that oftentimes provides real relief and healing to this condition. When working with such patients at our clinic, we incorporate acupuncture, bodywork, psychological, and medical advice about dietary changes needed. Natural herbs can also be an important adjunct to treatment.[3]

What Bodymind Healing Psychotherapy, or any psychotherapy, adds here is a supportive place for arthritis sufferers to come to terms with the social, interpersonal, and intrapsychic dimensions of the effects on their lifestyle. Some of the relevant components of effective psychotherapy are using cognitive restructuring to change cognitive distortions, working through patterns of learned helplessness, becoming aware of issues of secondary gain, increasing a sense of self-control and self-efficacy, using the symptoms as teachers to learn from the body, seeing illness as an initiation onto the path of the wounded healer, and countering self-blame with self-love. In conjunction with these components of psychotherapy, using a blend of cognitive therapy and energy psychology interventions can be helpful. For example, repeating the phrase of *even though I* _____, *I can still love and accept myself* can be a key component of the healing relationship to one's Self that has corollaries in the biochemistry, energy, and neurophysiology of the patient. The breathing, visualization, and self-soothing methods of BMHP can also be useful adjuncts to the integrative treatment approach. Further research is needed to substantiate these methods and explore the parameters of which, when, with whom, and how, these methods work best.

Carpal Tunnel Syndrome

In the Introduction I discussed the case of one of my turning-point patients who suffered with carpal tunnel syndrome (a syndrome associated with repetitive motion of the hands/wrists that causes chronic pain). To review, the following are some of the key issues regarding how the Commencement movement in Tai Chi helped to alleviate his carpal tunnel syndrome:

1. Qigong is not a one-time fix, but instead, it is a method of practice that usually needs to be continued to maintain healing results.

2. When integrating Qigong movements into the context of psychotherapy, the therapist needs to be aware of the transference issues so that the patient will feel free to address any limitations of success.

3. The way in which Qigong is integrated into the psychotherapy is important in order for the therapist to avoid making false promises, as well as to protect the patient from disappointment. Therefore, Qigong should be introduced as a scientific experiment rather than a promised cure.

One Tai Chi movement that was helpful for this patient, is the first movement of the Tai Chi set called Commencement or Raising and Lowering the Qi (Mayer, 2004b, p.158), which involves exhaling and pressing the hands down slightly at the level of the belly, bending the wrists just to the point where there is no-force, as if the practitioner is pressing a ball slightly down into water. On the inhalation the hands float up as if in water. This practice gets Qi to move through the joints without strain or force.

It is an established fact that mind-body interventions can often be helpful in alleviating the symptoms of carpal tunnel syndrome (Garlinkel et al., 1998). Also, it is becoming an established fact that various aspects of Chinese medicine can be helpful in the treatment of carpal tunnel syndrome. In a study, by Chen (1990), all but one of thirty-six acupuncture patients attained excellent pain relief from carpal tunnel syndrome after treatment. In the study's long-term follow-up, according to Pelletier (2000, p.144), twenty-four patients showed two-and-a-half years to eight-and-a-half years of pain relief.[4] In China, Qigong is often used to complement acupuncture treatment.

One basic thing to keep in mind if you are suffering from carpal tunnel syndrome is that usually your body is giving you a message to alter the behavior that is causing the problem. Altering the ergonomics of your work situation, changing the way you put your hands on the computer keyboard, changing your seating, taking more breaks, massaging your wrist with various ointments—such as Traumeel (www.healusa.com)—are important parts of everyday care.

According to Gach (1990), using the Qigong self-touch methods of acupressure should be a basic part of self-care for those who suffer from carpal tunnel syndrome. Try using the acu-point on the middle of the inner wrist (P-7) and also breathing and massaging with the circle, stop, breathe, and feel method on points up this meridian line (Pericardium) up the inner arm. Similarly, messaging a point on the middle of the outer wrist (TW-4) and points on this meridian line (Triple Warmer-5) up the outside of the arm can be beneficial.

People often inappropriately focus on the area of the symptom, rather than expanding the focus to include the whole body. Generally there is a constriction in the shoulder muscles around the spine, or even in the hips, that is correlated with the constriction of the nerves and the tightening of the tendons in the wrist. The points listed above are some of the most common points used to heal carpal tunnel syndrome. However, from the perspective of Qigong and the River of Life practice, it is important to focus both "upstream" and "downstream" from the apparent point of energy blockage. For carpal tunnel syndrome, imagine opening the river of life with self-massage on points upstream in the shoulder muscles, then let your intuition guide you downstream and explore points there. For instance, massage the meridian line down the outside of the hand, ending at the base of the pinky finger where the crease appears when you make a fist (Small Intestine-3).

When your body is crying out for help, it is also a great time to reach out for help from a loved one or bodyworker for a nice massage. Remember the principle from the chapter on chronic pain that sometimes it is best not to force touch in areas where there is inflammation. Instead, try touching adjoining areas in order to move the Qi to balance excess and deficient energy and also explore using the appropriate element of touch (fire, earth, metal, water, and wood) referred to in earlier chapters (Lam, 1999).

Joint Problems

Regarding Qigong movements for joint problems in general, the first principle is that before moving, learn to experience filling the ball of Qi through Microcosmic Orbit Breathing and visualizations. In addition to the preceding principles for carpal tunnel syndrome, the Yin-Yang Balancing Method (see Chapter Seven) can also be helpful.[5] To open the energy of the heart and to get the spiraling energy of the whole body into the meridian lines of the wrist and shoulders, try this sequence: Moving a Snake through the Joints, Dipping Your Hands into the Waters of Life, and Opening Your Heart to the Heavens (see illustrations in Chapter Twenty-one). These movements helped quite a few people, in our clinic, when used along with the recommended methods of other health professionals, such as diet, acupuncture, chiropractic, and light therapy (photon emission). Depending upon their finances, some patients would see one or more of these health professionals.

Locking of Joints Due to Stroke—My Father's Physical Therapy

Regarding joint problems, I would like to share a story about my father: For quite a few months after experiencing a stroke, he was lying in bed and unable to straighten his leg. During one of my visits, a physical therapist was trying to help my father straighten his leg by pulling it in the direction that would straighten it. She said to my father, "Come on, Mr. Mayer, you know it needs to be exercised to build its strength." Let's do it ten times. Then she began to pull on it and started to count. My father was unable to do this, and the physical therapist and my father were becoming frustrated.

So I asked her if she would mind if I tried something. She disgruntingly said, "Go ahead." I then said jokingly to my father, "Dad, you know that breathing and Qigong stuff I've always been trying to get you to do? Well, now I have a captive audience; how about doing an experiment with me?" My father agreed. I asked him to inhale as I moved his leg in the direction that it could move, then I asked him to exhale as I moved it right up to—but no further than—the place it was stuck. The physical therapist impatiently interrupted and in a demeaning tone, thinking I must be pretty stupid, said, "Of course, he can move it in that direction, sir; we're trying to get it to move in the other direction." I told her I understood what she was saying and asked her to be patient and just watch for a moment. Then I continued to have my father inhale as I bent his leg in the direction that was easy for him; with each exhalation I moved his leg a little further as it was beginning to regain its flexibility. Eventually after a few minutes, the leg was almost completely straight.

It was an important moment in my life to give this gift back to my father, and to see the physical therapist's amazement as she asked where I had learned this technique, because she had never been shown it in physical therapy training. I explained to her it was not a technique as much as it was a Taoist principle called *wu wei*, or effortless effort.

I explained to her that the Eastern viewpoint on healing is to not fight the current, but to go along with the natural forces of life. Using the body's natural movements the way it wants to go, synchronizing breath and movement, and not forcing are key principles of Taoist healing.

Fibromyalgia

Patients with a variety of conditions are appearing in doctor's offices and hospitals, and the cause of the condition remains unknown. One of these conditions is fibromyalgia (FM), a pain disorder in which the pain occurs at multiple locations accompanied by widespread stiffness, fatigue, weakness, and irritability. About four million Americans (about two percent of the population) suffer from FM, and ninety percent of those are women (Selfridge, 2001). Unfortunately, many in the medical industry do not take the sufferers' complaints seriously; and they often minimize sufferers' pain by suggesting they are imagining their pain. Taggert and associates report in an article on fibromyalgia in the *Journal of Orthopedic Nursing*, "The cause of this complex syndrome is unknown, and there is no known cure" (Taggart, Arslanian, Bae, & Singh, 2003, p. 353).

Some researchers in the field look at FM and other related disorders as sympathetic nervous system overload diseases. From the perspective outlined in Chapter Eight on Trauma, one way of looking at this disorder is that it may actually be our body's way of communicating that we have not listened to its expressed limits.

These types of somatization disorders may be the body's way of enforcing relaxation, setting limits, and asking for new lifestyle modifications to be made. However, the term *somatization disorder* does not do fibromyalgia justice, because there is a complex array of biochemical, energetic, and stress-related factors that are correlated with this disorder. To reduce FM to "nothing but psychosomatic" is not helpful.

Numerous research studies indicate that a combination of physical exercise and mind-body therapy is effective in symptom management (Taggart et al., 2003). In this same article in the *Journal of Orthopedic Nursing*, the effect of Tai Chi on FM was investigated in a pilot study with a one group, pre-test/post-test design. Thirty-nine participants with fibromyalgia formed a single group for six weeks of Tai Chi classes for one hour, twice a week. FM symptoms and health-related quality of life were measured before and after exercise. Twenty-one participants completed at least ten of the twelve exercise sessions. Although the dropout rate was higher than expected, measurements on both the Fibromyalgia Impact Questionnaire (Buckhardt, Clark, & Bennett, 1991) and the Short Form–36 (Ware & Sherbourne, 1992) revealed statistically significant improvement in symptom management and health-related quality of life.

Even though the research methodology of the above study lacks a control group and follow-up research on the dropouts, its findings on Tai Chi and FM offers some hope in an arena where little hope is given. In addition to this article in the *Journal of Orthopedic Nursing,* there are quite a few articles in professional journals that point to the healing effects of relaxation and exercise methods, like Tai Chi and Qigong on fibromyalgia (Mannerkorpi & Arndorw, 2004; Mannerkorpi, 2005; Creamer, Singh, Hochberg, & Berman, 2000).

There have even been randomized controlled trials supporting the efficacy of Qigong and Mindfulness Meditation in the treatment of fibromyalgia (Astin, 2003). Of interest, in terms of energy psychology in particular, is a randomized study in Sweden of self-administered Emotional Freedom Techniques (EFT) of women aged twenty to sixty-five years with fibromyalgia. Dr. Brattberg (2008) found statistically significant results favoring the self-administered treatment group using EFT compared to a waiting control group. However, these results need to be interpreted with caution because the drop-out rate from the study was high. All these studies are particularly significant due to the fact that pharmacological treatments produce unwanted side effects. When I attended a training session with Dr. Selfridge, at the 2005 energy psychology conference in Baltimore, where I also led a training session, it was reconfirming for me to find that such a leader in the field was promoting the beneficial effects of a mind-body-energy approach to healing fibromyalgia. Author of *Freedom from Fibromyalgia: The Five-week Program Proven to Conquer Pain* (Selfridge & Peterson, 2001), Dr. Selfridge spoke, during her presentation, about how the common pharmacological treatment of anti-inflammatory medication does not usually work. Not only is Dr. Selfridge a medical doctor and chief of the Complementary Medicine and Wellness Center in Madison, Wisconsin, but she is also someone who healed herself from this disorder. Dr. Selfridge indicated how she believed that fibromyalgia is a "disharmony of the spirit," and she used Chinese medical terms to describe the disorder. In *Freedom from Fibromyalgia*, Selfridge and Peterson speak of the need to identify triggers to one's symptoms, such as anger and shame; to do emotional house cleaning; and to use cognitive approaches and journaling to work with dysfunctional beliefs. They advise meditation and breathing exercises as key components of her treatment approach. In addition to those who have found a healing pathway through this approach, another place where behavioral treatment methods have proved effective in treatment of FM is at the Matthew Thornton Health Plan's Behavioral Medicine Pain Program in Nashua, New Hampshire (Pelletier, 2000, p. 85).

Discovering a similar pathway as these leaders in the field, I also developed a body-mind-energy approach to helping those who suffer from this disorder. In my experience with FM patients, I have found that their symptoms often developed during a time of great stress—outer or inner. Some patients did not listen to their body's need to relax; others did not pay enough attention to recharging their batteries, expressing their needs, or setting appropriate limits. It was as if each of their bodies were screaming out in multiple locations the message of *I'm in pain, I'm not going to let you overwork/overstress me anymore.* For other patients, I have found that some common denominators were inner stressors, such as holding in various feelings like anger or having internalized perfectionistic messages from their families of origin. Identifying beliefs that are relevant to the creation of their symptoms, like the person believing that he or she cannot rest until everything is done, is an important part of treatment. As I discussed extensively in *Bodymind Healing Psychotherapy* (Mayer, 2007), and is standard knowledge in the field of mind-body psychotherapy (Gatchel & Blanchard, 1993), the roots of somatization disorders often seem to come from the body expressing what the voice cannot. So, expressing the unique words and meanings underlying the "somatization" is crucial for each person.

Normally we think of symptoms as something we want to eliminate at any cost. However, symptoms sometimes serve a purpose that our conscious mind may be unaware of. Sometimes an unconscious secondary gain comes from the symptoms, that is, loved ones finally offer desired attention when they see the sufferer's pain. In such cases, an important part of the path toward symptom reversal is for the patient to express his or her needs to loved ones and to accept their love and attention. The body's wisdom delivers the symptom of pain for still another reason, as if it is like a boundary-setting parent . . . to stop a person from engaging in the detrimental, self-destructive behavioral patterns that may have created the FM in the first place.

At our clinic and in my private practice, the BMHP methods discussed in earlier chapters have been a helpful component in an integrated treatment approach to this disorder. For example, I use Focusing to find the felt meaning of the pain, identify the dysfunctional beliefs that led to taking on more stress than the body could handle, and clear the obstacles to expression. Solid clinical evidence in the field has shown hypnosis is helpful for fibromyalgia.[6] My patients often report that using the particular breathing and hypnosis visualization methods contained in the BMHP process, such as the River of Life, have been a valuable practice that stays with them in their everyday lives. Particularly helpful have been the components of BMHP that involve self-soothing by putting one hand on the heart combined with the energy psychology method (Craig & Fowlie, 1995) of saying aloud, or repeating to themselves silently with compassionate intention, *even though____, I can still love and accept myself.* Other key factors in healing include finding ways to change dysfunctional lifestyle choices, noticing dietary exacerbations, limiting caffeine intake, and setting appropriate limits with work and family members. Because even light touch or moderate exercise can oftentimes be painful, an adjunctive program of Tai Chi and Qigong can be ideal methods to keep the patient's circulation active and energy alive while not overstressing his or her body.

Many think of fibromyalgia as a modern disease, but Dr. Xiao-Ming Tian says the symptom complex now called fibromyalgia has long been known about in Chinese medicine (Selfridge & Peterson, 2001, p. 19). Because exercise is a key element of activating immune system response, Qigong is a natural practice to try in conjunction with advice from medical professionals. Practicing static Qigong first, until the ball of Qi is filled, and then moving from stillness to movement and back to stillness is a general principal to be honored. Some of the Bodymind Healing Qigong methods that FM patients have reported to be helpful are cultivating Qi through Microcosmic Orbit Breathing (see Chapter Four), Standing Meditation, finding the Circle That Arises from Stillness, Walking Meditation, and Dispersing Stagnant Qi (see Chapter Twenty-one).

For fibromyalgia patients (and all of us with body symptoms), the axiom is to listen to your body to find the method that is best suited to your individual needs. For example, one patient could not lift her hands above her shoulders to do Dispersing Stagnant Qi exercises. By using Microcosmic Orbit Breathing to fill her ball of Qi, pressing down instead of forcing up, and using self-hypnosis to imagine herself in water, she was eventually able to feel her hands spontaneously floating up until they passed her shoulders, as tears of joy came to her eyes.

Diabetes

The technological advances of Western medicine in the ability to monitor and bring into balance insulin levels has helped many diabetes patients deal with their disease. Psychotherapy in general, and Bodymind Healing Psychotherapy in particular, can also help Type I and Type II diabetes sufferers to find a self-accepting attitude to the difficulties and limitations that diabetes has on their lifestyle.

At our clinic, Qigong and BMHP together represented one spoke of an innovative wheel of treatment. Our treatment included leading-edge treatment methods for balancing our patients' insulin levels. For example, acupuncture was used to balance the patient's energy; and in addition to the standard Western treatment protocols, the doctor at our clinic introduced an experimental technology called *photon emission therapy* for diabetic neuropathy. I heard of many cases and spoke with quite a few sufferers whose symptoms of lack of feeling and pains in the legs were healed after Dr. Saputo treated their legs with this "light machine." Further research is needed to determine just how long these effects last, what types of patients this treatment works best for, how much placebo effect is involved, and more.

The Effects of Qigong Walking on Diabetic Patients

Qigong can also be a useful complement to Western medicine's contributions. A study (Iwao et al, 1999) in the *Journal of Alternative and Complementary Medicine* reported on an examination of "The Effects of Qigong Walking on Diabetic Patients." Here is the abstract from this study:

Objectives: The present study was designed to evaluate the advantages of Qigong Walking—a mild and slow exercise that uses all the muscles of the body, in comparison with conventional walking in patients with diabetes.

Interventions: Ten inpatients with diabetes mellitus and associated complications were studied on three different days. One day the patients did Qigong Walking, one day conventional walking, and one day they did no exercise. On the walking days, patients walked for 30–40 minutes, 30 minutes after they ate lunch. Plasma glucose levels and pulse rates were measured 30 minutes after lunch, and again, 20 minutes after exercising; that is, 90 minutes after lunch. These data were compared to those obtained on a day with no exercise after lunch.

Results: Plasma glucose levels decreased during both exercises (from 228 mg/dL before to 205 mg/dL after conventional walking and from 223 mg/dL before to 216 mg/dL after Qigong Walking). In both walking situations, the patients' glucose levels decreased more after exercise than when they did no exercise (229 mg/dL; P<0.025). The pulse rates increased after conventional walking (from 77 to 95 beats per minute; P<0.025), and were higher than those in the group with no exercise (70 beats per minute; P<0.01), and those after Qigong Walking (79 beats per minute; P<0.05).

Conclusions: Qigong Walking reduced plasma glucose after lunch without inducing a large increase in the pulse rate in patients with diabetes.

After hearing about this study and in response to a couple of my diabetes patients asking about my suggestions for exercise, I suggested that, in addition to following their doctor's advice, they might consider practicing the Yi Chuan Qigong Walking from my DVD. After a doctor at our clinic gave her enthusiastic approval, both patients reported that they enjoyed doing the exercises and found them helpful in experiencing a sense of relaxation and empowerment at the same time (*fongsung*).

The Bodymind Healing Psychotherapy Integral Approach to Diabetes

The bulk of my work with diabetic patients has involved standard psychological treatment for issues involving self-esteem, decreased sexuality, anger at having lifestyle limitations, and so forth. I have used the Bodymind Healing Psychotherapy methods listed in the previous chapters, particularly focusing on methods of cognitive restructuring. I have also found energy psychology methods beneficial in helping patients establish anchors to self-accepting states. For example, I used this method with one male patient whose negative cognition was *God must not exist, or I must have done something evil in a past life to deserve to carry this burden and encumbrance on my lifestyle. I'm a weakling who'll never get married.* The new constructive cognition for this patient was *we all have our crosses to bear and this is mine. The empathy for human suffering and other lessons I've learned have made me a better person, and the person with whom I am meant to be will accept all of me.* (Concomitant with this statement he reported a shift of SUDS level from an 8 to a 2.) Interestingly, when this diabetic patient said these words, he held an imaginary ball in front of this heart in almost exactly the way it is practiced in Yi Chuan Standing Meditation, which you can see in the illustrated practice Opening the Golden Ball of the Heart in Chapter Twenty-one. We were able to use this posture as an anchor (see Chapter Sixteen) for those times when he fell into his old, self-despairing voice; and we used the holding of the ball and walking with it as a metaphor for walking through life holding a ball of self-acceptance. When doing this posture along with the cognitive restructuring, his SUDS level went down to 0.

Headaches

There is now established literature regarding how inappropriate coping mechanisms are correlated with many headaches and how mind-body healing methods can be useful in the treatment of headaches (Pelletier, 2000).

After a health professional has done a differential diagnosis, and dietary considerations (such as excess caffeine), medications ingested, and severe medical disorders (like tumors) have been ruled out, mind-body healing methods come to the forefront.

Research in the field of clinical hypnosis shows that when a person imagines a stream coming down his or her arms and imagines it warming the hands, this can be an effective treatment for migraines (Andreychuk & Skriver, 1975). The basic principle regarding headaches and all somatization disorders is to wonder about the metaphorical meanings of the symptom so that the symptom becomes a symbol . . . but for what? A skilled psychotherapist, or your own process of self-reflection and focusing, can help you find out what is making your head ache in your life.

Once an answer is found through focusing on the felt meaning of the symptom, an opportunity arises to shape-shift into another way of being that could cope with this situation and the old habitual pattern. For example, one of my patients, a fifty-year-old female teacher named Abby here, suffered from severe headaches. After tracking when these headaches happened, she discovered that they most often occurred when her husband did not help with the housework. While Focusing on her anger during one of our sessions, an image and phrase came up from her childhood when her mother said to "grin and bear it." This felt shift and felt meaning led Abby to change her old life stance and begin to communicate, assert herself, and bargain with her husband.

In an integrative energy psychology approach for treating headaches, if making the hands warm can be of help as medical hypnosis has shown, why not use the many-thousand-year-old knowledge base of a tradition that has studied ways to make the hands warm. Chinese medicine offers a treasure-house of treatment methods. In addition to acupuncture—the best-known Chinese method for headache treatment—other branches of Chinese medicine can also prove to be of great help. For example, one randomized controlled study with adults with tension-type headaches showed that the Tai Chi group, compared to a wait list control group, had significant improvements in pain and other health-related quality of life measures, after fifteen weeks (Abbott et al., 2007).

Qigong static postures, breathing methods, knowledge of meridian lines, and movement methods are ways to tap on a somatic knowledge base spanning the centuries. One of my Qigong students who often had tension headaches said he enjoyed practicing the Tiger Qigong Animal Frolic while making angry faces after he got home from work; he said this was his favorite way to release the tension.[7]

Acupressure is also an important part of an integrated treatment approach. Depending upon the type and location of the headache certain acu-points can be touched, such as the points below the base of the skull in the hollow between the two vertical neck muscles (Gall Bladder 20) or points in the indentations on either side of the nose where the bridge of the nose meets the ridge of the eyebrows (Bladder 2). For a list of types of headaches and suggested acupressure treatment points, refer to *Acupressure's Potent Points* (Gach, 1990). Or using the principles in Chapter Seven, the Yin-Yang Balancing Method can be useful for self-treatment of headaches.

Raynaud's Syndrome

According to the *Merck Manual of Medical Information* (1997), "Raynaud's syndrome or phenomenon are conditions in which small arteries usually in the fingers and toes go into spasm, causing the skin to become pale or a patchy red to blue . . . Most often it is triggered by exposure to cold, the fingers and toes turn white, usually in a spotty fashion" (p. 136).

Medical hypnosis has also been proved beneficial to healing Raynaud's syndrome through suggestion procedures whereby subjects imagine that their hands are becoming warm (Braun, 1979; Jacobson, Hackett, Surman, & Silverberg, 1973). Again, the many-thousand-year-old methods of hand warming that stem from Qigong can supplement the behavioral health treatment of Raynaud's syndrome.

I personally suffered from this syndrome, and Standing Mediation and Qigong breathing methods that I learned from Master Han Xingyuan helped to cure this disorder (Mayer, 2004b, p.3). Standing with Master Han was an intense ordeal, like a trial by fire—or I should say a trial by extreme cold. During two summers in 1976 and 1977, Sifu Ha's Qigong class practiced Yi Chuan Standing Meditation with Master Han, standing in the freezing cold in San Francisco at 6 a.m. for up to one hour at a time. By staying with my sensation of being cold and just experiencing it, the coldness gradually changed to smoothness—my skin felt like baby's skin. Red blotches appeared on my hands; and then my whole body became warm. Now I had finally experienced one of the practices that I had disbelievingly read about in my scholarly research during my doctoral years—practices that are common in shamanic initiation traditions to cultivate "inner heat" (Eliade, 1956, pp.79–86).

Since then I have helped a few patients lessen and heal their symptoms through the use of the River of Life breathing methods. In these cases I changed the visualization to imagine warm water coming down the river to the hands. In addition to this method, focusing (Gendlin, 1978) on the particular issues that are stuck in the river (ice blocks) and allowing the compassionate light of the sun to melt them has been helpful to some patients; and others, have benefited from the practice of Qigong and Tai Chi.

Stomach Disorders

For all disorders of this area of the body, it is particularly important to have a differential diagnosis by your physician. You may also want to refer to the *Merck Manual of Medical Information*.

Crohn's Disease

Crohn's disease is a chronic inflammation of the intestinal wall. Like other diseases of the stomach area, Bodymind Healing Psychotherapy (BMHP) is well suited as a complementary treatment for treating this disorder because this disease is often rooted in stress and psychosomatic issues. One doctor who suffered from Crohn's reported no further symptoms after our Bodymind Healing Psychotherapy alone, with no Qigong or Tai Chi practiced. This example is not provided as evidence of success, because many times Crone's is known to remit after short-term episodes. In fact, her symptoms did reoccur later in our long-term therapy when a significant stressor arose in her life. Again, by using BMHP methods, she was able to alleviate the symptoms with no need for her usual medication. Further research is needed regarding how the specific methods BMHP can become part of an integrated treatment approach.

Irritable Bowel Syndrome

It is a well-researched fact that mind-body-spirit issues are inextricably connected with irritable bowel syndrome (IBS) and other functional gastrointestinal disorders (Salt, 2002). These disorders affect 35 million Americans and comprise ten percent of visits to medical doctors. It is important to have a differential diagnosis by your physician to approach your treatment in the best way because many gastrointestinal disorders can be mistaken for IBS.

Bodymind Healing Psychotherapy is one of many psychological approaches that can be helpful for this disorder. Somatization disorders, like IBS, are often related to a difficulty in differentiating and expressing feelings. The body seems to express "its irritation" by saying *I'm irritated by* ___. Understanding the psychodynamic roots of why a person holds onto feelings rather than expressing them is one step on the path to healing; another step is to examine the beliefs that are in the way of self-expression. Using cognitive restructuring along with somatic anchors is one important part of treatment. Qigong and Tai Chi are also natural ways to substitute a relaxation response for a stress reaction. In particular, the patients I have worked with enjoy using the Tai Chi Ruler exercise while they imagine putting down a ball of tension on their exhalation and re-empowering their hearts on the inhalation, as the Tai Chi circle moves back into the body (see illustration in Chapter Twenty-one). Moreover, doing self-applied Chi Nei Tsang (Chia & Chia, 1990) can be helpful for some people, that is, using gentle circle, stop, breathe, and feel movements, pushing into your belly as you exhale. Before pushing into your belly this way, check with your medical doctor to ensure that you have a correct diagnosis.

One patient, named Edith here, was the daughter of a medical doctor and was extremely skeptical of any mind-body-spirit connection to her IBS. But through "scientific" exploration and her journaling, she realized that every time she had a flare-up there was something serious going on with her son or husband. As soon as she and her husband made up, all of her symptoms disappeared. Through these realizations, she was able to attribute the roots of her inhibition to multiple rapes in her early adulthood; and from this trauma, she had internalized the belief that *it's best to not be visible*. Substituting a more balanced cognition was an important part of her process of change. When Edith said, "I know when to express myself and when not to, due to my wounds; and I'm going to allow myself the pleasure of expressing myself from my center in appropriate situations," she assumed a posture in which she held her hands in front of her belly. This posture became her anchor (see Chapter Sixteen) to be able to activate this state-specific state of consciousness. While talking about this gesture, I suggested that she might like to practice the Tai Chi Ruler exercise. Edith liked doing this as a way, not only to hold her power in her belly center, but also to let go of the ball of inhibition on her exhalation that had been so much of her previous pattern.

CHAPTER FOURTEEN

Qigong Psychosis

Qigong is not a panacea, nor are spiritual practices in general. As with any spiritual technique, when Qigong is practiced in an overly obsessive way, it can lead to psychological imbalances and at worst a disconnection with reality. This is an era when the importance of blending the psychological and the spiritual is apparent. In this spirit, Bodymind Healing Psychotherapy (BMHP) honors the deep, emotional, transformative journey to the underworld and the raising of our spirits through the treasure-house of the cross-cultural spiritual traditions of humankind. The following case illustrates the importance of integration in the realm of psychospiritual inner work.

Case Illustration: "I'm Going to Cut My Wife's Head Off with My Samurai Sword"

This patient, whom I will call Mitch, was referred to me by another Tai Chi teacher, who said Mitch was one of his most dedicated students. Mitch reportedly practiced up to ten hours a day and believed he was an advanced Taoist master. He was convinced that his one remaining obstacle was his wife, and he explained in our first session how his sword techniques were so developed that he thought he could behead her with no anger, just a centered samurai slice. I learned that this was not an exaggerated expression of feeling, but something Mitch was really considering doing. When I asked him what led to his wanting to do this he told me his story.

Mitch was secretly financing a woman friend who was in dire straights. This other woman was one of his closet friends from childhood (he assured me that there was nothing sexual between them). He said that his wife would never approve of him giving money to another woman, and that it was essential to his integrity that he be a giving "master" and not be controlled by a woman's narrow material concerns that went against the flow of the Tao.

This is a clear example of how a "spiritual" training without psychological inner work can create dangerous imbalances and delusional thinking. I was concerned that this patient could be a "danger to self or others," and I was getting ready to activate Tarasoff procedures.[1] But in our very first session, Mitch experienced a shift of perception as I spoke to him as a fellow Tai Chi practitioner. I questioned why, as such an advanced follower of the Way of the Tao, did he not at least trust "the Way of the universe" enough to ask his wife how she would feel? And even if she reacted negatively, I challenged him, "Don't you have the power to sink your Qi into your roots and hold your ground and work out a way both of your needs can be met? Doesn't an internal martial artist use the least force necessary?" At the end of the first session, Mitch agreed to try this, not to overreact, and not to "act out" his feelings before our next session.

To his surprise, his wife was not as upset with him as he thought she would be. She understood how he wanted to give to a long-standing friend. However, she did not want to finance this and suggested that they create two separate bank accounts so he could take his gift money out of that account.

This circumvented the immediate threat of danger. In the next sessions, Mitch and I explored the roots of his reactive pattern. His wife's not being there for his needs felt just like his mother who was "always hassling me about the amount of money she was giving me." Mitch's father had died suddenly when he was a child, and his mother was now financing his nonworking lifestyle. To make a long story short, in the next sessions, Mitch worked through his rage about his father's "abandonment" of him. Mitch also realized that he had made a decision to do whatever he wanted with his life, because he felt God and others had abandoned him. Mitch's inner work, on his entitlement issues and his narcissistic rage from having to be there for other's needs, helped him to commit to a new stance in life. Mitch eventually saw how it was to his advantage to hold a job in addition to his training in Tai Chi in order to develop his root in his Self and in everyday life and work. As he moved on from the feelings regarding his father's death, Mitch found a job he liked. He saw his relationship with his wife, and others, as an opportunity to practice being as centered in his emotional body, as he felt he was in his physical body. Mitch realized that due to his wounding and lack of emotional education in his family, he had never learned to "modulate his affects." Additionally, he now understood that doing "emotional" Tai Chi Push Hands with his wife and his life could help him learn to respond more appropriately and to avoid being overreactive. In Chapter 17 there is further discussion of affect modulation and Tai Chi; and Tai Chi Joining Hands practice as a Self-development practice is discussed more fully in *Secrets to Living Younger Longer* (Mayer, 2004b, pp. 172–180).[2]

Using Ancient Sacred Wisdom Traditions and Western Bodymind Healing Methods in Your Everyday Life

. . . Classical man saw psychological sickness as the effect of a divine action which could be cured only by a God or another divine action. When sickness is vested with such dignity, it has the inestimable advantage that it can be vested with a healing power. The divina afflictio then contains its own diagnosis, therapy and prognosis, provided of course that the right attitude toward it is adapted.

—C.A. Meier
Ancient Incubation and Modern Psychotherapy

Overview of Section III

Each of the chapters in this section is interwoven into a quilt. Each patch (chapter) of the quilt helps to form the whole, and many of the patches are repeated in other areas of the quilt. For example, in the psychotherapeutic process of changing one's life stance, the therapist may incorporate a patient's gestures to anchor desired state-specific states and may help the patient to gain affect modulation skills. As patients developmentally mature in their self-expression, develop affect modulation skills, exercise appropriate self-assertion, and learn to banter, they may embody some of the deepest principles of internal martial arts and not use any more force than is needed. Thus, in each chapter many of the principles from other chapters are coexistent, but one or more of the principles are highlighted to illustrate the issue in focus.

CHAPTER FIFTEEN

Changing Your Life Stance

*What is the work of works for man if not to establish in and by each one
of us an absolutely original center in which the universe reflects itself
in a unique and inimitable way and those centers are our very selves
and personalities.*

—Tielhard de Chardin

Shape-Shifting and Changing Your Life Stance

Earlier in Chapter Three I spoke of the Aesclepian temple rituals that involved
sending those who needed healing to the Dionysian theater. This cathartic experience, which could lead to the embodiment of a new life stance, was an important part of people's healing journey in this first holistic healing temple of the
Western world. There, people wore masks of different characters in order to
help change their identification with attributes of the character that was associated with their state of "dis-ease." You read earlier how the idea of shape-
shifting into different ways of being has been a fundamental aspect of shamanic
traditions the world over—a part of initiatory traditions that were helpful to
hunting, empowerment, and healing. In those sections I also discussed topics,
such as modern quantum biology, multiple personality research, mind-body
medicine, hypnotherapy, and a "state-specific" understanding regarding how
consciousness affects physical structure.

Case illustrations in this chapter will show specifically how, from the perspective of Bodymind Healing Psychotherapy (BMHP), the psychotherapy
process and our lives can be viewed as changing our life stances. The state-
specific states of consciousness that can be activated by integrating Western

bodymind healing methods and Qigong-related practices can aid the transformative process of shape-shifting to healthier ways of being.

Case Illustration: Social Phobia

Among those cases in which a combination of Standing Meditation, Qigong practice, and psychotherapy combine to help a person change his or her life stance, perhaps none are as poignant as the stories of those who gain the strength to stand up to someone who has abused them during their childhood. As a young boy, "Stan" was the smallest of all of his classmates as well as a gentle and sensitive child. When other kids engaged in cruel jokes and hitting contests, Stan shied away. Because he was so small, kids enjoyed bullying him when he would not fight back. Stan's stance was, in part, constitutional—his mother remembered that he was a gentle child even in his first few years of life.

Contributing to the fixation of this stance into a characterological pattern was Stan's physically abusive brother, who had told Stan, "I'm better than you at everything." By the time he was in his late teens, Stan felt so paralyzed that he developed a social phobia and feared contact with authority figures. He dropped out of college once and complained of multiple somatic issues including developing arthritis in his fingers. In his current occupational setting, Stan could not assert himself to his boss to ask for the raise he felt he deserved.

Stan was first a student in my Bodymind Qigong classes, which emphasize Standing Meditation and include some self-defense training. Then he decided to leave our student/teacher relationship to do Bodymind Healing Psychotherapy with me.[1]

A major turning point in Stan's life was when he found a stance to stand up to his brother through his internal martial arts practices. Though Stan's martial arts practices were important in giving him sensitivity and power, the verbal dimension of his power was equally crucial and needed to be developed through psychotherapy. One of the more significant moments during therapy occurred after Stan went to his family's home for Thanksgiving and his brother greeted him, "So, after all these years, I bet you're still not better than me at anything. Let's go out play some basketball one-on-one."

His brother's demeaning messages had always made Stan cower with anxiety in his stomach. But during this Thanksgiving visit home, after much inner work in therapy and a year of Standing Meditation practice, Stan found his verbal stance to address his brother's abusive message. Stan said, "You know something, you're not better than me at everything." His brother paused for a moment and said, "What do you mean. Give me an example. I'm still better at basketball and at every sport, and I make more money than you." Stan found the stance he had always wanted in his childhood at this moment and continued, "You're not better than me at everything—you're not better at being a kind brother." According to Stan, when he said this to his brother, it stopped him in his tracks and left him speechless for a moment. After apologizing for the way he had treated Stan in his childhood, a new relationship developed between them.

With a combination of his study of the internal martial arts—which emphasize the power of softness—and his therapy, Stan eventually transmuted his identification with being an ungrounded, wimpy male. He was able to work through his lack of self-confidence and asked for a raise at work, which he received. He learned to affect his arthritis in his hands with the power of his mind and through the use of acupressure points and the visualization methods that are a wider part of the practice done in Bodymind Healing Qigong.

This was no "total cure" but "a healing." Issues still arose; but through our work, Stan had cultivated a new stance toward his issues, and he had found a way of working with and through them. He now had a clear vision of the path ahead of him, whereas before, his primordial ground was paved over. Stan now recognized that just as his internal arts work takes practice, so does finding his psychological stance. He learned to be aware of how the abusiveness of his brother fragmented his energy. And Stan learned to practice cognitive restructuring when negative thoughts arise. Instead of his old thought of *I'm no good and can't stand up for myself*, his new restructured thought and stance became *I don't deserve to be treated badly despite any of my short-comings; and I will stand up for myself.* Then he breathes and practices returning to his grounded stance of power and self-assertiveness. It also helps that he is now able to use his Tai Chi Push Hands practice to play with his brother and demonstrate the power of his softness.

Case Illustration: Impulse Control—
The Exploding Karate Kid

"Arnie" was a thirty-year-old night-shift worker at an industrial firm. He was not one of my Tai Chi students; but during the course of our therapy, I referred him to another teacher in order to keep our therapeutic relationship unencumbered by two different types of relationships.

Arnie came to me on referral from his company's employee assistance program for exploding on two separate occasions—one time he put his fist through a window, another time he threw a vial of industrial fluid across the room.

Various forms of meditation may complement psychotherapy by providing ways for patients to develop an observing self, enhance equanimity, self-regulate and therefore improve self-control, and cultivate affect tolerance and emotional resilience in the face of provocative stimuli (Walsh & Shapiro, 2006; Mayer, 2007, pp. 24–31). So, as part of our psychotherapy, I introduced various meditation methods to Arnie. After trying the River of Life meditation method during our sessions, I suggested he practice it at home and at work. I hoped that it would help Arnie to develop some of the qualities known to be associated with Qigong meditation, such as constellate his observing self, change his emotional reactivity, help him to learn to sink his Qi to his belly to find a center there, discover his central equilibrium, reduce fragmentation, develop affect modulation skills, reduce sympathetic nervous system overarousal, and change his life stance. As part of this meditation practice, Arnie visualized the situations that triggered his loss of impulse control, then he noticed the waves of emotion, thoughts, and beliefs that arose; then he returned back to his breath in the River of Life exercise. When Arnie was reactive, he said he was not aware of his body. Because of this, he reported that it was particularly beneficial to learn to follow the river of his breath down into his body and become more mindful of kinesthetic sensations and bodily holdings. This practice was a first step toward helping Arnie learn to avoid capsizing and to maintain his central equilibrium in the crosscurrents as he set sail on his journey of transmuting old introjected bodymind patterns of response. To help further develop his observing self, I added a dis-identification method from Assagioli's *Psychosynthesis* (1965) to this practice, that is, "I have a body; but I am not my body. I have sensations; but I am not those sensations. I have thoughts; but I am not my thoughts. I have impulses; but I am not those impulses. What am I then? I am a pure center of awareness that notices all these things; but I am more than them."

A key moment in therapy occurred when Arnie was practicing the transmuting dimensions of the River of Life practice and focusing (Gendlin, 1978) on his body sense. He tried to identify the tightness that was there and noticed how puffed out he was in his chest. A memory surfaced of being in gym class as a child and noticing that his chest was caved in and his posture was slouched, whereas other boys' chests were more filled out and their postures more erect. The belief that ruled Arnie's life for the next ten years was forming: *a man is one who doesn't slouch, and a real man's chest is pushed out proudly.*

This was Arnie's way of expressing a common male theme that a man does not show his vulnerabilities and does not cave in to the pressures of life. Many people gave Arnie validation for being able to tolerate more than other guys could. For instance, he worked longer hours than any of the other workers. When anyone needed someone to take over one of the late-night shifts, Arnie was the one who would readily volunteer. He was very well liked for his willingness to help out anyone who had a problem.

Because Arnie would never "stoop so low" to admit his vulnerabilities or to ask for help on his late-night shift, when things bothered him, he would often build up resentment and explode. Also, Arnie started to realize that he had little true intimacy in his life in which he could express or show his real feelings.

Arnie had been a longtime practitioner of Karate; and at first, he balked when I suggested he might try Tai Chi—the best-known method of Qigong that helps to develop the qualities listed earlier and specifically emphasizes balancing strength and softness. I did not push this idea on him; but when he saw a man practicing it in a park one day, Arnie was struck by its grace and asked me for a referral. I gave him the name of a local teacher whom I respected. After six months of practice, Arnie began to discover a new type of strength. On one occasion he told me of the insight he had just gotten from his practice of Push Hands with another student—Arnie had discovered that *the softer you are, the stronger you are.*

The insights Arnie gained complemented our psychotherapeutic work. Arnie realized how he was never given any opportunity in his family of origin to speak of his vulnerabilities. His father was a Marine captain with a very stoical view of what it meant to be a man, and he "trained" Arnie in this attitude.

Arnie began to develop a new stance in his life of *A man is one who balances strength and softness. A man is one who can be with his whole Self—vulnerabilities and all.* Identifying and working with both his old and new life stance was a significant part of a larger psychotherapeutic process. Arnie learned to become more aware of the feelings in his body, and he became better able to differentiate and regulate his affects. He was able to identify when he was caught in his "son of the Marine captain stance," and he was able to be aware, as stressors arose, of his abilities to activate his softer, balanced "Tai Chi stance." Arnie was able to activate his observing self when stress arose, which led to improved impulse control, enhanced coping skills, and affect tolerance and proved particularly useful in the long hours of his late-night shift. The psychotherapeutic process along with the various meditation methods discussed previously led to better containment of his feelings and the ability to express them more often in an appropriate way. At a later point during therapy, Arnie was proud of himself on one occasion for expressing to a coworker that he was exhausted and irritable on his late-night shift. He asked the coworker to help him out by letting him nap for twenty minutes and wake him. To the best of my knowledge, Arnie never exploded at work again.

Case Illustration: Finding the "Right Man"

"Rachel" was a bright, vivacious student in her early thirties, who learned Standing Meditation as part of a psychological training process I offered at a local university. The following is a synopsis of a term paper she wrote and discussions I had with her.

Rachel had a history of many short-term relationships. During the time of her training, after a boring evening with her current partner, she thought, *he's not stimulating enough for me.* Crosscurrents of feelings then took her away from her own center of gravity, and she began to think that *life is depressing. There must be something wrong with me to be in a relationship that's not more alive. Maybe I shouldn't stay in this relationship any longer.*

After two months of practice, Rachel reported that Standing Meditation was helpful to ground her on her own "island of being" in the midst of waves of conflicting thoughts and emotions—waves that in the past made her criticize her partner with derogatory remarks. On this island Rachel had room to cultivate her awareness with some of the methods of Bodymind Healing Psychotherapy that I had given the class to practice.

When Rachel felt that her current partner was not stimulating enough, she focused on the bodily feeling that emerged as she reflected on the above issue and asked herself the question *what's this feeling all about?* As she did the River of Life exercise, Rachel felt the loneliness that arose from not being met in the way she wanted to be. She felt a closed door in her heart. She felt deadness there and desperately desired to be saved from the feeling. She became aware of the thoughts, and precisely how they disrupted the flow of her Qi. She reported having difficulty going back to her breathing.

Specifically, when Rachel noticed the thought arise that *he's not enough fun,* she become aware that her Qi went up into her head and an angry flushed feeling came into her face along with a contorted turn of the side of her mouth.

In Standing Meditation with psychological intent, we connect the feelings that arise while Standing with our family of origin issues. Self-psychology and object relations theorists believe that many of our core patterns develop from introjected representations of early objects, such as our parents. Our parents' beliefs, or lives, live in us as object-representations that need to be transmuted in order for us to be our real Selves.

Rachel associated the roots of her feelings with her unhappily married mother. Her mother thought her husband was boring and passed along the message to Rachel of *be careful not to get involved with a boring man.* Rachel became aware of the replaying tape of her early family experience, then she went back to breath, back to center, back to her own ground. This insight, and the resulting shift that happened in her body, led her to begin therapy with a therapist that I recommended. She began the process of differentiating her own life from that of her parents; and she began to take responsibility for making things fun in her relationship, instead of "expecting the man to do it."

In the third quarter of her training program, Rachel reported that while practicing the Opening the Golden Sphere of the Heart exercise (see Chapter Twenty-one), she found a sense of her own ground and a sense of her Self as a golden ball of energy that was sending out love to her mother. She realized that her mother's message was just a well-meaning attempt to save her daughter from a similar fate. Rachel's resentment of her mother started to melt away as her therapy continued, and Rachel started to take responsibility for initiating humor-filled interactions with her boyfriend. The last time I heard from Rachel she reported that once she began to let go of her internalized mother's fear, she was able to see that her boyfriend actually had a dry sense of humor with which she could play.

Enhance Your Stance: Transforming Your "Depressive Position" with Qigong

According to Melanie Klein's concept of "depressive position," as a person develops and matures, a realization comes that the hated mother is also the mother whom one loves. The depressive position takes place when we accept the mother as a whole person. We inhibit our need to attack and contain the feeling in ourselves, thereby tolerating the pain of our loved one's limitations. Klein's theory is insightful regarding ambivalence—one can love and hate the mother or any person and still have a relationship (Grosskurth, 1986).

To add to Klein's ideas of the depressive position as being a way of holding the opposites of good/bad and right/wrong in order to resolve splitting, Body-mind Healing Psychotherapy suggests adding a Qigong posture to practice this stance. While doing the Yi Chuan Qigong practice of Holding the Golden Ball of the Heart (see Chapter Twenty-one), imagine holding a yin-yang ball that holds all opposites—good and bad, right and wrong, and the ideal versus the denigrated self. There is a dot of the complementary partner in each. While holding the ball, allow a half smile to emerge and express itself on your face. Derived from meditation traditions, this half smile expresses *I'm not overjoyed because I'm in touch with the dark side and limits of life. Yet it's good to be alive, and to be able to hold all this.* Thus, we have what I call (with a half smile), "the Taoist depressive stance."

Just as acupuncturists sometimes suggest Qigong postures to their patients, so do I suggest, when appropriate, that a patient practice holding this Yi Chuan Golden Ball, Depressive Stance posture as homework, with the intent of resolving splitting.

I have spoken about stances as one of the keys to ancient traditions of postural initiation. As we hold "the Taoist depressive stance," we have a practice for "re-membering" and reintegrating the soul work that is part of a modern primordial psychotherapy. This includes finding a stance that helps to cultivate the "transcendent function" (Stein, 1982, p. 19) that unites opposites.

CHAPTER SIXTEEN

Your Everyday Gestures: Activating the Healing Energy of Your Primordial Self

Once upon a time a young man decided to go on a quest to the Taoist sacred mountain of Hua Shan to see if his life's meaning could be restored. Although he vowed to fast from all food and wait until a vision came, after three days, nothing happened. Weak from starvation, he fainted in the middle of his prayer circle and gave up his effort.

As he let go of trying, it was then that the founder of Tai Chi Chuan, Chang San Feng, appeared and offered to teach the young man how to move like the animals to restore his vital energy, and how to find his primordial Self by filling his body with the powers of the heavens and the earth.

And so this initiate learned how to move like a Snake Creeping Low. In addition to learning the physical movement, the snake taught him to descend into his darkness and find the way through his pain. Another week was devoted to watching and imitating the movements of a White Crane Spreading Its Wings. Mimicking the crane, the initiate put one foot in the water, and spread his not-so-imaginary wings. Into his awareness came a vision of how to step into his pain, and yet find a Transcendent Self that could observe his emotional process with nonattachment.

After forty nights on the mountaintop, learning from the animals, studying the ways of nature, and being visited by the spirit of various Taoist masters, he knew it was now time to leave. As he traveled down the mountain, he was very excited about all he had to teach.

The first person he passed was an old lady who was washing off a glass window with a circular motion. The initiate felt a wave of disenchantment come over him as he realized that she was doing the Tai Chi movement *Making a Circle between the Heavens and the Earth* (also called *Taoist Immortal Paints a Heavenly Rainbow*), just like he had learned it from Yang Luchan, the founder of the Yang lineage of Tai Chi.

"Maybe everyone knows what I know already and will not want to learn anything from me," he thought.

After walking a little further, he saw a man drop something on the ground and bent down to pick it up. "How does this man know the secret movement called *Grasping the Pearl at the Bottom of the Sea*, which I learned from Yang Cheng Fu? It's supposed to be a secret way to open the lower Tan Tien and ground the body's energy. What I know is nothing special, everyone knows it," he said to himself dejectedly.

Walking a little further, he saw a couple having an argument. The woman's arms were outstretched in the shape of a ball in front of her heart as she exclaimed to her husband, "Why can't you just listen to me?" The young initiate now reached his limit, for she was doing the special *Holding the Golden Ball of the Heart Meditation* posture that he learned from the founder of the Yi Chuan system, Wang Xiangzhai.

Just as the initiate was ready to give up and fall back into the sea of depression he knew so well, he came to a realization that, yes, everyone he saw was doing sacred movements, but most were unconscious of their sacred character. Then he realized that his path was to teach people to appreciate the meaning and beauty of what they were already doing in their everyday lives ... that our human movements, and our very Being, are divine gifts—if we could just see them as such.

—Michael Mayer
  Adapted and Retold from Shamanic Oral Teachings

The Taoist Initiate Who Sees the Sacred in Everyday Movements

When I tell this teaching story in workshops, I ask people to notice how their body is positioned, and to appreciate its sacred meaning. For you, I advise the same. Maybe your feet are crossed at the ankles, preventing your life energy from dissipating out your feet. Maybe you are touching your head at the temples, unconsciously instilling some idea further into your mind through touch. What *is* the sacred purpose of your current posture?

Tapping the Metaphorical Wisdom of the Bodymind Using Internal Martial Arts

Similarly, I began to notice my psychotherapy patients, particularly at key moments of change, move in ways that represent deep, often-unconscious transformative aspects of their psyches. There is a metaphorical wisdom of body language that is expressed at these moments. From my training in the internal martial arts, I noticed that the movements a martial artist uses to confront physical danger are often the same as, or similar to, the movements my psychotherapy patients expressed when dealing with emotional dangers. The ancient art of Qigong, of which Tai Chi is the best-known system, contains some of the best and most primordial of these empowering movements. The psychologist who is attuned to those bodily expressions can help to bring to awareness the bodily expression of the primordial Self as it moves toward empowerment and change. The clinician who is aware of these movements and their multifaceted meanings can help to grease the wheels that facilitate movement in the direction toward where the patient's psyche is already moving in its natural healing journey. To illustrate this incorporation of patients' gestures, I will use key moments in three different patients' bodymind healing process.

You read earlier how modern energy psychology uses the tapping of points to move energy and to anchor state-specific states of consciousness associated with new constructive beliefs that emerge in psychotherapy. At times, Bodymind Healing Psychotherapy (BMHP) also uses tapping techniques from meridian-based psychologies. However, I prefer to use a patient's own gestures that emerge at the moment a new healing, state-specific state of consciousness is expressing itself through the metaphorical wisdom of body language.

In medical hypnosis, "ideomotor signaling" (Rossi & Cheek, 1988; Hilgard, 1965) is used to have the patient communicate various things to the therapist; for example, for a patient to communicate when a trance state has been achieved. Many times, following the therapist's suggestion, the patient moves various body parts when he or she achieves a certain state-specific state of consciousness; for instance; the patient raises a finger or nods his or her head when in a relaxed state. The patient notices that these body movements seem to happen all by themselves following the therapist's suggestion. A therapist might suggest, "Your hands will come together when your creative unconscious is ready to begin therapeutic work." Or, "When your unconscious has resolved that problem in a satisfactory manner, your arm will come to rest on your lap." These ideomotor signals are interpreted as "objective proof" that patients can call upon the help of their creative sources whenever they need to (Rossi & Cheek, 1988, pp. 38–39).

Adding to this tradition of ideomotor signaling, BMHP proposes that natural movements of the body be noticed at the moment a felt shift occurs, and that we view this process in line with the knowledge base of Chinese medicine, Qigong, and internal martial arts traditions. Then, this "whole body, naturally arising, postural signaling" (without prior suggestion on the part of the therapist) can be interpreted as revealing the primordial pathways of the movement of the life force (Qi) as it opens new ways of being and new life stances. Whether or not the therapist knows Chinese medicine or Qigong, the therapist can help the patient to be aware of these body movements so that the patient can further anchor these state-specific states of consciousness for self-healing. And any of us when we have a new insight (Gendlin's *felt shift*) and a new potential pathway emerges on a stuck life issue—whether or not we are in therapy—can use the awareness of our bodily expressions at this key moment in our lives to anchor a new life stance.

The Healing Power of Psychological Metaphors Hidden in the Internal Martial Arts

Case Illustration: Sexual Abuse and Fist under Elbow

A forty-year-old woman, named Elaine here, was a psychotherapist and wanted to do a single session with me after one of my workshops. Elaine told me how she had been molested and raped by multiple family members in her childhood. She said she had done much work with many psychotherapeutic methods, including the tapping techniques of energy psychology. But she still reported being overly hypervigilant and a long way from developing adequate verbal affect modulation skills.

I like to explain *affect modulation* to my patients through the metaphor of having the ability to regulate the quantity of affective charge on the dial of one's feelings. At the lowest setting on the dial (0 on a 10-point scale), a person would be nonexpressive; and at the highest setting on the dial (a 10 on a 10-point scale), a person would be totally uninhibited in his or her expression. Modulating affect has to do with turning up the dial to the amount of force appropriate to the situation. There are striking parallels between the internal martial arts tradition where the practitioner is trained to use only the least amount of force necessary when confronted with an attack and psychotherapy's concept of affect modulation.

In Elaine's practice of affect modulation skills, she used the example of a man who was "coming on to her" in a workshop she had attended in the past. The old patterns that became activated were feeling like a victim, withdrawing in order to survive in the world, and holding on to overreactive anger about being intruded upon. She told me that in her current therapy, she was working on boundary setting and felt disappointed in herself that she was not able to follow through on the work she was doing with her current therapist. She said if she had been "more together," she would have said to the man, "Stop coming on to me, this is a workshop." I asked her how she felt about that response. She said that that type of boundary setting felt a bit extreme to her. I asked how she would ideally like to handle this man. Elaine paused for a moment and said she would rather just flick him off as if he were a fly bothering her. At that moment she unconsciously embodied this stance with a gesture demonstrating how she would like to flick him off. She put her left hand in a fist under her elbow, and her perpendicularly raised right hand flicked to the outside. I pointed out this arm gesture to her and asked her what she felt it expressed. She said that the stance felt so powerful to her that she did not need to overprotect herself, and yet it made her feel she was not so vulnerable that she was at the mercy of someone who was coming on to her in what she felt was an inappropriate manner.

It was amazing to me that Elaine spontaneously moved like this, though she had never taken a Tai Chi class or seen the movement called Fist under Elbow (Ha, 1995). We role-played a few examples of unwanted men coming on to her sexually and began the working-through process of finding the words to match her new empowered stance. She came up with these words for the man at the workshop: *I appreciate your interest in getting to know me, but I'm trying to concentrate on the workshop, and I have a boyfriend.* Elaine felt that this was a more appropriate response from the center of her "dial of feelings." She said that she would take the work we did back to her regular ongoing psychotherapist, and use it as a new place to begin.

Case Illustration: The Absent Father and Karate Chop Point Patient

"Emma" was a liberal arts university student who had not spoke to her father for five years. After her parents divorced when Emma was twelve years old, she felt abandoned and rejected by her father and his new wife. Even before this traumatic event, there had been a series of times when her biological father had not stood up for her; for example, when she was eleven, one of his drinking buddies, who was drunk, made a remark about her budding sexuality and touched her on her buttocks. Another incident was when her father did not stand up to his new wife when she broke her word about letting Emma stay at their house. She felt betrayed by her father and felt helpless in a world where "no one will stand up for me." Also, stemming from her having a very large and angry biological father and a new physically abusive stepfather, Emma developed a pattern of helpless withdrawal when stressors arose in her life.

One of her reasons for beginning therapy was to see if she could change her pattern of "taking her marbles and going home," that is, withdrawing when feeling betrayed by a group of friends—as she did in her childhood when she felt helpless to do anything about people's uncaring actions.

A large part of Emma's therapy focused on developing affect modulation skills so that she could learn to gain better control of expressing the center point on her dial of feelings—not withdrawing and not attacking (as was discussed earlier and will be discussed further in Chapter Seventeen). But here, to make a point, I will hone in on one key therapeutic moment.

In many energy psychology approaches, various combinations of acu-points are tapped as part of meridian-based therapies. One common point chosen as part of a larger sequence of points is found on the outside side of the hand, in the middle, called in energy psychology the Karate Chop point. It is acupuncture point Small Intestine-3.

The following is an example of BMHP's more phenomenologically based energy psychotherapy, which favors using the patient's own movements and his or her unconscious expressed intent. In one session, when Emma was getting ready to see her father after five years of not speaking to each other, she was role-playing speaking up to him. Her negative belief was *it's no use speaking up, because no one cares about my feelings* (SUDS level of 8). Her constructive belief was *I need you to stand up for me and the truth*. When Emma said these words, without knowing anything about the meaning of this point, she put her hand down forcibly on the couch, hitting the Karate Chop point (SI-3). As we worked on her tone of voice, which she felt was somewhat blaming and not clear, Emma searched for the appropriate way to express herself to her father, using my three-step method for constructive clearing of negative feelings (see Chapter Nineteen).[1] During the course of this role play, she realized that her voice tone would be more constructive if she was simultaneously centered with her strength and her heart. Emma spontaneously touched her heart when she was talking about this, and put her hand down on the couch simultaneously hitting her Karate Chop point. Then Emma said the same words, "Dad, I need you to stand up for me and the truth." She described these words and her gestures, which brought her SUDS level down to a 0.

Rather than choosing a series of therapist-imposed meridian points, Emma's story exemplifies how a patient's own movements are so naturally healing. The meanings in the points and gestures that naturally arise in patients at key transformative moments are organically emergent expressions of primordial healing energies activated as part of the healing process. These meanings are amplified by the therapist's understanding and exploration of their healing intent. For the patient, the potential to incorporate new ways of being and the ability to shapeshift into new characterological pathways can thereby be increased.

In this case, the Karate Chop point is known by acupuncturists and Qigong teachers to be a point that activates the central channel that travels up the back (the *Ren* channel) and controls the yang meridians. Telling this to Emma helped to underline the power she had just felt and helped her to appreciate the natural intuition of her body's wisdom. The simultaneous action of touching her heart and hitting her Karate Chop point with her other hand served as an anchor, which she told me she used when she finally cleared some feelings with her father on the phone one day. Her inner work and the way she brought her heart and power together in her communication with her father led to a new father-daughter relationship.

When Emma finally met with her father, she became aware of why she had such a problem dealing with him in her childhood and adolescence. He was domineering and left little space for her feelings. She described this meeting as being like hot air blowing at her. An image from our anchoring work came to her mind of a mudra that came spontaneously in one of our sessions. Emma, who had never practiced Tai Chi, found empowerment in the stance of putting her right-hand palm out in front of her heart and her left-hand palm up right below her chest. It is the exact same movement as the Tai Chi movement called Repulse the Monkey, which you can see on the DVD *Stillness in Movement* (Ha, 1995). Emma reported that this posture felt as if her right hand protected her from the onslaught she felt, and at the same time, her left hand expressed receptivity to create a new relationship. Interestingly, the idea of repulsing a monkey's jabbering intrusion is an apt metaphor for what Emma needed: a naturally arising stance of her primordial Self toward empowerment and healing through a gesture long ago encoded in the Tai Chi set. In addition, Emma said it was helpful to imagine herself Standing like a Tree firmly rooted in the earth to withstand the assault of her father's forceful style of expression. This posture, which we had practiced in a session one day along with Macrocosmic Orbit Breathing, also helped her to find a new adult stance with her father. The affect modulation role plays she had practiced, along with boundary setting, helped Emma create a new relationship with her father, in which she felt more comfortable establishing limits and expressing her need for space.

It should be noted that the reality of psychotherapy process is that one-time fixes do not usually change most long-standing characterological patterns. Continued practice of affect modulation, as well as grounding a new life stance, is a significant part of psychological change, as it was for Emma. What posture arises in you as you imagine confronting a blocked issue in your life? How can you anchor this new life stance?

Case Illustration: The Placating Professor and the Sword Mudra

A university professor, named Trent here, suffered from being overly placating and was self-deprecating despite many years in psychoanalysis. Once, he let his sick niece, who was his favorite relative, nose-kiss him when she was sick, even though he knew better. He caught a cold that lasted through much of the winter, motivating Trent to look more deeply into changing his dysfunctional pattern—the cold from his niece became a blessing in disguise.

Trent was very insightful about his problems originating from an abusive alcoholic father who often beat him. When Trent finally stood up to his father in his teenage years, his father had a stroke, which almost killed him. At that point Trent unconsciously decided to shut off his power. "My fear of the 'oedipal victory' is behind all this, I know." He also got in touch with how his desire to be adored was behind his placating pattern, which stemmed from what he called his "abusive, neglecting family."

One current issue Trent was dealing with was taking on extra administrative work for another professor. While he was talking about this, his fingers naturally went into a clawing position (which had also happened at other points during therapy); but this time he was touching his thumb to his ring finger. I explained to him that in Chinese medicine this ring finger was associated with the triple warmer meridian, which has to do with the power of three vital centers in the body—the belly, heart, and third-eye. This meaning was empowering to Trent as he then role-played asserting himself to the office mate who had been taking advantage of Trent's kindness. I also explained to him how this same hand gesture was called (two fingers up with the thumb holding the ring and pinky fingers) *the sword mudra*. He felt excited and empowered to begin exploring various ways to assert himself using variations of this mudra as a "hypnotic anchor" to bring him back to this state-specific state of consciousness when his old dysfunctional pattern emerged.

During another session, sweet, placating Trent role-played standing up to his father and told his dad to stop calling him a no-good loser. While holding his fingers in the sword mudra, he was more assertive than I had ever heard Trent be, in two years of our therapy. When I asked him what he would do next time a cute, sick child wanted to kiss him, he said this mudra would be inappropriate there; and it felt more appropriate to do a flick off of the ring finger as if to say, "I'm flicking off my old pattern."

Trent's old belief was *I need to do whatever I can to get adoration because I am unworthy of love.* Along the lines of asserting his newfound power to me, Trent refused to give his SUDS level, but said he felt a deep, pervasive feeling of sadness. Next, the new belief emerged of *I am worthy of love, and I don't need to whore myself.* As Trent focused on this new feeling that the felt shift produced, he experienced a sense of power, like anger, but more like holding a sword of power.

During subsequent sessions it was interesting to see how much Trent, who had been through years of psychoanalysis and was a very intellectual professor, had deep *chthonic* (meaning "deriving from the depths") bodily elements arise in his process. The activation of bodily processes is not limited to emotional types, and in my experience seems to happen across the spectrum of personality types. Once, while we were working with his shut-off power deriving originally from his fear of hurting his father, Trent became aware of his chronically cold hands and cold feet and how they symbolized his cutting off his power to hit his father. At this moment he again instinctively touched his ring finger with his thumb and described an intense heat arising in his belly. Then his hands shaped into claws as he became aware of his anger, and a buoyant feeling arose along with an image of an eagle. At that instant Trent's inhibitions regarding his promotional work for a new business he was starting came to mind, and along with this rising heat, a new belief emerged of *I deserve to express confidence and have heat in my life.* Then he said, "Even though there are dangers in putting myself out there, it's worth it to soar and enjoy life."

So, in Trent's case you see how the primordial elements of the psyche—elements of the body and elements of the imaginal realm—arise in everyday process in psychotherapy. These body movements and symbolic images became pathways to help anchor Trent to his primordial Self in situations when he needed to reclaim the power he shut off to protect his father.

Why Tap on Points on the Body When You Can Tap on the Wisdom of the Primordial Self?

In the cases in this chapter, you have read how body movements and hand gestures that naturally arise during the course of a patient's therapy can be used to ground, anchor, and amplify the new emerging patterns that arise in transformational psychotherapeutic processes. In Trent's case it is noteworthy that he instinctively touched the meridian line that energy psychology views as particularly vital. Donna Eden (1998) describes this meridian as key in developing aggressive, defensive strategies for maintaining the body's integrity (p. 244); and energy psychologists use the triple warmer point, TW-3 or the gamut point, as one of the main points in their healing algorithms.

Rather than choosing unknown acu-points to give the patient or having algorithms as a first-line intervention, I propose that the somatic unconscious wisdom of the patient can lead the astute clinician to harness its primordial wisdom. Standardized points can feel artificial to some patients and may take others away from their experience. BMHP is not adverse to tapping points or introducing them to patients to anchor new beliefs and awareness—because tapping on the empirical, proven power of acu-points has its merits. However, BMHP advocates as a first-line intervention, tapping on the natural arising bodily wisdom of the primordial Self, whether you are in psychotherapy or are using these energy psychology practices in everyday life.

Harnessing Your Natural Body Movements to Heal One of Your Life's Issues

The following is an example of how you can learn how to harness the natural body movements or gestures that want to emerge when you are dealing with a difficult life issue. For example, if you are a shy person who is afraid of expressing yourself, you can begin with formulating a negative belief behind your inhibition. Then continue with your process using the following example:

Negative belief: He/she probably won't be interested in me anyway so I may as well not reach out for contact.

More truthful or constructive belief: I don't know whether this person is interested in me or not. I will have the courage to reach out.

New gesture: Notice the posture that naturally wants to arise for this new life-stance. For example, maybe it is putting one hand on your belly and one hand is reaching out.

Anchor and new life stance: Use the above anchor to imagine reaching out to the woman or man you want to approach. Use the felt sense of this gesture/new life stance to shape-shift into a new way of being.

Following along the lines of humanistic and phenomenological philosophy, it is empowering to honor our own experience. Somatically oriented therapists believe that honoring the wisdom naturally arising from the body can fill us with a sense of awe regarding the mysterious source of healing within; and transpersonal therapists believe that this source of healing derives from that unfathomable power of the universe that some call "the nameless one." BMHP's approach to energy psychology draws from these traditions, adding that such instinctively arising movements are manifestations of the love of the primordial Self and its life energy (Qi), which seeks to restore equilibrium to a damaged world.

In the words of Ralph Waldo Emerson, "What lies behind us and what lies before us are small matters compared to what lies within us."

CHAPTER SEVENTEEN

Centered Emotional Expression: The Embodiment of Tai Chi

Health, well-being, and long life can only be achieved by remaining centered with one's spirit, guarding against squandering one's Qi, using breath and movement to maintain the free flow of Qi and blood, aligning with the natural forces of the seasons, and cultivating the tranquil heart and mind.

—Han Dynasty (200 BCE–222 CE)
The Yellow Emperor's Classic Book of Medicine

The Tai Chi of Emotional Expression

Centered emotional expression is fundamental to living a life in good relationship with others. In Western psychology today, this key to interpersonal harmony is talked about using the concepts of affect modulation and affect regulation (Schore, 2003). Modern psychological research has shown that those individuals who have suffered less childhood trauma may often have a better functioning prefrontal cortex and can modulate their emotional responses more easily than populations who have suffered a variety of traumas early in their lives (van der Kolk, 1994). Secure attachment to a primary caregiver early in life fosters a sense of self with affective competence (Briere, 1992). The healthy self has the ability to self-soothe, self-stimulate, tolerate being alone, and tolerate criticism (Pearlman & McCann, 1992). Psychological research in "the era of the brain" has shown how disruptions in early attachment sets the stage for many problems later on, including difficulties managing our feelings (van der Kolk, 1987).

Long before psychological research saw the importance of affect modulation and finding a balanced expression of the self in everyday life, Tai Chi practitioners were finding ways in their movements not to be overly yin or yang. For example, in the posture Single Ward Off, the practitioner is instructed not to be too far forward or too far backward. The instructions for this position are very exact: do not let the knee or the forward arm extend over the toes or you can cause knee injury and you will be aggressively leaning off-center; similarly, the initiate is instructed not to allow the forward arm or knee to move too far back so that you are constricted into an overly withdrawn position. The right palm is facing the chest as if holding a ball, and the left hand is at the level of the belly, palm facing downward.[1] This posture is also called Grasping the Bird's Tail and was reported to be used by the legendary Chang San Feng. The mythological tale says that though Chang was one of the greatest martial artists, he had such gentleness and receptivity that a bird could not take off from his hand. This was due to his having let go of so much, that when a bird tried to push off of his hand it could not, because there was nothing of substance to push off from.

Case Illustrations: Balanced Emotional Expression Is Enhanced by Tai Chi Postures

Healing Trauma with Fist under Elbow

How can modern affect modulation theory and the practice of Tai Chi join hands for each other's benefit? In the past two chapters, you have read examples of the way that Tai Chi and Qigong can aid in the process of affect regulation, though that was not my focus. For example, in the case of Elaine in the previous chapter, you read about the importance of affect modulation and finding the center of Elaine's dial with an interested man in a workshop. Instead of saying "stop coming on to me, this is a workshop," Elaine found the place in the center of her "affect modulation dial" and said, "I appreciate your interest in getting to know me, but I'm trying to concentrate on the workshop, and I have a boyfriend." In Elaine's case illustration, you read how a spontaneously arising internal martial arts posture of Fist under Elbow helped her to find the centered power to regulate her emotional expression so that she could set a boundary in a kind, yet firm way.

Balancing Boundary Setting and Welcoming with Repulse Monkey

Likewise with the case example of Emma, discussed in the preceding chapter, you read how an overbearing father contributed to Emma's belief that *it's no use to speak up because no one cares about my feelings.* After years of not talking to her father, she realized that a more modulated approach would serve her and her family better. During the course of trying to find such a balanced stance, you read how a naturally arising Tai Chi posture/mudra, Repulse the Monkey, emerged in which her outstretched, right-hand palm expressed the power of boundary setting and the left-hand palm up expressed a welcoming gesture. Even though Emma had never practiced Tai Chi or Qigong, this spontaneously arising movement helped to anchor her at a key moment in her life. When she met with her father, she later reported that keeping this stance in mind helped her not to verbally attack him for leaving the family; yet at the same time, she was confrontational about asking why he left and why he did not stand up for her with his new wife. By Emma being balanced in her approach with her father, she was able to fill in many of the missing pieces of her childhood. Though her father appeared as very strong on the outside, Emma grew to see her father's limitations in standing up to women. This helped Emma interpret his not standing up for her less personally—his inability to stand up for her was not about Emma's worth. Taking back her power and withdrawing her projections helped her to reestablish a relationship with her father.

Warding Off with Love: Grasping the Bird's Tail (Single Ward Off)

Another example is the case of a patient I will call Eve. After her parents divorced in her teenage years, Eve resented having to take care of her chaotic mother and a younger brother. Eve spoke about how she came from a very refined family where expressing limits about taking care of others in the family was frowned upon.

When Eve came to therapy, one of her issues that led to significant relationship problems was that she resented taking care of others' needs. Yet she had never made the connection between her current pattern and her parent's divorce and the early caretaking role that was forced upon her in adolescence. In addition, Eve was a regular at the local bodyworker's table, as she somatized her held-back feelings so that her body ended up expressing the issues that her voice had difficulty with. Neck pain was a common symptom for Eve.

Eve practiced Tai Chi with another Tai Chi teacher, and sometimes we would use the metaphors from her Tai Chi practice to communicate about affect modulation issues. Eve had a group of friends she enjoyed socializing with. Though Eve had warm feelings toward one of her friends, she described this friend as very emotional and needy. On one occasion Eve wanted to go away on a retreat with another member of their close-knit group with whom she shared a particular spiritual path. Her emotional friend started crying when Eve told her about this on the phone. Eve felt guilty about setting boundaries and her old neck blockage became activated. In our BMHP sessions, as Eve "journeyed to the underworld," she realized that the feelings she had now paralleled her feelings about having to take care of her mother and brother after the divorce. Eve was made to feel wrong when she did not help in her family and now a similar guilt was arising. During the course of our work together, I expressed this basic axiom of BMHP and other forms of therapy: *life is a school and everyday life stressors give us the lessons to learn.* Adding to this idea is the metaphor: life is a spiral, and if there is a block at one turn of your spiral, the same block will emerge at a later curve on your spiral (in your life) when you have acquired more developmental abilities to find better coping skills to resolve the issue.

During our first role play with her newfound strength, Eve said about her friend's disappointment, "It's not my job to fix it." Her old belief was *others aren't strong enough to be there for me* (SUDS level of 7). Her new belief was *others are responsible for taking care of themselves.* Tapping on her belly to ground that statement, Eve shifted to a SUDS level of 3 with a renewed sense of power; but her neck still felt twisted. I asked her to imagine expressing this to her friend, and Eve said, "I feel twisted in my neck when you cry and beg me to have you come along. It's not my job to shield you."

Eve realized that though this helped to release tension in her neck, she did not feel that this would be appropriate to say to her friend. This is where the meeting of affect modulation skills and Tai Chi helped Eve. She realized that at the top of her affective dial was rage at her friend for crying. At the bottom of her dial was her desire to leave the relationship so she would not have to take care of her any more.

At this point Eve used the metaphor of her Tai Chi posture Single Ward Off (discussed at the beginning of this chapter) and said that this posture—particularly her out-stretched upward right palm facing her heart and the back of her hand warding off an aggressive force—helped her to ward off her feelings of projected guilt. In the Tai Chi literature, this upward hand is described as turning over slightly as if something is spilling out from the heart, which helped Eve search for a compassionate response to her friend. The downward facing left hand by her belly helped her feel grounded. This posture served as a state-specific anchor for Eve when she spoke to her friend the next day. Eve found the middle of her dial and said to her friend, "I'm sorry you're hurt and feel touched you want to be with us. But I'd like uninterrupted time with you, and it wouldn't be that way with our other friend on this particular retreat. Let's do it another time later this summer." Saying this to her friend led to a deep conversation about the things they shared and the things they did not, and it helped Eve to hold her ground in her separation/individuation process with her friend.

Standing Up for Your Self and Your Dog: Single Ward Off

Another example was after Eve's dog was put to sleep and the veterinarian was giving Eve a lot of specific information about the type of drugs used and how the vet had done the best she could. Eve's old placating pattern began to come up in this situation with the vet. This feeling was accompanied by a smiling response that we had identified as related to her false self who had to pretend that she was happy taking care of her mother and brother. Eve reported that in this situation with the vet the memory of her Tai Chi Single Ward Off stance helped her transform her placating ways. We discussed how her outward right hand expresses holding on to the ball of her heart's truthful power, and how this stance also anchors her in not overextending herself while at the same time being compassionate toward another. Eve proudly told me that something clicked for her at that point. She knew she had to find a different stance to honor her memory of her dog and what he taught her about being with her natural instincts. Eve's observing self was then activated as she noticed that one part of her wanted to smile to make the vet comfortable so she would not feel guilty and another part of her wanted to scream at the vet and say, "Shut up, I need to mourn." However, remembering her affect modulation dial and her Tai Chi Single Ward Off posture, she said instead, "Thanks for your help and knowledge, but right now I need some space to myself."

In this manner, affect modulation skills and various Tai Chi postures are a natural complement to developing the ability to regulate our emotional expression and be appropriate to the situation. In the next chapter, you will read about another variation on the theme of how the marriage of internal martial arts and psychotherapy can help patients in their process of modulating emotional expression and developing self-assertion skills.

CHAPTER EIGHTEEN

Everyday Life as an Internal Martial Art

Tai Chi, the Supreme Ultimate, the immense absolute is the expression of the Great Harmony—the balance and mutual support of Yin and Yang. Whether boxing with your shadow or engaging in the complexity of life and things, The Supreme Ultimate within and around you secures the potential for harmony and ease in every moment of the eternal present.

—Wu Wei, legendary Qi master

Broadening Our Psychological Repertoires with Interdisciplinary Somatic Practices

In the previous chapter, you read how Tai Chi can enhance our emotional expression in everyday life. In this chapter, by hearing about the way some of my patients have benefited from Tai Chi principles, a pathway is opened for us all to consider how Tai Chi principles can help us in a variety of other ways, including how to banter with a bully, be self-assertive with your intimate relationships, and change your life stance.

In Chapter Eight on Trauma, you read what psychiatrist Dr. van der Kolk, the medical director of the trauma center at Boston University School of Medicine, and his colleagues said about how the first task of treatment for trauma patients is to regain a sense of safety in their bodies. Dr. van der Kolk et al. further indicated that assault victims often benefit from "model-mugging" programs, Outward Bound programs, and therapeutic massages. He advocates appropriate use of methods from spiritual and religious traditions to aid in the healing of trauma (van der Kolk, 1996). Along these lines I propose that Qigong can be useful not only as an extrinsic adjunctive activity to be recommended to help trauma patients find a sense of safety in their bodies but also for its wider range of usefulness in everyday life.

Verbal therapy on the surface may seem to be an intellectual oral pursuit. But behind the words we use in psychotherapy and in everyday life are stances, body expressions, and internal martial moves. Through the following case illustrations, you will read how energy psychology with its roots in Tai Chi can be a way to activate our primordial Self in a variety of everyday situations.

Language, Tai Chi, and the Body

A number of psychologically oriented authors have questioned how much psychological language itself is responsible for a lack of soulfulness in our modern lives. Robert Bly (1990) has suggested that psychological thought has contributed to the effemination of men. In James Hillman's lectures, he has questioned whether the obsession with growth and focus on victimization by our parents has turned us into a cult of child worshippers. The language through which we describe ourselves colors the way that each of us sees ourselves. It becomes the lens through which we view our identity and the structure through which we experience our life's meaning (Mayer, 1984) and the language of myth and story is an anecdote [sic] for the language of "dry psycho-logeeze" used by the field of clinical psychology (Mayer, 1984; 1993).

How much does our psychological language and style of talk stop a naturalness of self-expression in our emotional lives? Are the waters of life being put into culverts that make expression civilized, yet take out some of the essential minerals in the process? Does politically correct psychological language take the Qi out of verbal intercourse?

When we use the language of Tai Chi to conceptualize our way of speaking we have a language that gives us room to be with our primordial Selves. We wonder what it means to respond from our Tan Tien (the center below our navel), or our heart center in our verbal interactions. Words come from our bodies, and each of us can feel it when we are responding from our disconnected heads—our words lack power.

Part of the initiation into the Taoist art of Tai Chi Chuan is to practice bringing the embodied metaphors of these arts into our everyday interactions. Using only the amount of force necessary to deal with an oncoming force in order not to inflict unnecessary damage is one basic rule of the play of Tai Chi Push Hands. Psychotherapists will notice the similarity between the concept of using only the least necessary force and the concept of affect modulation, having control of the dial of one's emotions so that a person does not turn his or her emotion up too high in rage or down too low in inappropriate withdrawal. Tai Chi gives an embodied practice for activating the affect modulation dial of the body-mind; psychotherapy provides practice in "emotional Push Hands," that is, appropriately expressing one's emotions.

Often in my psychotherapy practice, I do not even use the language of Tai Chi—instead the metaphors become translated into the language that is most appropriate for a given client. For example, I may use the language of tennis or another sport. But the important question is how do we be with our primordial Selves in the difficult encounters of everyday life?

Verbal Tai Chi and the Subtle Art of Bantering: Case Illustration of Obsessive-Compulsive Disorder

"Bob" was a young man who suffered from an obsessive-compulsive disorder. He was addicted to being a perfectly refined good boy and was like the proverbial centipede, who when thinking about his next step was often frozen into inaction. He was continuously the butt of coworkers' jokes, at his job as a phone intake worker at a local company because he believed he was "such an easy target." When a coworker who continually took great joy in mocking Bob said that a sandwich he was eating "looked like it came out of someone's ass," Bob did not know how to respond. He reverted to his old standby that he had done all of his life—playing the part of a fool, pretending to enjoy being the butt of everyone's joke. He held his nose and acted out eating his sandwich of feces. Everyone laughed, but inside, Bob felt humiliated and wished he could find a way to stand up to this verbal bully's continuously demeaning remarks.

Bob had been the butt of everyone's jokes since high school. His inability to banter with his high school buddies led to feelings of shame and a self-identification of being a man unable to fend for himself. We may all underestimate just how much the ability to banter is crucial in psychological development to keep our power with others.

The word *bantering* etymologically derives from the old English "to cook properly, not overcook and not undercook." This meaning shows psychologists the early roots of *affect modulation* in verbal intercourse. The *Oxford English Dictionary* (1979) says that the first known use of *bantering* may have come from "bullies in White Friars," in old England and that etymologically it relates to the word *roasting*. Indeed, finding a defense against aggressive language does involve the ability to take some raw insult and roast it over a fire. This requires "cooking" the comment in such a way that we do not quite "burn the other," but instead transform its rawness into something palatable and more easily digestible. The process of roasting in early times required turning a piece of meat around on a spicate, which needs a careful turning so that the meat comes out "just so." When we attack back, we are just as raw as the attacker. We have not yet added the civilized element of bringing it into contact with our inner flame where our inner alchemical vessel contains it and subjects it to heat for the purpose of transforming the substance of the remark into something of great value. Bantering is a civilized art of using the heat of aggression in a playful manner. "Indulging in good humored jest," the *OED*'s definition of *bantering* is exactly this. It has the potential of bringing people closer together if we can alchemically process the heat.

There was a psychodynamic aspect to Bob's pattern of holding back his aggression. Early in his therapy, Bob realized that his early inability to respond to insults was rooted in his relationship with his father. When he would respond assertively to his Dad's put-downs, his Dad would just walk away. Bob felt castrated, abandoned, and learned to hold back his aggressive impulses. From many years of therapy during his adolescence, Bob learned to respond to insults by expressing his feelings and saying how that hurt him or made him angry. His father still withdrew and said, "Well if it hurts you or makes you angry, I just won't say anything. Have it your own way." This sulk-withdraw pattern further added to Bob's fear of self-expression and lack of natural aggressiveness.

But how does a person take such an insight and turn it into fire? Certainly Bob's uncovered anger at his Dad was part of the recovery process, but Bob was suffering from "a bantering disability" that made him feel crippled with his father and with his coworkers. Bob wanted to joust verbally with his Dad, and others who put him down, in order to find "just so" remarks that would make his point.

To help Bob explore how his natural style of expression actually felt, we set up a 10-point affect modulation scale: 10 feeling like a hit in the center of the target and 0 being a miss. He imagined expressing to his coworker *I don't like it when you say those kind of things to me. It makes me angry, and I wish you'd stop it.* This expression of true feelings that therapists often suggest may be highly appropriate with someone you are in an intimate relationship with, but not with everyone. As Sly and the Family Stone would put it, "Different strokes are needed with different folks." Or to continue the "roasting" analogy, each occasion requires turning the expression around the spicate on the fire to find the right amount of heat. Communication of real feelings is only one of the many forms that the "fire" of our expression can take.

Bob imagined that his coworker would respond to his real feelings of hurt and anger with *I was just kidding when I made the remark about the food, why do you take things so seriously?* These are the kinds of things this coworker had said to Bob in the past when he tried to stand up to him, and it had left Bob even further humiliated. Due to numerous years of psychotherapy with a number of therapists, Bob had learned how to express himself in psychologically real ways, but he had not learned how to use his fire in such a way that he had bantering skills. In his interactions with others, he often felt "roasted," rather than the other way around. Therefore, in this case, Bob rated his psychologically real response as a 1 on our 10-point affect modulation scale. It felt good to be real, but it left him feeling ineffective and humiliated.

Bob realized that this situation called for firmer boundaries around "the ball of his Self," rather than being so open and vulnerable about his feelings. Bantering was what was needed. Bob used the metaphor of the ball of his Self, though he practiced no internal martial arts, nor did he know I was a practitioner. Because Bob was an avid tennis player, we used the analogy that he did not want to hit the ball softly into the net, letting his coworker win the point, he wanted to hit the ball in the center of his racket back to his coworker.

Bob's first attempt at bantering in my office was to express his feelings in curse words, but he felt it did not hit the center of the racket. Bob felt that using that language would be like throwing the racket at the other player because he did not like the other person's shot. Bob tried on another response that felt a little closer to center: *Do you always put down what others are eating like that? I wonder how often you go out with people to eat, and how many have puked on you.* Bob felt that this rated a 6 on the 10-point scale because it released some of his aggression but still might be too aggressive for this particular work situation. The response that felt closest to the center of his tennis racket was to say in a light-hearted, humorous, but semi-real way: *Thanks for your comments. Now that I've lost my appetite, will you pay me for the sandwich I'm not going to eat, or should I take you to small claims court?* Bob gave this a 9 on the scale because he liked the fact that this let the coworker know that it upset him, he felt it was not inappropriately aggressive, and was assertive enough to "roast" the coworker. It would tell his coworker that the raw, uncivilized remark should cost him something.

Another example of something that happened to Bob took place when a woman called up his company, where he answered the phones. She asked him what was going on with a story about his company that had been on the nightly news two months earlier. When Bob responded that he did not know, she replied, "How could you not know about that? Do you come from Mars or something?"

"No, do you?" This was Bob's first reactive attempt to practice bantering during our session the next day. This a rated low 2 on his 10-point scale. Even though it did put the statement back on the other person, it was overly defensive; and he felt it was immaturely "tit for tat." When he responded with *last time I checked, I wasn't* or *yes I am, but please don't let anyone know,* Bob felt a little better and rated those responses a 6 due to adding in some humor to break his tension. A psychologically real response of *it hurts me and makes me angry when you put me down that way. I can't know every story that every member of the public wants to know* rated slightly worse. Bob rated that response a 4, commenting that though it might feel good with an intimate other, it was inappropriate and too self-disclosing in this situation.

Bob's favorite response was *sorry I don't know everything that you want me to, but I am very much an earthling, and like many of us from this planet I have many things going on in my complex life. I can't keep up with every story. Since I'm a fellow earthling and care about your needs and other's needs, I'd be glad to find the latest on that story for you.* Bob also wanted to add this clause to the last statement: *even though by your attack on my limitations, it seems like you may be from the red planet of war.* But though this last clause felt good to say in therapy, Bob felt the first part of his response had the appropriate amount of caring for others required by his phone intake job. However, it felt good to him that he was developing his bantering ability so he could come up with remarks that allowed him the pleasure of letting out some of his anger through sarcasm, turning the caller's attack back to her.

What Bob was practicing is very much like Tai Chi Push Hands—using the other's force to circle the energy back to the other practitioner. Tai Chi teaches using the least amount of force necessary to achieve one's desired result. In Bob's case he found the amount of force that fit his job and used a tennis metaphor to describe his sense of achievement. The way Bob put it was, "I don't need to throw my tennis racket at her;" instead saying *we are both earthlings* he felt he made his tennis point.

Each of us has our own 10-point scale on which a particular remark feels like it hits the mark, given our needs and the appropriateness of the situation. When reading the above practice, in affect modulation each of us may not find Bob's scale fitting with our sensibilities; each of us has our own dial of affective and effective bantering. We know when a remark is "just right"—like a tasty morsel, an oral treat that tastes good as we put our tongues around our palate. It is this that heals our "bantering disability."

Where do we go to learn the art of bantering? Maybe we are lucky, and our rivers of Qi are flowing freely enough so that our instincts allow bantering to come out naturally. If not, we may pick it up in our early schooling from interactions with and modeling from our peers or parents. Bantering involves the subtleties of communication; and because it is so vital to a healthy life, like communication in general, we would hope it would be part of our "education," which means "to draw out" what is deep inside. Unfortunately, in a culture that emphasizes the three Rs and with cutbacks in school counseling programs, there is often not enough education about the psychological needs of sensitive or emotionally blocked youngsters. They may get As in English but get wounded in their interactions with peers. Education of the heart, and of activating the primordial Self, would be a blessing to our children and our society.

I am reminded of a story in the "Spirit Rock Meditation Newsletter" about how a six-year-old girl named Mattie was teased by her schoolmates by being called "four eyes" because she wore glasses. After speaking to her mother—a meditator—about this, Mattie went to school armed with the words she needed and finally said to her abusers the next time they insulted her, "Having 'four eyes' isn't such a bad thing. You might do better if you had four eyes: two eyes to see the world, a third eye in the middle of your forehead for wisdom, and another eye in your heart. If you had four eyes instead of two, you probably wouldn't be putting me down for my limitations."[1]

From the mouths of babes and from the eyes of the six-year-old inside of each of us, like Mattie, we are all on the path of learning and practicing the heartfelt art of bantering. Where can the lessons of Bob and Mattie benefit you in the internal martial arts of your everyday life?

Finding Verbal Power in the Ring of Life: Case Illustration of the Wife of the Verbally Adept Salesman

As part of teaching patients how to recapture the long lost art of bantering, a therapist can role-play the important characters from the patients' lives to help them recover aspects of their primordial Selves that may have been damaged or not developed in childhood. One woman, named Rebecca here, was in the midst of a divorce and complained that she could not stand up to her husband during the divorce proceedings. She complained about his arrogant, unyielding style of communication. The psychodynamic root of Rebecca's falling into a victim stance was that she was repeatedly hit in childhood. One vivid memory came from when she was eight years old and was hit and pulled out of bed for not cleaning her room. From this and other traumatic experiences, she developed the belief that *nice girls don't get hit.*

During the course of the divorce, Rebecca's husband wanted to see the kids on Wednesday nights. The problem was that this was the only fun night she had available to spend with her kids. As she focused (Gendlin, 1978) on her bodily felt sense, Rebecca realized that her fear of self-expression was rooted in her fear of being hit or judged: *if I don't give someone what they want, I feel that I'm bad and selfish.*

During our therapy Rebecca often went into a victim stance complaining about her husband being too good of an arguer because he was a salesman and being able to "convince anyone of anything;" and she indicated that he usually demeaned her in the process. I role-played with her and asked her to stay in touch with her body as I said some things to her. I then role-played her salesman husband asking her to buy my office chair: "What's wrong with you that you won't buy my office chair for $500? It's a great deal. You must be a terrible business woman and have no sense."

Some of the purposes for this role play were to teach Rebecca to do the following:

- *Learn to shift from a victim stance to one of expressed power.* Often called *response-ability,* this is the ability to effectively respond to another rather than put the emphasis on the other's expression.

- *Differentiate between when someone is merely angry or raising his or her voice versus when someone is blaming her and making her wrong.* In this regard, I differentiated between raising my voice in anger because I was upset that she would not buy the chair versus being abusively demeaning to her and making her wrong for not buying it.

- *Learn to modulate the dial of her emotional expression appropriate to the intent of the other person.*

During our role play, Rebecca was able to stand up to me and say, "If I don't give you the money you are asking me for, there's nothing wrong with me; and I don't deserve to be treated badly or be blamed. I resent you making me wrong to manipulate me into giving something I don't want to give." Our role playing helped Rebecca stand up to her husband and negotiate various key points in her child custody and divorce agreement.

Both Bob's and Rebecca's cases show how the clinician who wants to use the essence of Tai Chi as a verbal martial art in psychotherapy can do so with no Tai Chi training.

Role Playing: To Activate Our Vital Energy

Choice of Clothing

As in Rebecca's case, attacking a patient's clothing in a role play can provide a way for the patient to learn how to shift from a victim stance to an empowered stance, to differentiate various voice tones and intentions of the attacker's dysfunctional communication, and to learn to modulate affect with an appropriate response. So, instead of attacking Rebecca for not buying my chair, I could have role-played criticizing her choice of clothing. After a clinician assesses a patient's ability to handle such role plays, the clinician's aim is to find some less-charged life sphere that can give the patient a chance to get some distance from the everyday life issue that triggers a defensive or overly reactive response. Similar to a boxer being coached on how to use a punching bag or to respond to a punch while wearing protective gear, "practicing one's moves" in psychotherapy gives a person the chance to develop skills to use later when entering into the "ring of life." Such methods give patients the opportunity to learn to breathe when attacked or criticized; to reverse their instinctual fight, flight, or freeze response; and to develop new response patterns thereby. Qigong and BMHP can add key elements to such role plays. For example, Qigong can add relaxed breathing methods that help patients sink their Qi to the belly center (Tan Tien) rather than hold their breath in fear; and these combined methods can add the use of self-touch to anchor the place in the patient's body that is activated in the new life stance.

Tai Chi Practices to Enhance Empowerment and Change Your Life Stance

There are other dimensions of how to use the interface of Tai Chi and energy psychology together to enhance our well-being. For those who have been victims of abuse, for example, you can take a Tai Chi class. In my Tai Chi classes, I have taught other therapists' patients who have been sexually and physically abused[2] and watched them benefit from Tai Chi Push Hands to regain a sense of safety in their bodies.[3] There are a variety of considerations when deciding which type of martial art to choose. Some prefer model mugging or a hard style martial art, like karate. Not as cathartic or as physically oriented to self-defense as certain other martial arts, Tai Chi is better suited for those who wish to find a gentle approach to discovering their internal power. Again, it is important not to be overconfident in your abilities when viewing Tai Chi or any other martial art as a method of self-defense.

You have read numerous examples about the integration of psychotherapy with Tai Chi, Qigong, and Standing Meditation to help a person shape-shift into new life stances. These stances enable a person in psychotherapy, or any of us, to access state-specific states of consciousness that help the individual cope with external and internal stressors and develop the ability to self-assert, modulate affect, and banter better. For instance, you read how Stan was able to respond to his brother's long-standing derogatory, castrating comments of "I'm better than you at everything" with "You're not better at being a kind brother." You will read in Chapter Twenty how Roberta's passive-aggressive "ostrich behavior" was transformed through a combination of psychotherapy with another therapist, a Mythic Journey Process, and the practice of certain animal form movements to help her recover her primordial Self-assertion abilities.

CHAPTER NINETEEN

Healing with the Elements and Transpersonal Hypnosis

Oh, what a catastrophe for man when he cut himself off from the rhythm of the year, from his unison with the sun and the earth. Oh, what a catastrophe.... This is what is the matter with us. We are bleeding at the roots, because we are cut off from the earth and sun and stars.... We plucked it from its stem on the Tree of Life, and expected it to keep on blooming in our civilized vase on the table.

—D. H. Lawrence

Transpersonal Psychology and the Energies of the Wider Whole

Energy psychology can be looked at as a subset of transpersonal psychology. When I was training graduate students in transpersonal psychology programs over a twelve-year period, I defined *transpersonal psychotherapy* this way: "Transpersonal psychotherapy is an integrative approach that combines traditional psychotherapy with ancient sacred wisdom traditions; it emphasizes how healing comes from the wider whole of which we are a part."

Transpersonal psychology has been called the fourth force of psychology along with the humanistic/existential, cognitive-behavioral, and Freudian/neo-analytic psychologies. However, those in the field of transpersonal psychology do not look at their tradition as separate from mainstream psychologies. Body-mind Healing Psychotherapy (BMHP) builds, in part, upon a foundation in transpersonal psychology.[1]

The shift from traditions that honored the elements and energies of the wider whole of life to modern culture's anthropocentric focus has been part of the ongoing march of civilization. Historically, the disconnection of humanity from nature has roots in the shift from the worship of goddesses in the second and third millennium BC to the worship of a deity of the heavens (Stone, 1976). Consequently, the archetypal image of the sacred in Western civilization has become a disembodied one: a male God living in the upper stratosphere on a throne. Adding to humanities' disconnection from reverence of the earth, the philosophy of atomism growing from seventeenth-century Europe put forth the case that a human being is an isolated fragment in an alienated universe. Central to this viewpoint was Descartes error of *I think therefore I am*, as contrasted with *I feel, therefore I am* or *I am a child of God* (a higher spiritual power in the universe), *therefore I am*. Virgil, author of the *Aeneid*, said, "We make our destinies by our choice of gods;" and therefore, we create our own chosen "reality bubble" by worshipping the mind, feelings, or our view of the Creator of Life.

The rise in Western technologies and philosophies are all part of the benefits and detriments of modern civilization. On the positive side, we have created comfort and safety from some of the elements of nature with air conditioners and heaters. The chemical elements of the earth have been harnessed to fight malaria, polio, and other health conditions. Yet many of civilization's advances have repercussions and have led our healing efforts away from trusting the elements of natural life in our bodies and in the surrounding universe (such as natural herbs).

Recently there has been a balancing of this disconnection from our roots in nature and the universe. The new physics is at the forefront of showing how human beings are in fact condensed light and how the separation of our physical bodies from the surrounding universe is an illusion. Many authors and others have shown the modern world the reality of this knowledge in the area of quantum physics (Capra, 1975; Peat, 1997). And members of the new biology movement, such as Bruce Lipton (2005), have shown how our human connection with the wider universe is even true on a cellular level.

The need to reconnect with the wider whole of which we are a part is a key element for healing our psyches, as well. As I have mentioned before, according to ancient Chinese medical philosophy, the universe, the human body, and mind were composed of the energies of the five elements: fire, earth, metal, water, and wood. In premodern medicine, when a person was ill and out of balance, an analysis was made regarding which element was in excess or was lacking. Then herbs were given and points on the body were either needled with acupuncture or touched with acupressure to return the energies of mind, body, and spirit to harmony with the natural balance of life. In Western esoteric traditions, the initiate was tried by the four elements: fire, earth, air, and water. The ancient Greeks believed that the soul itself was composed of a vaporous substance formed out of the four elements, and that healing the soul took place when these elements were in balance.

Transpersonal Hypnosis and Healing with the Elements

Case Illustration: Writer's Block

Honoring this idea of healing with the elements, I developed the concept of transpersonal hypnosis in the 1980s, which was a step in the direction of bringing the use of the metaphors of the energies of life into transpersonal psychology. A patient, named Marcy here, found the metaphor of the elements of nature to be particularly transformative in treating her writer's block. A student in her early twenties, Marcy was enrolled in a program for young screenplay writers. After she took a workshop of mine, I had a chance to work with Marcy for only two sessions because she lived out of state.

When Marcy came in for our first session, she told me she had not been able to add to a play she had been working on for three months, and she was considering leaving her program. Her closest friends were also writers, who seemed to be turning out articles and producing plays without any of the problems Marcy was experiencing. She felt like a failure.

First, Marcy described, in detail, how hard she had tried to find a way through her writing blocks. She felt defeated and was coming to the conclusion that she just did not "have it" and that she needed to recognize she was an awful writer.

Marcy was expecting me to tell her she was a good writer, as all of her acquaintances had; so she was taken aback when I told her that she was overlooking just one thing: that, of course, she was a terrible writer—everyone is. I told her that her problem was fighting this basic truth. She was startled at first, because everyone else was trying to comfort her by attempting to convince her that she was a good writer. This paradoxical intention method (Frankl, 1967), used in psychotherapeutic healing and clinical hypnosis, is also fundamental to Taoist healing—by not trying to make things happen, things happen. By being "nothing special," a very special human quality emerges.

Marcy came to me as a psychotherapy patient partially because she knew that I had written a prize-winning book and that even though she would not have enough time to do depth psychotherapy with me, she had heard that sometimes results could be achieved in a shorter time and that I could give her some advice. Creating a bond with her as a fellow writer who is also often blocked, I told her the story of how I learned about writing blocks from writing my doctoral dissertation, which later turned into my book *The Mystery of Personal Identity* (1984). I told Marcy how I had been blocked for a period of six months about how to start my writing. I saw a sign of relief wash across her face as if she were thinking *if a prize-winning writer can be blocked for six months, maybe it's not so bad that I'm blocked for three months.*

Drawing on the old tradition of using the transformative energy of stories to heal, I told Marcy the following story about writing my dissertation:

One day, completely depressed, I gave up and walked outside for a breath of fresh air realizing that I just did not have what it took to write. As I breathed in the fresh air, all of a sudden an idea came to me; and from there, my dissertation grew. I realized that the idea came "from the air" and I started to joke around with myself that this is how the expression of "the idea came out of thin air" arose. Maybe, I thought, other writers had discovered what I had: that they could not write either and that ideas come from the air. I further wondered whether in ancient times astrologers knew this, and that's why they said that knowledge is associated with the air element. I got so invigorated by this hypothesis that the energy carried over into my writing and ideas started flowing forth for a chapter or so. I would just go out for a breath of fresh air when I got stuck and an idea would come to me.

I was becoming relatively self-assured, thinking that I could just call on the air element to write. When one day, working on the second chapter, it came again. I was completely blocked. I went outside and nothing happened as I tried to invoke the air element. Day after day I would go for walk and nothing came. I gave in to the belief that I was just no good at writing and decided to take a shower to get away from it all. While I was in the shower, I started to relax and realized how critical I was of myself. I became more aware of how I was unable to let my writing flow because my inner critic was so perfectionistic. I realized that I had done this all of my life and mourned how difficult my schooling had been for me. I realized that I needed to keep my critic out of the first draft of my writing and let it in only with later drafts. As my tears merged with the water and I let go, an idea emerged for a blocked section in my writing. I realized the great healing power of water, and I appreciated that by my letting go in order to be with the power of the water element that it could write through me.

Then I thought, all I need to do is take showers when I get stuck, get in touch with the water element, and I will be healed. But eventually I got to the place that even a shower would not help. I went to the refrigerator took out a piece of bread to escape the fact that I could not write at all. As the bread grounded me, I got in touch with how a grounded experiential flavor was missing in the theoretical section that I was working on in my book. I realized that the earth element was speaking to me and helping me to be more grounded in my approach.

It was only after all of this—and many more writing blocks, even though I breathed fresh air, took showers, and ate bread—that I fully recognized my foolishness as a writer: I now knew that I could not write at all and that it was the elements of creation that wrote through me—in their own time and in their own way. I realized that my attachment to being able to write was similar to my attachment to having a given element heal me. Like my attempt to control the writing process itself, I had become attached to trying to control the elements of creation to write through me. I then deeply realized that it was only in letting go of trying to control the elements of writing—and being open to what comes—that the appropriate element of the universe could come to my aid and help in my healing.

In our two allotted sessions, Marcy and I also touched upon the roots of her blocks in her inner critic, and we worked as much as possible along the lines of Bodymind Healing Psychotherapy to work through these energy blocks regarding writing. We identified one of her family of origin issues of being an overachiever to please her parents. By practicing cognitive restructuring, she learned to change her negative belief from *I need to be a great writer to be worthwhile* to the belief of *my destiny as a writer is waiting to be drawn out of me by the elements of the universe around me.* Marcy's SUDS level significantly decreased with this new belief, showing that her bodymind was beginning to metabolize the new way of seeing her path as a writer. She also appreciated the self-soothing she experienced when she touched her heart, because she had always been self-described as "such a mental person."

Marcy also requested some Bodymind Qigong movements to help her with the tension that accumulated when she was writing. I was able to show her briefly some movements, such as Opening the Shoulder Well, the wood element of BMHQ (Mayer, 2004b, p.104); Tai Chi Ruler, for general relaxation and balancing of energy; and Moving a Snake through the Joints, to release common body areas that accumulate tension while writing.

After our two sessions, I did not hear from Marcy for about a month, then I received a phone call from her saying that she had broken though her writing block one night while looking into her fireplace. Marcy told me that the metaphor of "fire" had created a felt shift for her. She said that while looking there, she realized how she had always tried to be a bright light in her parent's eyes, and how comparisons with other relatives had stifled her own natural internal fire from burning. Looking into her fireplace, she had gotten in touch with the natural fire she had left behind as a child. I only heard from Marcy one last time when she graduated from her writer's program and thanked me for the influence that our sessions and the elements of life had had on her writing.

How is transpersonal hypnosis different from traditional hypnosis? For one, they have different philosophical foundations: In traditional hypnosis a story is used to reframe a current life experience and create a new way of seeing the world. In transpersonal hypnosis there is an explicit opening to a reality that is connected with the energies of the primordial powers of the universe and respect for its inherent powers.

However, it is not so much the method that is important here as the experience of being "called" by something—some power greater than our egoic selves. When we experience our life as "a calling" and the problems that arise in everyday life as an initiation by the elements, purpose enters into our lives, and a calling is indeed undertaken.

We now know that reactivation of the center of our brains, where the meaning centers such as the amygdala lie, is an important part of healing trauma and restoring energy to the Self. Anyone who is a writer knows that mini-traumas are a part of the writer's everyday life. As Thomas Mann said, "A writer is one for whom writing is more difficult than it is for other people."

Many of the dimensions of Bodymind Healing Psychotherapy can be helpful to clearing writing blocks. In addition to the elements of nature, and the psychodynamic and cognitive distortions needing to be cleared, the movements from Bodymind Healing Qigong listed above can help to clear the body of encumbrances that block the muses of writing. These all are necessary tools for the writer's toolbox—just as much as pens and paper.

Case Illustration: Flying Phobia

The following case shows how by being aware of synchronistic happenings in a therapist's office, or in our lives, can be integrated into our lives for healing—another example of how sensitivity to the healing elements of the universe, as they synchronistically intercede into our lives, can become hypnotic anchors to aid the process of transformation.

A corporate manager, "Barry" had never before had a fear of flying, but he developed a phobia after the infamous wave of terrorist attacks on September 11 and after he was on a plane that hit an air bump and dropped "what must have been one thousand feet." As he imagined going on his next speaking engagement, Barry described his SUDS level as an 8. Barry's process further illustrates the multilayered approach of BMHP (outlined in Chapter Five) as he explored his "journey to the underworld." Some of these layers coincide with the steps of BMHP, and some are broader in scope.

STEPS TO HEAL A FLYING PHOBIA WITH THE TRANSPERSONAL DIMENSIONS OF BODYMIND HEALING PSYCHOTHERAPY

1. **Breath and Imagery:** First, we did the BMHP process of using Microcosmic Orbit Breathing and the River of Life visualization. As Barry reexperienced being on the plane, he focused on a body sense that felt like an ice block in his upper stomach and said, "We're going to die." Then doing cognitive restructuring, a more-balanced belief arose as he said, "There's a small chance of dying." But this created an unexpected rise rather than a fall in his SUDS level, which he reported to be 6.5.

2. **Focusing:** On the next level down in the underworld, as Barry focused on his body sense while he imagined flying, he became aware of a lack of control and not trusting many aspects of life, including trusting the airplane. From this, his SUDS level raised even higher to a 7.75.

3. **Psychodynamic:** He said this feeling of fear felt similar to when he was a child and was afraid of going to a playground due to killings in his neighborhood.

4. **Self-Soothing:** The self-soothing that had been helpful to Barry in the past did not seem to work for him as he attempted not to try to change this inner child's feeling, but to accept himself as he is.

5. **Energy Psychology:** Barry tried out the statement *even though I have this phobia, I can love and accept myself,* but this intervention from the Emotional Freedom Technique did not produce a lower SUDS level because he still needed to do more work on the psychodynamic layer. His father's message had been *buck up and get over it.* Measuring himself by his father's expectations hindered Barry's ability to relax and find a compassionate relationship to his issues.[2] Paralleling his process of measuring himself against his father's standards, Barry also measured himself against other managers in his company "who didn't have such fears."

6. **Teleology:** Once the psychodynamic layer was brought into awareness, the teleological level could be explored, which involves the forward-oriented purpose of a symptom. Barry became aware that his sensitivity to the fearful realities of life, such as planes crashing, was both his talent and his curse. As he accepted his path as a wounded healer, a felt shift happened and a real self-acceptance and self-soothing could begin. Then the use of self-soothing touch brought him to a SUDS level of 1.

7. **Practice:** Barry became aware that his upcoming plane ride was an opportunity to practice reparenting and self-soothing as he accepted his very nature of being a sensitive individual.

8. **Synchronicity of the Healing Elements:** Just as we were doing this inner work, we heard the synchronistic sound of a dove cooing right outside my office. Barry interpreted it to be saying *I fly every day and though there are hawks and potential dangers, I find peace.* Barry's SUDS level had dropped to 0.

This well-respected manager now flies to speaking engagements around the country; and although anxieties arise, he uses his self-soothing touch, the various layers of BMHP, and his power symbol (medicine animal) of the dove to aid him in his process of "re-membering" his primordial Self.

Barry's process illustrates how the various dimensions of a person's "journey to the underworld" are implicitly part of the realm of everyday clinical practice and psychological healing; however, many clinicians may not explicitly describe their work this way. This multilayered way of conceptualizing the patient's journey adds a psychospiritual depth to the process. Barry's case shows how certain energy psychology methods, though helpful, do not always result in one-session cures. Healing the primordial Self often involves not only incorporating the relaxation response, self-soothing, self-touch, the cognitive layer, the psychodynamic layer, and time; but sometimes it also it involves a little help from the synchronicity of some higher power that lies behind the workings of this wonder-filled universe.

Anchoring State-Specific States Using the Five Elements of the Internal Martial Arts

There are three styles of internal martial arts: Tai Chi, Pa Kua, and Hsing-I. Body movements for specifically activating the five elements are contained in Hsing-I (Smith, 2003); and the focus on healing with the elements is part of the "healing the internal organs" set of medical Qigong.[3] Movements from these sets can be used as hypnotic anchors in BMHP as suggested throughout this book. When appropriate, I suggest that patients practice a movement from these sets to help anchor an element that is helpful for their healing and cultivate a missing aspect of their primordial Self. For example, in one session with Barry, I chose the metal element to help him to cut through his introjected father's message to "buck up." Interestingly, the movement in Hsing-I involves bringing the right hand down like a knife in a slicing motion, leading with the side of the hand. This point is the same point used in energy psychology (SI-3), the Karate Chop point. Barry felt empowered when doing this movement along with saying, "I can cut through my father's bullshit and finally be compassionate with myself." When his father's voice came to mind on plane trips, Barry used his right hand in this mudra to anchor this new state-specific state of consciousness.

Four Elements of Constructive Communication of Negative Feelings

The ancient idea of using the energies of the elements of life to heal can be applied today to psychotherapy with individuals, as well as couples. The following is the four-step method that I have used with couples for the last twenty-five years. It takes the four elemental energies of premodern Western psychology—fire, earth, air, and water—and shows how they can be brought together as healing elements of constructive communication (Mayer, 1993).

- **Fire:** *First express your intent in communicating your feeling.* For example, "There's something I want to clear up with you because I care about you, and this issue is affecting my feelings about our relationship." (Fire raises the intentionality to a higher level, like fire ascending.)

- **Air:** *Distinguish between the whole person and the behavior you do not like.* For instance, "I love you and care about you deeply, but the mess you leave in front of the closet is really getting to me." (Air distinguishes between the whole and the parts.)

- **Water:** *Express your feelings as "I feel" statements not as blame or name-calling "you are" statements.* For example, "Dealing with this mess is really making me angry. I notice myself walking around feeling resentful for hours after coming into the room, and I don't like being this way."

    Water expresses the hot and cold of your inner river of experience. A way to get in touch with and deepen "the river of your communication" comes from first focusing on your body sense (for example, your clenched jaw). Then you resonate a word with this sense until it feels like a match ("I feel . . . angry"). To get the felt sense, ask yourself what gets to you so much about this issue or what makes you so angry . . . and wait for an answer. For instance, "What gets me so much about the mess is that it makes me feel out of control. It makes me feel scattered, like the way I am when I'm messy. And just like I'm impatient with my own scatteredness, I get that way with yours. I guess I have to admit that I have a hard time with not having my own way, and it scares me to reflect upon whether I'll ever be able to make it long term in a relationship because of my issues with this kind of thing."

- **Earth:** *Ask for what you want.* Frame the issue as a problem that the two of you have. For instance, "I wonder how we can work this whole thing out. I'd like to be able to find a solution to this together because I'm at the point of tearing my hair out." This is the bargaining phase. Remember, you are not necessarily entitled to get what you want, but you do deserve to be able to ask for and talk about it. Then you might suggest, "How about agreeing to at least put your clothes over there, out of the way instead of in the middle of the room." (Earth involves finding practical solutions to the problem.)

The above elements are common ways to encourage healthy communication between two people. Bodymind Healing Psychotherapy puts such elements of effective communication back into connection with the elements of the wider whole of which we are a part in order to enhance interpersonal communication further. For example, if we start off by saying to our partner, "I'm angry with you for leaving your clothes out in front of the closet," he or she may become defensive. There is less of a chance of evoking or provoking defensiveness if you say something like, "I'd like to clear something with you because you are my partner, and I'd like to tell you something so I can stop holding on to it, and we can find a way to work with this dynamic in the future" (Fire). This prepares your partner to receive the feeling. Likewise with all of the other elements, by operating together, each element is enhanced by the wider whole.[4]

The following is a chart of this process that shows how both parties can use it to communicate. It is important to note how Person B, the responder, first needs to listen empathically to all that Person A, the initiator, has to say until the initiator feels heard. After the initiator is heard, then problem solving and bargaining can occur (Earth).

STEP	PERSON A *The Initiator*	PERSON B *The Responder*
1	Express your intent in communicating your feeling.	*
2	Distinguish between the whole person and the behavior you do not like.	*
3	Express your feelings as "I feel" statements, not "you are" statements.	*
4	Ask for what you want.	*
5	*	Empathize with PERSON A's feelings until you are sure they been heard accurately. Make sure you see PERSON A's acknowledgement that they feel empathized with.
6	Respond to PERSON B, letting them know if you felt they "got" what you felt in step 3. If they are missing something, let them know what's missing. (PERSON A and B go back and forth between steps 5 and 6 until PERSON A feels heard.)	*
7	*	Respond to what PERSON A asked for in step 4, and tell them what you are willing to do with regards to that issue.
8	Problem solve together, propose and discuss possible solutions, come to a conclusion.	Problem solve together, propose and discuss possible solutions, come to a conclusion.
9	Close the circle. Tell PERSON B how you feel about the process.	Close the circle. Tell PERSON A how you feel about the process.

© Dr. Michael Mayer, from *Trials of the Heart* (Celestial Arts 1994)

Figure 4. The Four Elements of Constructively Expressing Negative Feelings

CHAPTER TWENTY

The Mythic Journey Process: Transforming Your Demons with a Qi-Filled Story

We have not even to risk the adventure alone, for the heroes of all time have gone before us; the labyrinth is thoroughly known: we have only to follow the thread of the hero path. And where we had thought to find an abomination, we shall find a god; where we had thought to slay another, we shall slay ourselves; where we had thought to travel outward, we shall come to the center of our own existence; and where we had thought to be alone, we shall be with all the world.[1]

—Joseph Campbell

If you are wondering how storytelling has anything to do with energy psychology, as Carl Jung pointed out, symbols have the capacity to awaken healing energy, as all of us have experienced when we hear an uplifting story.

Throughout this book I have indicated that there is more to energy-based psychologies than the technologies of tapping and muscle testing. The whole realm of Qigong (including breath, movements, postures, and awareness) as well as symbolic process modes of inner work can be included under the emerging "re-membering" of the ancient roots of modern psychology. Ancient sacred wisdom traditions are key elements to unlocking the treasure-house that is the human psyche.

During the 1970s and 1980s, my work in integrating psychotherapy and the Western mystery traditions culminated in the development of the Mythic Journey Process (Mayer, 1993) and is now updated here. Among the various psycho-

mythological and symbolic process methods used nowadays to facilitate healing, the Mythic Journey Process is unique in how it is not as tightly structured as
guided imagery, and therefore, it allows one's own tale to freely emerge. However, the method also has a structure to it that provides riverbanks through which
one's unconscious stream of imagery can flow and be guided.

Mythology: The Key to the Door of Your Psyche

Ancient myths are becoming new resources for the human venture. The written works and interviews of Joseph Campbell gave the study of world mythologies increasing respect. James Hillman (1975), Sam Keen (1989), Robert Bly
(1990), and a vast number of Jungian-oriented authors have shown the importance of ancient myths and storytelling to bring soul to modern culture.[2] It
seems that we are in an age of mythological renaissance. It is a time when the
mythic Sword of Excalibur can rise again—a time for reviving the gods and
goddesses of imagination to give meaning to modern life.

Throughout the ages, mythic stories have been passed down describing the
deep inner transformations of the psyche. We have seen how these legends can
show us oceans of possibilities within us and help us begin the odyssey that
will transform our souls. Today, with the many different religious and mythic
traditions, we are in a unique position—we are able to set sail and find our own
myths on an even larger ocean. We can create our own mythic journeys from
all the past mythic literature and our imaginations.

Our very lives are mythic journeys; and when we depart, it will not be our
bones that will be left, it will be our stories. They are our link to immortality. Yet
the importance of stories and myths have not been integrated as a formal part
of our education.[3] We are told stories by our parents and teachers, but we are
not trained in their deeper mysteries: their ability to soothe the soul and transform, awaken, and heal us.

To understand the essence of the healing power of myth, we must first explore
its primary ingredient—symbol. A symbol is to a story what a note is to a song.
Edward Edinger has pointed out that the early use of the Greek word *symbolon*
referred to a stick that was used in a trading agreement.[4] To mark the transfer of

ownership of an object from one person to another, a stick was divided in half to symbolize the sale. Just as these sticks were reminders of a greater unity, symbols today help reconnect us with something larger than ourselves.

Everything is part of a greater whole. Just as a lung is part of a human body and its identity must be understood within that whole context, we as human beings in order to fully comprehend our identities must connect ourselves to a wider whole. The secret of myth's healing power comes from how it helps us to create a likeness between us and an aspect of the surrounding universe. This likeness is a particular use of symbol—a metaphor.

In the Mythic Journey Process, we create a likeness between our current life situation and a person or situation of ancient times, and we make room for the power of imagination to enter through this likeness.

Identifying and Overcoming Our Inner Demons

Whether you are the most positive, rational thinker in the world or a traditional religious person who is against iconic pagan imagery, we all have our problems, obstacles, and demons lurking under the veneer of our lives. It is these archetypal aspects of the human condition that the Mythic Journey Process brings forth. By facing the particular "demons" behind our psychological problems, we can deal with suffering at its root (Hillman, 1975). Picturing the form of the demon and how we will address it changes confrontation into adventure. The demon may turn out to be the monster of our fear. The giant may be our inertia or suppressed power. By directly facing and dealing with the demon, we can rediscover our lost selves and gain access to the treasure of our inherent nature.

Throughout time, myths have recorded the numerous ways that heroes have confronted various demons. Whether it was by attacking, wrestling, or feeding them, each encounter offers us an approach to a present-day demon.

Petrifying Fear: The Story of Perseus and Medusa

Hearing a story that contains a problem like ours helps us face our demons and feel less alone in our suffering. For example, maybe our partner continually gets angry when we come home late from work. Perhaps we fear that the relationship is endangered because we need our freedom, or perhaps we feel smoth-ered but are too petrified to discuss it because our partner reacts so strongly.

A mythic analogy to this situation can be found in the tale of Perseus and Medusa: in which each of us is Perseus, and Medusa represents our angry part-ner. In this myth, Medusa's face was so horrifying that it had the power to pet-rify into stone the people who dared look at it. Using the example above and reading this story, we may see that maybe we are not dealing with our own personal neurosis, but with a wider, universal issue—the petrifying fear of a powerful figure. Instead of feeling alone and isolated, we can feel linked with those ancient heroes who struggled with monstrous embodiments of the same forces that we are now coping with. What once felt like neurotic suffering becomes an adventure as we explore how our problems were dealt with in the mythic past.

In order to save Perseus from being turned into stone, Athena, goddess of wisdom, gave him a shield to reflect Medusa's image. By looking into the shield instead of looking directly at her face, Perseus was able to approach Medusa and behead her. We might look to the myth of Perseus and Medusa and ask ourselves *what in my life could function like Perseus's shield?*

We can reflect on our situation aided by the distance our own inner shield gives us. Imagine that we realized that in the past we felt petrified of hurting our mother or being rejected by her when she disapproved of and limited our behavior. As a child, we gave in to her demands in order to survive. And per-haps we developed a pattern of constantly giving in to others' demands for fear of hurting them or being rejected by them. Metaphorically speaking, we may have turned to stone inside, acceding to the demand, but with a stiff upper lip, resenting the restriction. A pattern may have developed to withdraw in other ways in our relationships.

Reflecting on our partner's image in the mirrored shield, we might be able to understand his or her issues better. Perhaps our partner was feeling a loss of control in the relationship or was not feeling needed or cared about. Reflect-ing upon what caused the anger rather than reacting to it, we can "behead the monster," that is, diffuse our reactivity.

Reflecting in such a way in the midst of seemingly monstrous emotions requires the proper implements. Perseus was given an adamantine sickle and winged sandals by Hermes and a helmet of invisibility by Pluto. We must learn what these implements mean and learn how to use them so that we are prepared when we meet the Medusas in our life. For example, perhaps the sword's parrying ability would be useful in its ability to point to the real issue, slice through the mire, and to find the truth of the underlying feelings.

Perseus's sickle was adamantine (made of the hardest stone). Today we know that the hardest stone is diamond, but any stone that is very hard has sustained years of pressure by the earth's forces. If it is a diamond, it has become clarified. Perhaps the myth is telling us that we must be patient regarding the hard-to-bear forces in our situation. There is a purpose behind the pressure—to create something that is clear and of great value.

The image of this sword tells us that we must combine the qualities of hardness (not being weak about the "hard truth") with the softness of a sickle's curve. On the one hand, we cannot passively cave into our partner's demands, we must be strong in our assertion that there is more here than meets the eye. But the soft lunar curve must also be present in the discussion, reflecting on both partners' underlying issues. A straight-edged-sword approach will not do. If we point our sword in a judgmental way, the mythic solution will not be found.

The imagery tells us that at a certain point in exploring our different viewpoints, Hermes's winged sandals might be useful to help us walk lightly into the underworld to examine our own issues—our feelings of being smothered and our partner's difficulty with feelings of neediness. Discussing these feelings can give us winged sandals that transport us to the upper regions, as Hermes's sandals transported Greek heroes to that place of compassionate perspective. This takes place only if we are able to keep our ego under the "cap of invisibility." If we are enraged by our partner's neediness, or we withdraw in anger, the hero's goal will not be accomplished.

In one version of the myth, after Medusa was beheaded, Pegasus the winged horse emerged; and as he ascended, he kicked a mountaintop from which sprang the fountains of the Muses. Indeed, when two people work through issues such as these, wellsprings of creative energy are released. We may learn to use humor to dramatize our issues or be awed by the insight they bring. Love may be reborn.

Remember that Perseus's quest was for Andromeda, his beloved who was chained to a rocky cliff. Medusa's head and the weapons that he accumulated in his quest were used to free her from the dragon. Often it seems that our beloved is chained to a rocky cliff and that the relationship is tottering on the edge. Ultimately it requires a quest like Perseus's to rescue the feminine in us and in our partner. The feminine symbolically represents that lunar quality of inner reflection that must be rescued from the hard rock of rigidity.

Myths record the tests and trials of the human spirit. They are keys to the psyche's secrets, which are brought to life by our imagination. Just as it takes a combination of factors to create a rainbow (light, water, and a person at the proper angle), so do myths provide illumination when we see a story from a particular angle. There is no single correct angle to interpret a story from because each angle produces its unique vision that is meaningful to us at a given time.

In the Mythic Journey Process, when we feel lost, we can create our own stories and use the symbols that arise from our inner vision to help us find the way into the cave of our unconscious. There, we can meet the demon, wrestle with it, and find the jewel of our own Self.

Focusing and the Mythic Journey Process

The Mythic Journey Process is a way of harnessing the ancient power of myth to work through modern-day problems. It combines elements of the Focusing technique with archetypal psychology.

Eugene Gendlin is a present-day hero in the field of psychology who researched the factors that produced change in the psychotherapeutic setting. In his study at the University of Chicago,[5] Dr. Gendlin analyzed tapes of different therapies to discover what factors were present in successful therapy. His Focusing process (Gendlin, 1978) was developed from this research. Gendlin proposed a way to develop our body's felt sense as a guide to new meanings and fresh perspectives on life's problems. He found that a felt energetic shift (felt shift) occurred when a person found new meaning for a life problem. The Mythic Journey Process adds to Focusing the richness of symbolic language.

The Mythic Journey exercise consists of starting with our bodily felt sense of a chronic physical or psychological problem, and then telling a story about this problem, transposing it into ancient times as we did with Medusa. While the story is being told, we continually refer to the bodily felt sense, noticing how it changes along with the development of the story. We can eventually reach a point where the story begins to tell itself and experience a felt shift and new meaning regarding our problem.

The Mythic Journey Process is a contemporary embodiment of the ancient mythic journey to the underworld. Just as the mythic Greek hero Theseus used Ariadne's thread to find his way into and out of the underworld labyrinth to free the captive children from the monstrous Minotaur, so do we use our bodily felt experience as a thread into and out of our psychological underworld to liberate the energies of our inner experience. The steps of the Focusing process become guideposts along our path.

In the first step of Focusing, called *clearing a space,* we find a friendly relationship to a life issue by saying, "Everyone has their stuff to deal with and here's mine. If I had a friend, I wouldn't be hard on him for having this to deal with." Because we are often harder on ourselves than we would be on a friend with the same problem, we need to find a relationship to ourselves that is like the relationship that we would have to a friend with a similar problem.

Dr. Gendlin also found that an important factor in successful therapy was a person's ability to use his or her body's felt sense to create movement in therapy. In his book, Gendlin (1978) gives an example of a traditional couple (pp. 45–50). A wife at home cleaned the table. Her husband returned home after getting a job promotion; and in his excitement, knocked the milk onto the table that his wife had just cleaned. The woman became aware of her bodily feeling of anger and began the Focusing process. She resonated the word *anger* against the felt bodily sense of the issue surrounding her husband's promotion. She then stopped for a moment and said, "No, that's not quite right. I'm not sure what I felt, but it's not quite anger." For some people, this can be a difficult moment because they cannot identify specifically what they are feeling. In

Gendlin's Focusing process, we learn to trust an unclear felt sense and wait for something to emerge. While staying in touch with the unclear feeling of "a hole in my stomach," this woman realized, "It's not so much anger; what's getting me the most is the void I feel about being left behind in my life." At this point she sighed and there was a "felt energetic shift" in the way her body carried the problem. (In this example, we can see in Dr. Gendlin's work the phenomenological core of a primordial energy psychology.)

In the Focusing technique, our bodily felt sense can be used as a guiding light. We can imagine that the woman might be guided to express her feelings to her husband and be comforted or that she might look for a way to develop her life further.

The healing role of the body has long been recognized in mythology. Today's students of mythology, however, often fail to give the body due respect. Body feeling and archetypal image are mutually interdependent systems; they are isomorphic translations of each other into that other medium. Without the interweaving of body and myth, healing is not complete.

The insights gained from Gendlin's Focusing technique, coupled with mythology, can be an important next step in mythic voyages. Many of the subtle elements of the Focusing technique are integrated in the counseling setting but to describe these elements thoroughly is beyond the scope of this section.[6]

Prelude to the Mythic Journey Process

The inner journey in the Mythic Journey Process parallels journeys to the underworld that have been spoken of by the earliest healers of the psyche.[7] Shamans and temple priests of the mystery schools have spoken of it as a journey into the body of the earth or into the dark caverns of the unconscious. Myths suggest ways to prevent us from getting lost.

As modern people we can use Focusing on our experience and felt sense in combination with the Mythic Journey to follow Theseus's path. We can join these methods to serve as our thread through the psychological underworld to find and liberate the energies of the natural child within us.

The Mythic Journey Process starts with a grounding exercise that helps clear a space where we find our center, our inner pillar. Using a Taoist breathing technique, we can experience the Tan Tien center below the navel. When we do the breathing meditation properly,[8] this center can become a pillar to return to when we encounter fear in our inner labyrinth.

The Mythic Journey Process

The Mythic Journey Process begins with a breathing meditation combined with *clearing a space* step of Focusing and an imagery exercise:

Notice your exhalation ... the pause ... and how the inhalation comes naturally from this pause. After a few cycles, notice how your body feels different and notice the way you have settled down to be in contact with the ground under you. Are you held off the ground in any way? Feel how being with your breathing cycle can help you let go to the ground under you so that you are simply here.

If there is any residual tension in your body, just notice it in a way that establishes a compassionate, friendly relationship to it. If a friend of yours had a similar tension, you would find room to accept him or her in spite of the issue. Find this relationship to any tension in your body, letting the natural breathing facilitate the friendly relationship. During the following process, when something arises that you want distance from, just breathe this way and return to the relaxed place—your inner pillar.

One way to combine the breathing meditation with searching for an issue is to imagine that as you breathe out, it is like letting go of some of the tension in your body and lowering a bucket into the well of your Self, deep beneath the surface tension that you may be carrying at this moment. The bucket is tied to a secure pillar at the top. As you breathe out and lower it, you come to a place where your breath pauses before you take in the next breath. As you pause, it is as though the bucket is waiting for something deep within to fill it, some issue that stands in the way of you feeling all right. As your breath comes in, the bucket rises. It may take quite a few exhalations (lowering of the bucket) until something from deep within you comes into your bucket.

The first step of the Mythic Journey consists of finding an issue and an associated bodily felt sense of this issue, just as in the Focusing technique. For some people, the body sense comes first; for others, the issue emerges first. If the body sense comes first, do you know what this body sense connects with in your life? If the issue arises first, do you feel where this issue lies in your body? You might start by proclaiming *everything in my life is completely all right* and noticing what issues arise to contradict this. With each issue that emerges, you establish a compassionate, friendly relationship to it. Create enough distance so that you can acknowledge *I recognize you're there, but I'm not going to work on you right now. Maybe I'll come back later.* Imagining yourself somewhere else in the room, feeling the way you do when you are with this issue, is one way to clear a space.

As issues pop up, give yourself time to notice how they affect the subtle barometer of your body. It is from your body's reaction that you will know which issue to choose to work with. As you approach this "friend," you can get a felt sense of the issue.[9] For further aid in getting the felt sense, sometimes it helps to say to yourself, *I could feel completely fine about this whole thing.* When a voice inside contradicts this statement with the idea *no I couldn't feel fine about this,* that is the felt sense.[10] What is this sense all about? Wait for something to come up from the felt sense. See if you can distinguish between trying to think about it and just having something emerge from the sense itself. It may be a word or an image or a sound—trust whatever comes for you. To get a "handle word or image" for this felt sense of the issue, just wait as if you were a fisherman by an ice hole: You cannot rush a fish onto your hook. Just wait for what pops up from your body's sense of the issue as a whole.

What word or image seems to resonate with the sense of what this issue is all about? You will know that you have something that resonates by the response your body gives—the way its movement is facilitated when something gets to the crux of the matter.

What is the worst thing about this issue for you? At this point it helps to actually write down the issue on a piece of paper along with the bodily feeling you have noticed. Note bodily feelings in parentheses. For example:

- **Issue:**

- **Body sense** *(write this in parentheses):*

- **Handle word/image:**

- **The worst of it:** *(Ask the felt sense various questions, such as what is the worst of it and what is the crux of this issue?):*

Then the mythic dimension begins.

The Mythic Dimension

The first part of the mythic dimension of the Mythic Journey Process is to take your issue and the associated bodily felt sense and to create a story about a character in ancient times who had the same problem. Begin with the words: *Once upon a time . . .*

There will be three parts to the mythic dimension. First, describe the problem you are facing in mythic terms: Where does this mythic character live in terms of terrain, surroundings, and so forth? How did this problem come about? Was it created in a relationship with a young prince or princess's mother and father, the king and queen? Use your own characters and imagery. (The second two parts of the mythic dimension will be illustrated in the following case example.)

It is key to transpose the felt sense of your own obstacle into mythic terms: What created this problem in the character's life? Was a curse or spell put on you? If so, for what reason and by whom? Give an actual face or name to the "demon," and write it in capitalized letters to personify it, such as Fear, Blame, or Self-Doubt. Naming or "facing" the specific demon is very important (Hillman, 1975).

Case Illustration: A Critical Perfectionist's Mythic Journey Process

The issue for one patient, who was a perfectionist, was an intense criticizing that led to attacking his partners. The following Mythic Journey Process was written at a key point in "John's" long-term therapy:

- **Issue:** My difficulties with relationships

- **Body sense:** (clenched jaw)

- **Handle word/image:** Anger. He imaged his "demon" to be a Serrated Sword. Then John proceeded with part one of the mythic dimension and developed the felt sense of this demon into the following story.

- **The worst of it:** *No one is good enough; I'll never find anyone with whom to have a long-term relationship.*

Once upon a time ...

The Serrated Sword of Criticism was given to my father's father many generations ago when he was down and out. He sat on a mountaintop praying for power and the ability to support his family when a mountain demon came to him and gave him a serrated sword with a mountain emblazoned upon it. He said that the cuts made with it and the blood on it would proportionally increase the sword's power and would help him ascend the mountains of earthly life to be great, admired, powerful, and respected. He was told to make a family crest of it and begin practicing with his own family.

Indeed, great power and admiration came to this family of swordsmen and women through the generations. Though wounds occurred and blood was let increasingly, the sword's power was the key focus of the family. Applause was given at the family dinner table for the great swordplay of the day, whether it was against the bulls killed for dinner or the other swordsmen defeated. Even family wounds inflicted were respected if done in a skillful way.

The second part of the mythic dimension of the Mythic Journey Process describes how impossible it seems to defeat the demon, and the problems it has caused. What methods have you tried that have not worked to defeat it? Transpose those methods into mythic terms. For example, John added to his story:

Although our royal family attained a castle on a mountaintop and much power in the world through our fine discriminating cuts, the prince's life was not a happy one. As great a swordsman as he was and as admired as he was, he was alone most of the time.

The problem was the sword, the very one that had given him such pleasure in his youth, the one for which he and his family had been admired for generations. When it was handed down to him, it went out of control. Each time it would become unsheathed, it would cut anything he looked at in a discriminating way. It cut all of his lovers to bits. The prince tried to break the sword, but many generations of power made it unbreakable. He tried to get rid of it at an Eastern religious temple; he denounced it and tried to bury it. But he felt impotent without it and had trouble climbing the castle steps if the sword was not in his belt. (slumped chest, feeling of being defeated)

Accentuating how impossible it seemed to defeat the demon brings out the "soulful dimension" (Hillman, 1976) and can help prevent Pollyannaish solutions. Again, check back with your body's felt sense and note it in parentheses.

Concluding part two, make a statement that addresses the specific nature of the impasse and the specific obstacle or demon the character is dealing with. Indicate how you specifically feel knowing that nothing can be done to deal with it. This is "exploring the resistance" mythically. For example, from John's story:

The Prince of the Serrated Sword felt that he could not give up the way of the sword for he was too good at it, and it was too much a part of his nature. Yet at the same time, he could not live with it. There seemed to be no end to the loneliness and the guilt that the prince felt over cutting up his lovers. The Critical Sword seemed all-powerful. (depressed, hollow feeling in my chest)

The prince used his discriminating insight to see where the power of the sword came from. He relaxed and sensed the presence of the old mountain demon above him. Above him and to the right, he noticed a demon called Smug-Faced Pride.

It added an electric glow to the sword each time the prince said, "Look at what an adept swordsman I am." Upwards and to the left, the prince was able to sense the presence of another demon, Needy-Faced Expectation. It added a desperate, angry, warlike hacking motion to the sword each time the prince said to others, "If you aren't the way I want you to be, I'll cut you up to fit into the 'right' mold."

The third part of the mythic dimension begins with writing these words: *Then one day....* Then describe what happened one day. Let some solution to the impasse come to you. Give it time. If no solution arises in you to break the impasse, then think about who could deal with this demon: imagine some heroic figure, animal, or mythic creature and see what happens when it meets your demon. Use your creative story-writing capacity to let the story tell itself. Continuing John's story:

Then one day, while the prince was depressed and looking into a mountain lake, he began to reflect upon whether he wanted to be a swordsman if it meant having no love. (Something lets go in my chest area: a sense of openness comes there as I sigh.) At that moment a Maiden of the Lake[11] appeared with the golden sword Excalibur that had been thrown back into these waters many years ago.

Tears came to his eyes as the prince explained that he could not go on being a swordsman if there was no love in his life, and yet he could not give up his family's path either. He asked for her help.

With compassion, the Maiden of the Lake taught him the one movement that the mountain demon had neglected to teach his forefather many years ago. She instructed him to feel with his heart before he was about to use the golden glowing sword and caress it as if it was a beloved from whom he was asking guidance. Then he was to look at the polished mirror that the sword's metal became, reflect as he was doing at the lake when he met her, and ask for guidance on how to use the sword in the service of love and truth.

As the prince followed her instructions, he noticed that as he held this sword in front of him, a ray of light came from his heart and bounced off the sword. His eyes could direct it, but only when they were reflecting inward with clear intent. "This light," the Maiden of the Lake said, "had the ancient power to transform anything that he wanted to heal."

The Maiden said that this was the true power of the sword that had been lost through the ages. She explained that before the sword was used for fighting, it was used for directing energy to points on the body that were in need of healing. She told the prince stories of how her teachers of the Golden Age used this sword in daytime to bring the healing power of the sun, and at night to bring the powers of the stars to earth. All this was done with the same meditation that she had just given him—using the powers of reflection and the power of the heart's glow.

With the Maiden of the Lake before him, the prince felt his heart's desire to be a healer, and he reflected upon the mountain demon above him. A light went to the demon and transformed him into a beneficent mountain spirit whose purpose was to help others to climb to their own heights. (a feeling of fullness in my chest)

As he reflected on the electric light around Smug-Faced Pride, this conceited demon changed to a healing ally. The smug expression changed to a smile, like the Buddha's, as he realized that "skill" is not one's own but is borrowed from the powers of the universe, the stars, the sun, and the earth.

As the prince reflected upon Needy-Faced Expectation, he realized that much of the world's and his own suffering came from this demon's misplaced needs for power over others, for false security, ego recognition, and worldly success. With the sword's light on this demon, a new power came to the sword—a compassionate understanding of human foibles. A new form of sword dancing came from this transformed demon which gave the prince's movements a heartfelt, gentle, slicing motion, as when a person cuts a flower for a loved one and in the cutting wants the flower to suffer as little as possible. As when the sword masters of ancient times had cut a field of wheat with deep appreciation for the forces of nature that went into producing the growth of the plant, so would the prince try to appreciate that which went into the growth of all that he was to use his sword upon. The prince vowed to make it his new practice to have tenderness when he used his sword to point out the places that became uncentered in his own and other's everyday life.

When the prince returned home, he created a new family crest with the Golden Glowing Sword of the Heart over the Critical Serrated Sword. The

Maiden of the Lake's sword had the power to stir the prince's compassion. In the future when the Critical Sword came out, the Maiden's sword was there to help remind the prince that its sharp power was to be put to a healing rather than a destructive use. This was not easy work, but at least now the prince knew what the work of his kingdom was. When the old sword arose, his work was to reflect on it with the heart meditation that he had learned and thereby bring love and compassionate understanding to the kingdom. (Open-hearted, glowing feeling in my chest, and hope through my whole being—a feeling like I've found what my life work is.)

Your story does not have to have a happily-ever-after ending. Simply note your actual sense of the issue and transpose it into mythic terms. Often time is an important force to integrate into the story. Remember, it took Moses forty years in the desert to complete his destiny. What is the destiny, the purpose for which your character is going through his or her trials and tribulations? Sometimes this dimension of meaning and purpose can contribute to a felt shift.

After you reach a place in your story where it feels complete for the moment, notice your body's felt sense and note it in parentheses at the end of the story.

Bring the adventure of this character back into your own life now. Reflecting on his or her quest, ask yourself what you can learn form the character's adventure and how your own path feels different now.

Reflection on the Mythic Journey Process

Many people experience new meaning emerging from their story and note that at a certain point in writing, they find the story writing itself. Some report that it is as if something were overtaking their writing and giving them a solution. It is unimportant whether one calls this a muse, our higher Selves, right-brain function, the healing mind/energy of the universe, or intuition. The felt energetic shift that happens and the new meaning and perspective born on a blocked life issue help us to heal regardless of what one calls the source of healing.

When people are stuck in a critical part of themselves, as the Prince of the Serrated Sword was, there are a variety of ways to create a shift in life stance. When combined with Gendlin's Focusing, both Tai Chi Sword Dancing practice and Western psychotherapy with its symbolic process methods go right to the crux of the psychological issue and can create a felt shift in a person's life stance. All are paths that lead to learning to wield a sword with compassion.

In this example of a Mythic Journey Process, the prince had to find a new life practice to change his "critical serrated-sword way of being" to become a compassionate coach of his own and others' limitations. As you read earlier, Dr. Jung knew that body and archetypal image are two ends of a spectrum and that healing can enter from the infrared or ultraviolet end of that spectrum. Or as the ancient Taoist alchemist would put it, intention (Yi) follows energy (Qi), and vice versa. Therefore, working on our life energy involves working on all psychospiritual and bodily facets of ourselves. A person's life stance at a given moment, and the energy that goes along with it, does not change through the medium of the body alone.

Case Illustration: The Passive-Aggressive Ostrich— Healing Trauma and Withdrawal

In the middle of my five-day Bodymind Healing Qigong workshops, participants do a Mythic Journey Process, and then they have the option to incorporate a Tai Chi or Qigong movement that helps to anchor the felt shift that oftentimes takes place at the end of their mythic journeys. So, I invite you to do the same. Perhaps some Qigong animal form, sword dance, or some other posture or movement of your choosing will help you to embody the shape-shifting that may take place in your Mythic Journey Process. If you are so inclined, I invite you to do the movements in this book, use the movements from another Tai Chi/Qigong teacher, or create your own movements.[12] Though Tai Chi, Qigong, or other movements are not necessary for the Mythic Journey Process, they do help to bring out a somatic dimension, which has the capacity to increase the method's transformative possibilities.[13]

The combination of these different facets of BMHP can be seen in the case of a young female student who had a pattern of passive-aggressive behaviors at significant times in her life. "Roberta" was engaged in psychotherapy with another therapist to work on her passive-aggressive tendencies because they were getting in the way of her intimate relationships, particularly with her husband. She also did the Mythic Journey Process, Tai Chi, and the animal forms of Qigong with me as part of her Bodymind Healing Qigong certification program. Roberta's story illustrates how the Mythic Journey Process can combine to help heal trauma and enhance a healing experience of shape-shifting from one life stance to another.

- **Issue:** My husband's aggressivity and my withdrawal
- **Body sense:** (anxiety in my stomach)
- **Handle word/image:** Ostrich hiding my head in the sand
- **The worst of it:** *I feel like a weakling for not being able to stand up for myself.*

Roberta's Mythic Journey Process activated memories of her running away from severe stressors in her teenage and young adult years, including a rape. This running away produced a belief that *as soon as you sense danger, it's better to immediately leave.* In her Mythic Journey, Roberta pictured and felt the demonic forces as Attacking Giants crushing her chest, closing off her ears, making her body tense like taught metal, which resulted in her running away from these feelings, like a Fearful Ostrich. Through her Mythic Journey Process, she realized that this was an overreaction to many things that were not as dangerous as the rape of her youth. Her excessively reactive pattern resulted in her not listening to her husband when he was giving constructive critiques; instead, Roberta often withdrew with passive-aggressive behaviors, such as threats to end their marriage. In her Mythic Journey Process, her favorite movement from Hua Tao's set was Crane Opens the Door to the Heavens (Mayer, 2004b, p.131). This movement is used as a nonforceful way to split the force of an aggressor. As Roberta got in touch with an image of herself doing this posture, she felt a noticeable felt shift of her stomach loosening its tight grip, and she realized that her husband was often trying to be helpful. We discussed how one of the crane's powers was to peck and differentiate the good food from the bad and spit out what was distasteful. In alchemy this is called the *seperatio* phase (Edinger, 1985).

Roberta realized that as her mythic quest rather than withdraw, she must assert to her husband what she did not like about the way he expressed himself. She later told me that in psychodynamic therapy, she was learning affect modulation skills to express herself appropriately and avoid being overly reactive to each occasion. Roberta reported that the Crane movements were helpful in showing her how to keep her heart open yet appropriately defended when needed. Last I heard, her relationship with her husband was better and her "ostrich behavior" occurred less often. Roberta said that now she almost always caught herself when the body feeling associated with the Attacking Giants came up. She used her anchor of touching the backs of her hands together in the Crane Splitting mudra (Mayer, 2004b, p. 131) to find her Crane power and to differentiate between what was harmful and what she could deal with, as she cleared the way for her heart's grounded expression.

Case Illustration: The Desperately Grasping Parrot—Healing Abandonment and Neediness

The power of "naming," even without any internal martial arts practice, can be an important part of shape-shifting into another life stance. The significance and healing attributes of a mythic name can be seen with "Mary," a woman in her mid-twenties, who was in therapy for the guilt and desperation she felt from hanging out at various places as she looked for the man of her dreams. She described her disappointments going home each night without a man. She realized that the rejection she felt was similar to what she felt from her single mother who would often abandon her to go out on dates when Mary was young.

- **Issue:** Finding the right man
- **Body sense:** (hole / emptiness in my heart)
- **Handle word/image:** Needy, grasping for someone who isn't there
- **The worst of it:** *I'll never find a life partner.*

In doing her Mythic Journey Process, Mary took her needy felt sense and imagined being a huntress in ancient times. Her demon was a Desperately Grasping Parrot, who would try to hold on to desired objects with its weak claws. The grasping claws, though, would frighten its prey away. It would chatter, parroting back clichés that it had learned in order to impress, but all the chatter only frightened away all the beautiful, wild creatures of the forest.

The young princess was originally given the Parrot as a present by her mother, the queen, as she abandoned the princess to go off for greater adventures than could be had with a young child. (hole in my heart, emptiness)

Mary's single mother actually did go out on dates quite often in Mary's formative years, and Mary traced her first memories of this sense of neediness to these times in her early life. She learned to talk incessantly whenever her mother was there, to fill up the silence. Mary would try to say all the right things, parroting what her mother might like to hear so that her mother might stay with her more.

In her Mythic Journey Process, the curse was that the Parrot would emerge out of her needy stomach each time Mary went hunting for someone to love. The Parrot drove everyone away. The healing intervention came for her one day in her Mythic Journey Process in the form of Artemis, the Greek goddess of the hunt, who was Mary's favorite goddess in mythology.

One day when the princess was depressed in the forest because she had not caught anything, Artemis appeared and offered to teach the princess the secrets of hunting … how in primordial times the Master Huntress knew that love was something that came from our connection to the whole world. (a sense of rising excitement and a sense of purpose)

As if straight out of classical mythic literature, Mary was describing *anima mundi*, soulful love of the world. She was expressing, in her own terms, the classical idea that at a certain point in our evolution, we as human beings transposed this *anima mundi* into *anima personalis*, a love for one human being, hopeful that this one person could contain her love for the world and universe. A large task indeed!

Artemis taught the princess how to hunt by enjoying all that was around her. If no deer came to her, she could still feel love for all surrounding life—the way light bounced over the meadow, the colors at sunset, and her relaxed position against the tree while she waited. Artemis told the princess that it was only in modem times, when the cult of true hunting decayed, that hunters would be devastated if they returned home without a deer. In primordial times, through the quality of waiting, the Priestesses of the Temple of Hunting always returned home with something of value. Upon hearing this, the princess (stomach opened and relaxed) and her pet Parrot were both stilled as never before. (a melting sensation in my stomach)

A few months later, Mary related how she sat watching the interesting variation of light shine on the table plants at her favorite local bar. She described a new sense of "life as practice." Though feelings of loneliness still arose, Mary said that her "hunting" now had a felt sense of adventure to it. A new context emerged, one of practicing the ancient art of "true hunting." She became more aware of her desperate, needy chatter and began to practice being a Stilled Parrot Who Enjoys the World while Waiting—her new symbolic name.

Conclusion

Many people who do the Mythic Journey Process find a new name for themselves. As in ancient initiatory rituals, it offers a new identity, and a new life stance for the person. This new name defines a new path and a new practice in one's life.[14] It is much like the new name Native Americans receive in their initiatory rituals in that it holds a power, linking the person to a transpersonal purpose, a path to a sacred life, and a destiny worth pursuing.

The Mythic Journey Process is a *quintessential* energy psychology practice. By using Qigong postures to ground our psycho-mythological inner work, a vital pathway is opened to change our life stances. The Mythic Journey Process is a way of responding to those who might ask, "Where are our heroes today? Where are those mythic adventurers who were able to deal with the archetypal demons of their age and open a path for fellow sufferers?"

Perhaps if we follow Ariadne's thread into our own underworlds, our stories—like hers—will be placed in the night sky; they will be like the crown of Ariadne (the Corona Borealis constellation) that Dionysus put there to immortalize her as a guiding light for lost souls to find their way. By opening our mythic imaginations, each of our life stories can become a guiding light for humanity. For who are we, but stars in the making, hoping to shed light on the darkness of space and thereby give new life energy to ourselves, our planet, and to fellow travelers everywhere.

Healing the Healer in You: Bodymind Healing Qigong's Twenty-Minute Practice Routine

Bodymind Healing Qigong is a physical exercise system, a Self-healing pathway, a spiritual practice, a method of transforming your life stance, a way to find your ground in the midst of the emotional crosscurrents of everyday life, and an initiatory tradition. It is also grounded in psychoneuroimmunological and quantum biological research and may become a practice that will stay with you for a lifetime.

—Michael Mayer

CHAPTER TWENTY-ONE

Bodymind Healing Qigong's Twenty-Minute Practice Routine

The Qigong traditions are thousands of years old: The fact that Qigong and Tai Chi (the best known system of Qigong) have stood the test of time attests to their effectiveness. These fitness practices have been carefully refined over several thousand years. The various forms of practice can be categorized by their degree of activity, ranging from completely motionless to very energetic. They include techniques that are performed in total stillness as meditation or meditative breathing exercises. Qigong and Tai Chi also involve gradual movement, like a dance in slow motion. Martial arts such as Kung Fu are vigorous forms of Qigong.

—Roger Jahnke[1]
Getting Your Immune System in Shape (2002)

Oh, Healer, Replenish Thy Self

What do you do to replenish yourself after your healing work with others? Whether you are lovingly present for your friends and family or a health professional who spends long hours each day helping others, everyone's batteries run down and need recharging.

Qigong stems from a cross-cultural lineage of healers who developed methods over thousands of years to help people cultivate the energy of life. One form of Qigong, for example, was developed by Boddhidharma (the founder of the twenty-eighth patriarch in the tradition of the Buddha Gautama) after he saw how the bodies of monks were atrophying from sitting for so long (like our sedentary office workers). The story goes that Boddhidharma went into a deep mediation and stared at a wall to help solve the monks' problem. One version of the legend says that after thirty years of meditating in front of this wall, he came up with one of the systems of Qigong called the Qigong for Changing the Muscles, Sinews, and Bone Marrow *(Yin Jing Jing)*. Thus, it is no wonder that Qigong is associated with dissolving one's inner walls.

Many Qigong systems can help restore our vital energy. The one I developed synthesizes ten different systems of Qigong.[2] Because this system takes about one-and-a-half hours to practice, I have been encouraged by others—such as Dr. Wayne Jonas, former director of the National Institute of Health, Office of Alternative Medicine—to develop a shorter twenty-minute routine that is better suited to the busy modern lifestyle. I am grateful that he asked to include my twenty-minute routine in one of his upcoming books as an aid to others who desire a shorter method that still captures the essence of the many healing elements of Qigong. I now use elements of this shorter routine during breaks with my psychotherapy patients, and I am pleased to report, so do many other health professionals.

I developed this practice routine to activate some of the key types of energy that healers, and the healer in all of us, need to restore vitality. It includes first doing a prelude exercise of your own choosing, followed by these eight practices: (1) Standing Meditation practices—to return to the source of healing energy; (2) Dispersing Stagnant Qi—to clear blocked Qi and cleanse stress; (3) Tai Chi Ruler (also called Tai Chi Chih)—to restore equilibrium, soothe, relax, and revitalize, just like the poles of a battery or the rocking of a child by a mother; (4) Ocean Wave Breathing—to recharge the heart; (5) Moving a Snake through the Joints—to limber the joints; (6) Crane Walking and Flying—to lighten the felt sense of the heart, develop balance, and strengthen the legs; (7) Yi Chuan Walking Meditation—to stay connected to sacred awareness as you walk through life; and (8) Wuji Standing Meditation—to give you a chance to pause and experience the Qi activated by your previous practices and return to the source of healing energy (wuji). These eight practices are state-specific practices to restore vitality to various elements of the primordial Self.

The Bodymind Healing Qigong Twenty-Minute Routine

This brief routine takes you from stillness to movement and back to stillness, and it helps you find the stillness in movement and the movement in stillness. (As always, consult with your doctor or appropriate health professional before engaging in such physical activities.)

Prelude to Bodymind Healing Qigong

As a prelude to the twenty-minute set, activate your energy in your own chosen way, with your favorite exercise. One of my favorite ways to begin is to do the following:

1. Bring the Yang Energy Down from the Heavens:

   With your hands at your sides, open the palms to the outside, let the hands rise up the sides of your body above the crown of your head, then bring the heavenly Qi down the front of the body. Three cycles of this movement provide a nice centering practice and help begin to create sacred space. To see a pictorial representation of one of the parts of this practice see the Dispersing Stagnant Qi picture later in this section.

2. Bring the Yin Energy Up from the Earth:

   Start with your hands by your sides, then gather up the earth's energy with your hands, bringing your wrists together until they cross in front of the heart, palms facing toward your body as if you are holding a ball there. Then open your hands palm outward, spreading your hands apart, out and upward, as they open the energy you have just brought up from the earth to the heavens. Finish this movement by bringing your arms back down to rest at your sides. Three cycles of this movement provide a powerful, expansive opening of the yin energies, and your heart, to the sky—a nice prelude to generating some energy to be applied to the creation of an axis mundi, as you assume the Standing Meditation posture in the short set of BMHQ that follows.

The Eight Bodymind Healing Qigong Practices

I. Standing Meditation Qigong: Revitalizing Your Energy Bank Account

A. STANDING LIKE A TREE

Keep both feet parallel, pointing straight forward, about a hip and a shoulder's width apart. The knees are unlocked, approaching being over the toes. The pelvis is slightly turned forward as if you were getting ready to sit down on a stool. The lower back is slightly pushed out so that the lumbar curve begins to disappear, allowing the lower back to approach being straight. The chest and shoulders are relaxed, causing a slight rounding of the upper back. Imagine there is a cord descending from a star attached to the top of your head so that you are like a puppet dangling from the heavens. Your chin is slightly tucked. Your arms hang loosely at your sides. The tongue is touching the top of the palate just behind the teeth. The eyes can be open in a soft gaze—half open or closed. Notice the natural flow of your breath. Pay attention to how long and deep your breath is without trying to force it to be calm. Be aware of any sensations or thoughts that emerge during this practice, while continually returning to your breath.

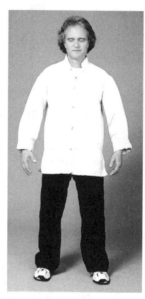

Figure 5. Wuji Standing Meditation

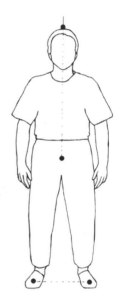

Figure 6. Puppet Dangling from Heaven

As you stand, feel the way your spine makes a connection between the heavens above and the earth below. After a number of breaths, imagine yourself as a tree with deep roots. Let your exhalation slowly descend down into your roots. What are you rooted into in your life—family, friends, loved ones, spiritual traditions? Let an image arise of what this root system is like. On your inhalation, imagine drawing in from those roots to strengthen your trunk. Then on your next inhalation, allow the Qi to rise up to your branches, reach out for the light, and transform that light into energy as you imagine giving your fruit to others.

The Circle That Arises from Stillness:

After standing for a while—since trees are not rigid nor are we—allow circles to emerge from your stillness by moving your weight fifty-one percent over your right heel, then over your right toes, then over your left toes, and then over your left heel. Imagine a snake or a vine spiraling up the tree, bringing the energy of the earth up and around the tree of your spine to the heavens. Stay in stillness for most of the time—practicing the Circle That Arises from Stillness occasionally and then returning to stillness.

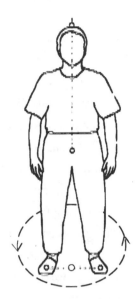

Figure 7. Circle That Arises from Stillness

Bodymind Healing Purpose: Research has shown that this "nonmovement" posture increases the coherence in the brain between the two frontal regions, between two occipital regions, and between the left and right temporal areas.[3] This practice is also called Wuji Standing Meditation. *Wuji* means "the void," or the mother of Qi, so this posture is considered one of the best ways to fill your "Qi bank account." Stillness is a powerful way to activate the Qi and is also a way of bringing up the psychological and physical issues that block the Qi. By being with our Selves, we initiate a pattern of alchemical transformation that over time dissolves chronic body blockages. During this process, tingling, vibrating, shaking, and sensations of asymmetry may occur as blocks in the rivers of Qi shake loose. Do not be alarmed, just breathe through these sensations, practice the Circle That Arises from Stillness, or take a break and come back to the practice when you are ready. All these Qi activation signs are ways that the Qi is healing old areas of blockage. Eventually this method

333

may lead you to experience the Sea of Elixir—an experience of dissolving into that sea of cosmic bliss (altered state of consciousness) spoken of in the Taoist text *The Secret of the Golden Flower* (Wilhelm, 1963).

B. HOLDING GOLDEN BALLS IN THE WATERS OF LIFE

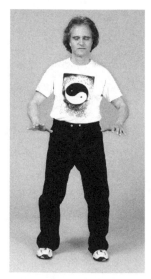

Figure 8. Holding Golden Balls in the Waters of Life

While using the same stance as in the previous Standing Meditation, allow your wrists to rise and then, with palms down, descend down to the belly area (Tan Tien). Then imagine that you are standing in a slowly moving river, your palms are slightly compressing two balls down into the water with just enough pressure so that they are steadied from floating downstream. The energy in your feet sinks down into the streambed, and your knees bend just so much that you take root, which prevents the river from moving you downstream. Stand in this posture for as long as is comfortable (initially two to four minutes). If it starts to feel difficult, listen to your body, allow another few exhalations, and return back to Wuji Standing Meditation Posture 1 to refill your Qi bank account.

Bodymind Healing Purpose: This stance comes from *Yi* (intention) *Chuan* (fist, or ability to hold the power of the five elements in your fist) Qigong. One way to use your intention while you are Holding Golden Balls is to imagine that you are sending healing energy from your palms (*Lao Gong* points) to some part of the earth that is in need of healing. Imagine that you are sending energy there on your exhalation and replenishing yourself on the inhalation. This is a favored practice of bodyworkers, acupuncturists (who use the posture to focus their intention on sending energy through the needles), and for healers in general. This posture is also a favored stance for developing *fongsung*—the Chinese term for relaxed alertness. This state of *fongsung* can be seen in cats when they appear simultaneously very relaxed yet ready to pounce.

C. FINDING YOUR OWN STANCE

There are infinite ways to discover your true Being, but love holds the brightest torch. If you follow it, you will be guided beyond the limits of age and death. Come out of the circle of time, and find yourself in the circle of love.

—Deepak Chopra
  Ageless Body, Timeless Mind

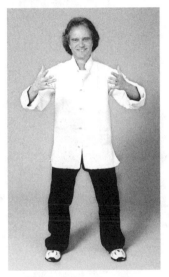 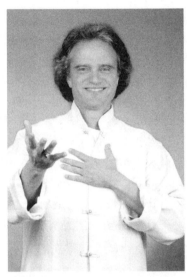

Figure 9. Opening the Golden Ball of Your Heart

Figure 10. Feeding the World with Your Heart (Wild Goose Says Hello)

Find your own Standing Meditation posture that expresses the stance you need at this moment. Two potential stances you can choose are pictured here. Both are good for replenishing your heart's energy.[4]

2. Dispersing Stagnant Qi

After Standing Meditation, it is important to disperse stagnant Qi. Begin with your hands by your sides as in Standing Meditation—while breathing in, raise your hands to the sides, palms up, until they are outstretched over your head. As your palms face the top of your head, stop and breathe nice long exhalations. Imagine that your right and left hands are like electromagnets with a yang (right hand) and yin (left hand) polarity. You might imagine that any stagnant energy remaining on your skin after standing is like iron filings. Very slowly and while you are breathing, allow your hands to gradually descend about six inches from your body while the iron filings jump onto the electro-magnet from the magnetic attraction.

When you reach the bottom, with your hands by your sides, turn off the electromagnet by letting go with a few long out-breaths.

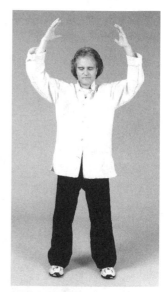

Imagine that the iron filings are turning into molten lava and seeping back to the iron at the core of the earth. Dispersing Stagnant Qi is done three times: first to cleanse the skin, second to cleanse the internal organs, and third to wash the bone marrow. Other Dispersing Stagnant Qi exercises include massaging and tapping the body, and tapping your toes against the ground—as hoofed animals do when they have stood too long in one place.[5]

Figure 11. Dispersing Stagnant Qi

Bodymind Healing Purpose: According to modern physics, human beings are condensed light. When the light of the universe condenses in our bodies and takes on our emotional and physical blockages, it acts like logjams blocking the free flow of a river. Standing Meditation can constellate and make us aware of these places of stagnant Qi. Dissolving and Dispersing Stagnant Qi exercises can loosen the logjams and allow the river of life to flow again, to evaporate into water vapor, and to transform into space. By moving back and forth from Standing Meditation to Dispersing Stagnant Qi exercises, we return to our source as the Beings of light we are. In this exercise, the movement of the hands down the body while focusing on the exhalation is used for those suffering from hypertension to help cleanse the body of stress and help sink the Qi. The sink-ing of the Qi is accomplished by focusing on the downward movements of the hands while exhaling with long-breath. Johnson (2000) suggests for hypertension that the practitioner imagines sending Qi down the Gall Bladder meridian. For more about Qigong and hypertension, see Chapter Eleven.

3. Tai Chi Ruler

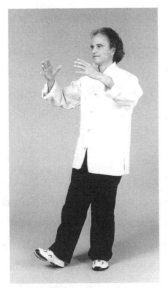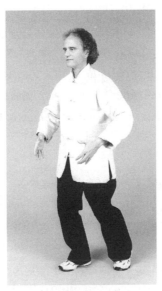

Figure 12. Tai Chi Ruler—Drawing in Healing Energy

Figure 13. Tai Chi Ruler—Releasing Toxic/Stagnant Energy

Place the right foot slightly in front of the left. The left foot is at a forty-five-degree angle and your left big toe is aligned with the middle of the right foot. Keep a fist's distance between the extended backward line of the right foot and the left heel, so there is sufficient width between your feet.

Slowly rock backward onto your left foot and inhale while your left knee bends and your right toes rise off the ground. Next, breathe out as you rock forward while your back, left heel rises naturally off the ground. Repeat until you feel the sensation of filling and emptying your forward and rear foot, in turn. Your weight, when forward, should be over your right foot, knee bent. When your weight is on your left, back foot, your bent knee approaches being over the front of your foot. Be careful not to extend your forward knee beyond your front toes.

Now integrate hand movements: Place your hands about six to eight inches apart, palms facing each other as if you have a ball between your hands. Your hands should be far enough apart so that the upper arms allow space for imaginary little balls to fit in the armpits. As you rock forward, allow the hands to come down to three fingers distance below the navel. As you rock backward, the hands come up and circle inward, toward the heart. As your hands rise up and inward, you might want to imagine bringing the loving energy of the universe into your heart, as you say I'm bringing in the fresh. As you exhale and breathe out, your hands come down, as if laying a ball filled with your troubles or dis-eases as you say I'm letting go of the stale. After about twelve repetitions on one side, switch which leg is forward and repeat the movement to ensure balance between the right and left sides of the body.

Bodymind Healing Purpose: As you practice on the right side, you can practice healing a life issue that has been difficult for you—recharging your Self on the in-breath and letting go of tension on the out-breath. As you practice on the left side, create a healing ritual during which you put a problematic body part or chronic disease into the center of the circle you are making that circulates the energy of the universe through you to lead you back into balance with the healing elements of the universe. This movement is also used for reversing the fear response of the body and balancing sympathetic nervous system over-arousal by focusing on sinking the energy of the body to the lower back (Ming Men) simultaneously with the hands raising up to the top of your circle of movement. For those suffering from trauma (or for all of us involved with the mini-traumas of everyday life), this movement can be helpful to help us let go of stress and re-empower ourselves when used in conjunction with other appropriate psychological healing methods.

4. Ocean Wave Breathing

After you have practiced Standing Meditation for some time, you will begin to feel a natural rocking movement that synchronizes with your breathing. You may notice that your weight shifts back to the heels as you inhale and that your weight naturally shifts onto the balls of the feet as you exhale. From our earli-

est experiences of being rocked in the cradle, rocking is a primordial way to energize, heal, and soothe
the bodymind.

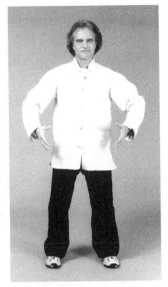

*Place your outstretched hands, palms facing each other,
in front of your belly. Experiment with synchronizing your hand movements outward and inward from
your belly with your breath. It is as if you are blowing
up a balloon and then allowing it to naturally inflate
and deflate. As the body rocks backward, the breath
goes in, and your hands go outward, expanding your
ball. As the body rocks forward, the hands come in
and the breath goes out, collapsing your ball. As you
continue to inhale and exhale, make the arm motions
larger and larger.*

Figure 14. Ocean Wave Breathing

Bodymind Healing Purpose: This practice can be done with hands in front of
the belly or the heart. The belly area (Tan Tien) is the physical center of the
body where heaven and earth meet. While practicing Ocean Wave Breathing
be aware of how you have been off center this week and allow this movement
to recharge and expand your center where heaven and earth join their creative
forces. If you do the practice with hands holding the ball in front of your heart,
imagine recharging "the battery of your heart" as you are doing your expanding and gathering motions.

5. Moving a Snake through the Joints, Dipping Your Hands into the Waters of Life, and Opening Your Heart to the Heavens

*Keep your legs spread wider than in other Bodymind Healing Qigong movements.
As you shift to the right side, your right palm faces out next to the right thigh
and the back of the left hand slides up your left thigh. Then shift your weight
back to the left side as your left palm faces up by your left leg while the back of
your right palm slides up the right side of your leg. Practice this movement with
focus on the hips first, then at the shoulder level. This exercise is paired with the*

339

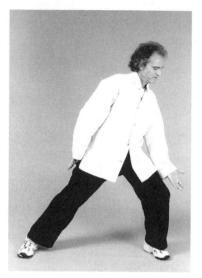 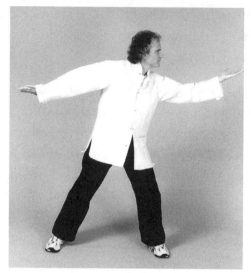

Figure 15. Moving a Snake through the Hip Joint

Figure 16. Moving a Snake through the Shoulder Joint

exercise Dipping Your Hands into the Waters of Life in which you bend forward, as your shoulders rotate forward and your palms face upward. Then bend backward, Opening Your Heart to the Heavens, as you face up toward the sky at about a forty-five-degree angle with your palms facing upward (for illustration, see Bodymind Healing Qigong DVD [Mayer, 2000]). Finally, return back to the hips, but this time focus on moving a spiral through any body part that is problematic. As you spiral a snake through your joints, imagine your spiraling movement going all the way up to the galactic spirals and all the way down to the spiraling forces in the molten core of the earth. Imagine your problematic body part is just a little point in the spiraling forces of life. At the end of this exercise, as your hands move up and down your legs, make smaller and smaller spirals until there is no movement at all. Can you experience the spiral in your stillness?

In the Taoist tradition it is said that when you can find the stillness in the movement and movement in the stillness that health and the experience of light in the body can be found. As you are residing in stillness, you might imagine the spiraling DNA that forms a double helix at the center of your cells vibrating though you are still and that your cells are electro-magnetic receivers and senders ("nano-

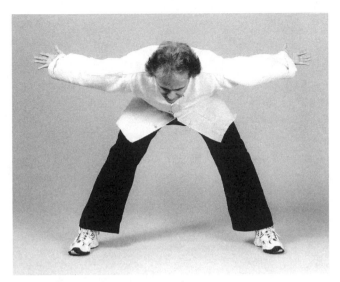

Figure 17. Dipping Your Hands into the Waters of Life

antennas") connected with the wider healing forces of the universe—modern science confirms both of these are facts (Lipton, 2005).

Bodymind Healing Purpose: This three-movement sequence (Moving a Snake through the Joints, Dipping Your Hands into the Waters of Life, and Opening Your Heart to the Heavens) is an excellent preventative and a complementary treatment for joint, hip, and shoulder problems. It is also useful for chronic diseases that relate to a sedentary lifestyle. The practice, in particular when you go back and forth from movement to stillness, is excellent for activating and filling the reservoir of your energy field.

6. Crane Walking and Flying

This is one of a series of Animal Qigong movements based on the Chinese five elements—wood, fire, earth, metal, and water—each of which corresponds to particular organs of the body. For this fire posture:

Step out at a forty-five-degree angle and cross your arms in front of your heart.
As your hands rise up and one leg rises up, keep your toe still touching the ground

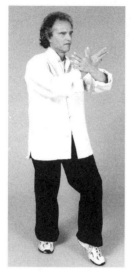

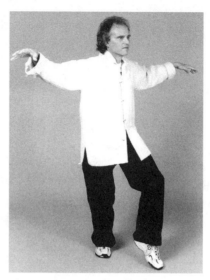

Figure 18. Crane Crosses Wings

Figure 19. Crane Walking

as you become a Crane Walking. When your hands descend they can come to your sides or all the way down (or cross over) in front of your belly where they gather Qi. Synchronize the movement with your breath and repeat on right and left sides approximately four times. (The Taoist method of training is to progress slowly to avoid injury or strain; therefore, we do Crane Walking before practicing the next movements.)

After sufficient strength is built up from Crane Walking, you can become like a Crane Flying: Again, step out at a forty-five-degree angle (as done in Crane Walking); but this time on the inhalation, lift your knee along with raising your arms, so that the knee begins to approach being parallel to your hip. Then as you exhale allow the hands to descend as if they are sinking down in water.

Practice on both right and left sides and allow the fingertips to flutter slightly as they rise up to activate Qi. Eventually to strengthen the legs more, hold your posture in the arms-raised position for one to five exhalations.

During these Crane exercises, experiment with using the sound ha (vocally or sub-vocally) on the exhalation to relax the heart (for hypertension), and to increase the energy of the heart (for hypotension) use the sound heng on the inhalation. While being in touch with the life issues in your heart, feel and imagine the healing powers of the Crane bringing your heart back into balance.

Bodymind Healing Purpose: The Animal Frolics were created in the second century AD by Chinese physician Hua Tuo who synthesized the shamanic knowledge of the healing power of the elements with Chinese medicine. In the Crane postures, we are given a way to feel the Qi rise from the earth to lighten

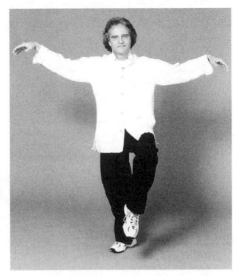

Figure 20. Crane Flying

the heart, and we are given a way to increase our balance. An article in the *Journal of the American Medical Association,* Province et al. (1995) showed that Tai Chi was a more effective system for preventing falls amongst the elderly than many Western exercise systems. For those with balance problems or with limitations in leg strength, move slowly in your lifelong cultivation practice of Crane Walking in order to develop the proper leg strength before moving on to Crane Flying. Listen to your body about how long to hold the Crane Flying posture with your hands raised. Follow the Taoist axiom "less is more" to avoid injury and to cultivate your Qi. Also, as we see from the descriptions above, the Crane is used to help heal the energy of the heart.

7. Walking Meditation Qigong

Start with your posture as in the Wuji Standing Meditation posture (see Figure 5) at the beginning of this chapter. While standing, slowly shift your weight from one leg to the other. First, your weight is equally balanced; then very gradually, shift your weight back and forth from right and left until you can support 100 percent of your weight on each leg as the other leg slowly comes in to join it. While sup-

porting all weight on one leg, move the other leg forward in a crescent moon step. Gradually put down your weight— putting first 5 percent, then 10 percent, until the weight is 100 percent over that foot. Then do the same with your next step. Breathe in as you bring one foot closer to the ankle of the other and synchronize your exhalation with step- ping down. The spirit of

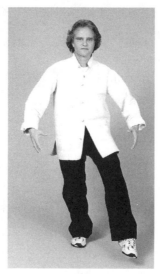

Figure 21. Walking Medi- tation Qigong—Holding the Golden Ball

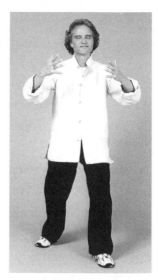

Figure 22. Walking Meditation Qigong— Opening the Heart

your walking is like a stalking cat. Walk as if there is sandpaper under your shoes and you are sanding a deck. For those who have difficulty walking, are recovering from sports injuries, or suffer from chronic movement disorders, try doing this Walking Meditation with a chair next to you for added support. Prac- tice walking forward and backward. Eventually you walk while imagining hold- ing a ball in various ways; for example, under your hands as in Holding Golden Balls in the Waters of Life posture (see Figure 8). While stepping down, exhale and press the palms down toward the earth and say, "I let go of the stale," or "I give to the earth." Inhale as you bring one foot closer to the ankle of the other and let the wrists rise as you say, "I take in the fresh" or "I bring in the healing energies of the earth."

Bodymind Healing Purpose: Walking Meditation is excellent for those who have difficulty walking, are recovering from sports injuries, or suffer from joint dis- eases or chronic movement disorders—such as Parkinson's disease or multiple sclerosis. Walking Mediation is an integral component of the Yi Chuan Stand- ing Meditation Qigong tradition. Walking Meditation is a self-healing and spir-

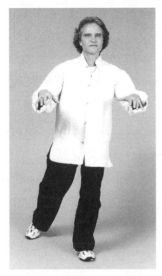

Figure 23. Walking Meditation Qigong—Drawing in Energy from the Earth

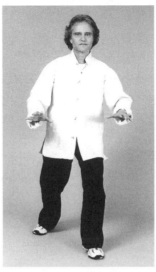

Figure 24. Walking Meditation Qigong—Giving Energy to the Earth

itual practice for carrying the Qi that you have developed in Standing Mediation to test *(shili)* whether your Qi "breaks"—a metaphor for keeping the centeredness that you have cultivated in the stillness of Standing Meditation.

8. End Your Routine with the Wuji Standing Meditation Posture

It is most helpful to end your routine returning to the Wuji Standing Meditation posture. In cross-cultural mythic terms, Wuji Standing activates "the myth of the eternal return" (Eliade & Trask, 1954); that is, renewing your Self by reestablishing a connection to the source of healing energy in the cosmos. After moving, we return to stillness to honor the Taoist precept: healing energy comes from progressing from

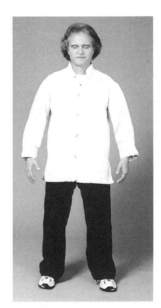

Figure 25. Wuji Standing Meditation Qigong

stillness to movement, then back to stillness. The key is to find the stillness in movement, and the movement in stillness.

I am often asked how long one should do each of these practices. The answer is that I do not know how long you should do each of them ... but you do. Please listen to your bodymind.

AFTERWORD

Reflections: At the Source of the Stream of Modern Psychology

Earlier, I told the story of how I learned in my master's degree program that psychology began in Wilhelm Wundt's laboratory in Leipzig, Germany, in 1879. This left me wondering about psychology's origins before that time in one man's laboratory.

I asked and explored the question: What is the source of the stream of thought that has become *psychology*? As I went on a journey upstream, I found a world-wide river system of ancient sacred wisdom traditions. I found that astrological metaphors were used to help people connect their personal identities with the universe of which we are all a part. I stripped the astrological language of its deterministic leanings in *The Mystery of Personal Identity* (Mayer, 1984). In the process of integrating this language with transpersonal psychology, I showed how this ancient tradition could be re-visioned in such a way that it could answer critics' concern that astrology could be used as an excuse for one's neurosis and lead to faulty deterministic thinking that would rob a person of his or her own will. By so doing, I showed how astrological language could become palatable even to skeptics. I demonstrated how astrological language could be incorporated into depth psychotherapy to help people find new meaning by seeing how personal identity is connected with the wider whole of which we are a part.

As I continued my journey upstream I found that ancient Greek mythology and the art of storytelling represented some of the oldest forms of psychological healing and could transform the way people look at their problems. The book I wrote at that time, *Trials of the Heart: Healing the Wounds of Intimacy* (1993), culminated in the Mythic Journey Process, which showed how to use ancient myths to heal modern-day problems. Throughout my journey, I was humbled and overwhelmed by the number of rivers of knowledge that could bring refreshing perspectives from the lands of our psychotherapeutic ancestors. I wondered why people downstream did not seem to know about these healing rivers, and why these methods were not more incorporated into the education of modern therapists.

For example, alchemy contains rich metaphors for the various phases of the metallic and psychological processes for turning lead into gold, and for the soul's journey of self-healing (Edinger, 1985). In the Kabbalah of the Jewish tradition, one of the earliest forms of energy psychology talked about how the energy of the universe that is expressed in the archetypes of the "tree of life" comes from *ain soph* (the void, the source of creation, similar to the Chinese concept of *wuji); and the Jewish prayerful *davening* tradition (rocking back and forth while praying) has songs to help virtually every affliction, such as loss of power and lack of being able to cope with life. Other Jewish sacred songs help the daveners to dissolve into the love of the universe and connect with the source of life's energy. Singing chants and songs from ancient sacred wisdom traditions can add to other psychological inner work similar to the way that energy psychology traditions use humming to help heal the present-day psyche. I have spoken about how the roots of Buddhism contained a tradition of postural initiation that combined "dissolving" practices and working with the *klesas* (emotional issues) on the path to psychospiritual health. In *Secrets to Living Younger Longer* (2004b), I showed how the traditions of postural initiation and energy healing are part of a worldwide cross-cultural river system of healing the psyche in Greece; Native America; India; as well as in China, through its tradition of Qigong. Among the deep, lost rivers of ancient psychological knowledge that I discovered on my journey were the ancient mythologies of shape-shifting, which contain metaphors for using the imagination to aid the process of psychological transformation. Combining somatic practices, such as Qigong, with these cross-cultural, shape-shifting healing methods helped my patients, students, and me to draw from the elements needed to heal our relationship with our primordial Selves.

And we should remember that beyond all traditions, at the source of all rivers and at the deepest origins of the stream of psychology is a fundamental truth that healing comes from the elements themselves, each of which are expressions of the awe-inspiring, loving energies of the universe ... that some call God.

The Deva That Sits at the Place Where Two Streams Become One

In the past, Western culture has looked at the practices and philosophies of indigenous cultures as "less than" Western medicine and psychology. We have treated these age-old practices with an attitude similar to the way the missionaries treated the practices of Native Americans. In midst of the current healthcare crisis, we may do well to investigate and incorporate the teachings of ancient lineages into our current medical and psychological methodologies. By doing so, we honor our ancestors and colleagues who learned to heal from traveling pretechnological pathways. By not including ancient sacred wisdom traditions into our approach to healing the psyche, we commit a crime analogous to our cultures' running over the Native Americans. We get to occupy the land, but we lose the sacred knowledge of how to be with its treasures.

One of the treasures coming from the land of ancient psychology—the psychology of the "soul"[1]—is the notion that there is a *deva* in every location in the natural world. Another name for devas are *elementals,* because they carry the healing powers of the elements of nature (Jung, 1974). It is said that every deva has a form, usually feminine, that communicates to those who listen. There are devas of the waters—*nereads*, devas of the air—*sylphs*, and devas of the earth—*dryads*. These devas are specific to locale, and not being "major deities," they are more humble, more down to earth, and have more intimate personal messages to give us. The male counterpart to devas are *daimons*, such as Eros, god of erotic love. Devas and daimons occupy a mythic place on the ladder of creation in that they are not gods, yet they are not human beings either—they are beings that travel between the two realms of heaven and earth. Being in touch with their attributes can help us humans to journey in that space.

On one level, this book is a communication from "the deva where two streams become one." Before you dismiss this notion as archaic or smile thinking this idea is quaint, instead, allow yourself to wonder about the places in nature that have drawn you to them and meditate upon what message is waiting to be drawn from that place in nature. We don't call our deepest ways of being "human nature" for nothing. We are inextricably connected with nature; and our own healing, our life energy, and our messages for humankind come from this connection with the wider whole of which we are a part.

REFERENCES

Abbott, R. B., et al. (2007). A randomized controlled trial of Tai Chi for tension headaches, *Evidence Based Complementary and Alternative Medicine*, March 4 (1), pp. 107–113.

Achterberg, J. (1985). *Imagery in healing: Shamanism and modern medicine.* Boston: New Science Library.

Achterberg, J., Dosey, L., Gordon, J. S., Hegedus, C., Hermann, M. W., & Nelson, R. (1992). Mind-body interventions in alternative medicine. *Expanding medical horizons: A report to the National Institute of Health on alternative medical systems and practices in the United States.* Washington, DC: USGPO.

Achterberg, J., Dossey, B., & Kolkmeier, L. (1994). *Rituals of healing: Using imagery for health and wellness.* New York: Bantam Books.

Ader, R., & Felton, D. (1991). *Psychoneuroimmunology.* San Diego, CA: Academic Press.

Alexander, C., & Langer, E. (1990). *Higher stages of human development.* New York: Oxford University Press.

Alexander, C., Langer, E., Newman, T., Chandler, H., & Davies, J. (1989). Transcendental meditation, mindfulness, and longevity. *Journal of Personality and Social Psychology, 58,* 950–964.

Alexander, C., Reinforth, M., & Gelderloos, P. (1991). Transcendental meditation, self-actualization and psychological health. *Journal of Social Behavior and Personality, 6,* 186–247.

Allen, J. J. B., Schnyer, R. N., & Hitt, S. K. (1998). The efficacy of acupuncture in the treatment of major depression in women. *Psychological Science, 9*(5), 397–401.

Almas, A. H. (1988). *The pearl beyond price.* Berkeley, CA: Diamond Books.

Alpert, R. (also known as Ram Dass) (1971). *Be here now.* San Cristobal, NM: Lama Foundation.

Altrocchi, J. (1994). Non-drug treatment of anxiety, *American Family Physician, 10,* 161–166.

American Psychiatric Association. (2000). *Diagnostic and statistical manual of mental disorders* (4th ed). Washington, DC: Author.

Anand, B. K., Chhina, G. S., & Singh, B. (1961). Some aspects of EEG studies in yogis. *Electroencephalography & Clinical Neurophysiology, 13,* 452–456.

Anderson, C. (2000). What's new in pain management? *Home Healthcare Nurse, 18*(10), 648–658.

Andrade, J., & Feinstein, D. (2004). Energy psychology: Theory, indications, evidence. In D. Feinstein, *Energy psychology interactive.* (Appendix, pp. 199–214). Ashland, OR: Innersource.

Andreson, J. (2000). Medicine meets behavioral medicine. *Journal of Consciousness Studies, 7,* 17–24.

Andreychuk, T., & Skriver, C. (1975). Hypnosis and biofeedback in the treatment of migraine headache. *International Journal of Clinical Experimental Hypnosis, 23,* 172–183.

Archart-Treichel, J. (2003). Efficacy evidence builds for vagus nerve procedure. *Psychiatric News, 38*(17), 26.

Arguelles, J. (1972). *Mandala.* Berkeley, CA: Shambhala.

Arkowitz, H., & Mannon, B. (2002). A cognitive-behavioral assimilative integration. In F. Lebow (Ed.). *Comprehensive handbook of psychotherapy, 4* (pp. 317–337). New York: Wiley.

Arthur, J. (2000). *Mushrooms and mankind: The impact of mushrooms on human consciousness and religion.* Escondido, CA: The Book Tree.

Asch, S. (1955). On the use of metaphor in the description of persons. In H. Werner (Ed.), *On expressive language.* Worcester, MA: Clark University Press.

Assagioli, R. (1965). *Psychosynthesis.* New York: Viking Press.

Assagioli, R. (1991). *Transpersonal development: The dimension beyond psychosynthesis.* London: Crucible.

Astin, J. A., Berman, B. M., Bausell, B., Lee, W. L., Hochberg, M., & Forys, K. L. (2003, October). The efficacy of mindfulness meditation plus Qigong movement therapy in the treatment of fibromyalgia: A randomized controlled trial. *Journal of Rheumatology, 30*(10), 2257–62.

Astin, J. A., Shapiro, S. L., & Schwartz, G. E. (2000). Meditation. In D. Novey (Ed.) *Clinician's rapid access guide to complementary and alternative medicine.* St. Louis, MO: Mosby. {As cited in Pelletier K. (2004), p. 28.}

Ausubel, K. (2000). *When healing becomes a crime.* Rochester, VT: Healing Arts Press.

Baer, R. (2003). Mindfulness training as a clinical intervention. A conceptual and empirical review. *Clinical Psychology: Science and Practice, 10,* 125–143.

Baggott, A. (1999). *The encyclopedia of energy healing: A complete guide to using the major forms of healing for the body, mind and spirit.* New York: Godsfield Press.

Baker, A. H., & Carrington, P. (2005). *A comment on Waite and Holder's research supposedly invalidating EFT.* Retrieved from www.energypsych.org/research-critique-eft.htm

Baker, A. H., & Siegel, L. S. (2005). *Can a 45 minute session of EFT lead to reduction of intense fear of rats, spiders, and water bugs?* A replication and extension of the Wells et al. (2003) laboratory study. Manuscript in preparation.

Bandler, R., & Grinder, J. (1975). *The structure of magic.* Palo Alto, CA: Science and Behavior Books.

Bandler, R., & Grinder, J. (1979). *Frogs into princes: Neuro-linguistic programming.* Moab UT: Real People Press.

Bandler, R., & Grinder, J. (1981). *Trance-formations: Neurolinguistic programming and the structure of hypnosis.* Moab, UT: Real People Press.

Barber, T. (1978). Hypnosis, suggestion, and psychosomatic phenomena: A new look from the standpoint of recent experimental studies. *American Journal of Clinical Hypnosis, 21*(1), 13–27.

Barber, T., & Meyer, D. (1984). Changing unchangeable bodily processes by (hypnotic) suggestions: A new look at hypnosis, cognitions, imaging and the mind body problem. *Advances, 1*(2), 7–40.

Barcia, R. C. (1972). Effects of rupture of membranes on fetal heart rate pattern. *International Journal of Gynecology and Obstetrics, (19)*, 169. In J. Robbins (1996), *Reclaiming our Health: Exploding the medical myth and embracing the source of true healing* (p. 47). Tiburon, CA: H. J. Kramer.

Barefoot, J. C., Dahlstrom, W. G., & Wiliams R. B. (1983). *Psychosomatic Medicine, 45*, 50–63.

Barnes, P. M., Powell-Griner, E., McFann, K., & Nahin R. L. (2004). Complementary and alternative medicine use among adults. United States: Centers for Disease Control and Prevention National Center for Health Statistics. Advance Data, No. 343, (2002, May 27).

Barring, A., & Cashford, C. (1991). *The myth of the goddess: Evolution of an image.* London: Viking Arkana.

Basmajian, J. V. (1963, August). Control and training of individual motor units, *Science*(2): 440–441.

Beck, A. T. (1979). *Cognitive therapy of depression.* New York: Guilford Press.

Becker, R. (1985). *The body electric: Electromagnetism and the foundation of life.* New York: William Morrow.

Becker, R. (1990). *Cross currents: The promise of electro medicine.* San Diego, CA: Jeremy P. Tarcher.

Becker, R., Spadao, J., Marino, A. (1977). Clinical experiences with low intensity direct current stimulation of bone growth. *Clinical Orthopedics and Related Research, 124*, 75–83.

Benor, D. (2008, in press) *7 minutes to natural pain release: WHEE for tapping your pain away—The revolutionary new self-healing method,* Fulton, CA: Energy Psychology Press.

Benor, K. J. (1992). *Healing research: Holistic energy medicine and spirituality* (Vol. 1). Munich, Germany: Helix Verlag.

Benson, H. (1975a). *The maximum mind.* New York: Avon.

Benson, H. (1975b). *The relaxation response.* New York: Avon.

Benson, H. (1983a). The relaxation response and norepinephrine: A new study illuminates mechanisms. *Integrative Psychiatry, 1,* 15–18.

Benson, H. (1983b, July). The relaxation response: Its subjective and objective historical precedents and physiology. *Trends in Neuroscience,* 281–284.

Benson, H. (1984). *Beyond the relaxation response.* New York: Avon.

Benson, H., Rosner, B.A., & Marzetta, B.R. (1973). Decreased systolic BP in hypertensive subjects who practice meditation. *Journal of Clinical Investigation, 52,* 80.

Bettleheim, B. (1977). *The uses of enchantment.* New York: Vintage Press.

Bingham, A. (2000). A phenomenological investigation of the experience of being under the influence of prozac. *A dissertation for The California Institute of Integral Studies.*

Black, A. (1994, December). The drugging of America's children. *Redbook.*

Blount, A. (Ed.). (1998). *Integrated primary care: The future of mental health collaboration,* New York: W. W. Norton.

Bly, R. (1975). *A little book on the human shadow.* San Francisco: Harper and Row.

Bly, R. (1990). *Iron John: A book about men.* New York: Addison Wesley.

Bogart, G. (1991). Meditation and psychotherapy: A review of the literature. *The American Journal of Psychotherapy, XLV(3),* 383.

Bohm, D., and Peat, F.D. (1997) *Infinite potential: The life and times of Davic Bohm.* New York: Basic Books.

Bowlby, J. (1969). *Attachment and loss, Vol. I: Attachment.* New York: Basic Books.

Brattberg, F. (2008). Self-administered EFT (Emotional Freedom Techniques) in individuals with fibromyalgia: A randomized trial. *Integrative Medicine,* Vol. 7, No 4 (Aug/Sept).

Braun, B. (1983). Psychophysiological phenomena in multiple personality and hypnosis, *American Journal of Clinical Hypnosis,* Vol. 26, pp.124–35.

Braun, B. G. (1979). Hypnotherapy for Raynaud's disease. In G. D. Burrows, D. R. Collison, & L. Dennerstein, L. (Eds.), *Hypnosis* (pp. 141–156). Amsterdam: Elsevier/North-Holland Biomedical Press.

Breggin, P. (1991). *Toxic psychiatry.* New York: St. Martin's Press.

Breggin, P. (2001). *The anti-depressant fact book.* Cambridge, MA: Perseus Pub.

Brennan, B. (1990). *Hands of light.* New York: Bantam.

Briere, J. (1992). Theory and treatment of severe sexual abuse trauma. An overview. Presented at the Orange County CA Annual Child Abuse Conference, Anaheim, CA.

Briere, J. (1997). *Psychological assessment of adult post-traumatic states.* Washington, DC: American Psychological Association.

Brown, J. W., Robertson, L. S., Kosa, J., & Alpert, J. J. (1971). A study of general practice in Massachusetts. *Journal of the American Medical Association, 216,* 301–306.

Bugental, J. G. (1978). *Psychotherapy and process: The fundamentals of an existential-humanistic approach.* Reading, MA: Addison-Wesley.

Burini, D., et al. (2006). A randomized controlled cross-over trial of aerobic training versus Qigong in advanced Parkinson's disease. *Eura Medicophys.* September, 42 (3), 231–8.

Burckhardt, C. S, Clark, S. R., Bennett, R. M. (1991). The fibromyalgia impact questionnaire: Development and validation, *Journal of Rheumatology*, Vol. 18.

Burr, H. S. (1972). *The fields of life.* New York: Ballantine.

Burr, H.S., & Northrup, F.S. (1935). The electro-dynamic theory of life. *Quarterly Review of Biology,* 10, 322–333.

Cahn, R., & Polich, J. (2006). Meditation states and traits: EEG, ERP and neuroimaging studies. *Psychological Bulletin. 132,* 180–211.

Cai, S. F. (1986). *Wujishi breathing exercise.* Translated by M. Den. Revised by T. Shen. Hong Kong, China: Medicine & Health Publishing Co.

Callahan, R. (1985). *Five minute phobia cure.* Wilmington, DE: Enterprise.

Callahan, R. (2001). *Tapping the healer within.* Chicago, IL: Contemporary Books.

Campbell, J. (1978). *The mysteries: Papers from the eranos yearbooks* (Bolingen Series XXX). Princeton, NJ: Princeton University Press.

Campbell, J. (1988). *Historical atlas of world mythology: The way of the animal powers* (Vol. 1). New York: Perennial Library.

Cannon, W. (1914). The inter-relationship of emotions as suggested by recent physiologial research. *American Journal of Psychology, 25,* 256.

Canter, P., & Ernst, E. (2003). The cumulative effects of transcendental meditation on cognitive function: A systematic review of randomized controlled trials. *Wiener Klinische Wochenschrift, 115,* 758–766.

Capra, F. (1975). *The tao of physics.* Boulder, CO: Shambhala.

Carbonell, J. (1997). An experimental study of TFT and acrophobia. *The Thought Field, 2* (3), 1–6.

Carbonell, J. L., & Figley, C. (1999). A systematic clinical demonstration project of promising PTSD treatment approaches. *Traumatology,* 5(1), Article 4. Retrieved from www.fsu.edu/~trauma

Carey, B. (2005, October 18). Can brain scans see depression? *New York Times.* Retrieved from www.nytimes.com/2005/10/18/health/psychology

Carlson, L. E., Speca, M., Patl, K. D., & Goodey, E. (2003). Mindfulness based stress reduction in relation to quality of life, mood, symptoms of stress and immune parameters in breast and prostrate cancer outpatients. *Psychosomatic Medicine. 65,* 572–581.

Case, P. (1976). *The great seal of the United States: Its history, symbolism, and message for the new age.* Santa Barbara, CA: J. F. Rowny Press.

Chambless, D. L., & Hollon, S. D. (1998). Defining empirically supported therapies. *Journal of consulting and clinical psychology, 66,* 7–18.

Cheek, D. (1969). Communication with the critically ill. *The American Journal of Clinical Hypnosis, 12*(2), 75–85.

Chen, G. S. (1990). The effect of acupuncture treatment on carpal tunnel syndrome. *American Journal of Acupuncture, 18,* 5–9.

Chen H. H., Yeh, M. L., & Lee, F. Y. (2006). The effects of baguanjin Qigong in the prevention of bone loss for middle-aged women, *American Journal of Chinese Medicine,* Vol. 34 (5): 741–7.

Chen, K., & Yeung, R. (2002). A review of Qigong therapy for cancer treatment. *Journal of International Society of Life Information Science* (ISLIS), *Vol. 20*(2), 532–542.

Cheney, R. (1996). *Akashic records: Past lives and new directions.* Upland, CA: Astara.

Cheung, B. M. (2005). Randomized controlled trial of qigong in the treatment of mild essential hypertension. *Journal Hum Hypertension,* 19: 697–704.

Chia, M. (1986). *Iron Shirt Chi Kung I.* Huntington, NY: Healing Tao Books.

Chia, M., & Chia, M. (1990). *Chi Nei Tsang: Internal organ massage.* Huntington, NY: Healing Tao Books.

Cho, Z. H., Chung, J. P., Jones, J. B., Park, H. J., Lee, H. J., Wong, E. K., & Min, B. I. (1998). New findings of the correlation between acu-points and corresponding brain cortices using functions MRI. *Proceedings of the National Academy of Science,* March 3, *95,* 267–73.

Chopra, D. (1990). *Quantum healing: Exploring the frontiers of mind/body medicine.* New York: Bantam Books.

Chuen, L. K. (1991). *The way of energy.* London: Gaia Books.

Chuen, L. K. (1999). *The way of healing: Chi Kung.* New York: Broadway Books.

Cleary, T. (1991). *The secret of the golden flower.* San Francisco: Harper Collins.

Clinton, A. (2002). Seemorg matrix work. In F. Gallo (Ed.), *Energy psychology in psychotherapy:A comprehensive source book.* New York: W. W. Norton.

Cohen, K. (1997). *The way of Qigong.* New York: Ballentine Books.

Cohen, S., & Herbert, T. B. (1998). *Psychosomatic medicine.* Paper presented at the annual meeting of the American Heart Association. Published 1993, Stress and immunity in humans: A meta-analytic review. *Psychosomatic Medicine, 55*(4), 364–379.

Colum, P. (1944). *The complete Grimm's fairy tales.* New York: Pantheon.

Conn, L., & Mott, T. (1984). Plethysmographic demonstration of rapid vasodilation by direct suggestion: A case of Raynaud's disease treated by hypnosis. *The American Journal of Clinical Hypnosis, 26*(3), 166–170.

Corbin, H. (2001). *History of Islamic philosophy.* New York: Kegan Paul.

Cortwright, B. (2007, in press). *Integral psychology.* New York: SUNY Press.

Craig, G. (2004). *Emotional freedom techniques manual.* From http://www.emofree.com.

Craig, G., & Fowlie, A. (1995; 1997). *Emotional Freedom Techniques: The manual.* Sea Ranch, CA: Author.

Crasilneck, H. B., & Hall J. A. (1985). *Clinical hypnosis: Principles and applications.* Orlando, FL: Grune & Stratton.

Creamer, P., Singh, B. B., Hochberg, M. C., & Berman, B. M. (2000). Sustained improvement produced by nonpharmacologic intervention in fibromyalgia: Results of a pilot study. *Arthritis Care Research, 13*(4), 198–204.

Crown, D. P., & Marlow, D. (1960). A new scale of social desirability independent of psychopathology. *Journal of Consulting Psychology, 24,* 349–354.

Cuthbert S., & Goodheart G. (2007). On the reliability and validity of manual muscle testing: a literature review, *Chiropr Osteopat* 2007, 15:4.

Damasio, A. R. (1994). *Descartes error.* New York: Grosset/Putnam.

Danaos, D. (2002). *Nei Kung: Secret teachings of the warrior sages.* Rochester, VT: Inner Traditions.

Dao, D. M. (1990). *Scholar warrior: An introduction to the Tao of everyday life.* San Francisco: Harper Collins.

Darby, D. (2001). *The efficiency of thought field therapy as a treatment modality for individuals diagnosed with blood-injection-injury phobia.* Unpublished doctoral dissertation. Minneapolis, MN: Walden University.

Davidson, R., Kabat-Zinn, J., Schumacher, J., Rosenkranz, M., Muller, D., Santorelli, S., et al. (2003). Alterations in brain and immune function produced by mindfulness meditation, *Psychosomatic Medicine, 65,* 564–570.

Deadman, P., Al-Khafarni, M., & Baker, K. (1998). *A manual of acupuncture.* East Sussex, England: Journal of Chinese Medicine Publications.

Deatherage, G. (1975). The clinical use of mindfulness meditation techniques in short-term psychotherapy. *Journal of Transpersonal Psychology, 7,* 133–43.

Deikman, A. (1982). *The observing self.* Boston, MA: Beacon Press.

Delmonte, M. M. (1984). Meditation: Similarities with hypnoidal states and hypnosis. *International Journal of Psychosomatics, 31*(3), 24–34.

Delmonte, M. M. (1985). Biochemical indices associated with meditation practice: A literature review. *Neuro-Science and Bio-Behavioral Review, 9,* 557–561.

Delmonte, M. M. (1987). Constructivist view of meditation. *American Journal of Psychotherapy, 41,* 286–98.

Deri, S. (1990). Changing concepts of the ego in psychoanalytic theory. *Psychoanalytic Review, 77,* 512–58.

Devine, E. C., & Westlake, S. K. (1995). The effects of psycho-educational care provided to adults with cancer: Meta-analysis of 116 studies. *Oncology Nursing Forum, 22*(9), 1369–1381.

Diamond, J. (1979). *Behavioral kinesiology.* New York: Harper & Row.

Diepersloot, J. (1995, 1999). *Warriors of stillness*. Walnut Creek, CA: Center for Health and the Arts.

Diepold, J. H. (2000). Touch and breath: An alternative treatment approach with meridian based psychotherapies. *Electronic Journal of Traumatology, 6*(2). Retrieved from www.fsu.edu/trauma

Diepold, J. H., Jr., & Goldstein, D. (2000). *Thought field therapy and EEG changes in the treatment of trauma: A case study*. Moorestown, NJ: Author.

Don, N. S. (1977). The transformation of conscious experience and its EEG correlates. *Journal of Altered States of Consciousness, 3*.

Dong, P., & Raffill, T. (2006) *Empty force: The power of Chi for self-defense and energy healing*. New York: Random House.

Dossey, L. (1992). But is it energy? Reflections on consciousness, healing and the new paradigm. *Subtle Energies, 3*(3), 69–81.

Dossey, L. (1993). *Healing words: The power of prayer and the practice of medicine*. New York: Harper San Francisco.

Dossey, L. (1994). Healing Energy and consciousness: Into the future or a retreat to the past? *Subtle Energies, 5*(1).

Dreher, H. (1998). Mind-body interventions for surgery: Evidence and exigency. *Advances in Mind-Body Medicine, 14*(3), 207–222.

Dunn, A. L., Trivedi, M. H., Kampert, J. B., Clark, C. G., & Chambliss, H. O. (2005). Exercise treatment for depression: Efficacy and dose response. *American Journal of Preventive Medicine, 28*(1), 1–8.

Durlacher, J., & Scott, W. (2002). An energy psychobiology trialogue: The physican's perspective. In F. Gallo, (Ed.), *Energy psychology in psychotherapy: A comprehensive source book*. New York: W. W. Norton.

Dusseldorp, E., van Elderen, T., Maes, S., Meulman, J., & Draij, V. (1999). A meta-analysis of psychoeducational programs for coronary heart disease patients. *Health Psychology, 18*(5), 506–519.

Dychtwald, K. (1977). *Bodymind*. New York: Pantheon.

Eden, D. (1998). *Energy medicine*. New York: Jeremy Tarcher.

Eden, D. (2008). *Energy medicine for women: Aligning your body's energies to boost your health and vitality*. Jeremy P. Tarcher/Penguin.

Eden, D., & Feinstein, D. (2008). *Energy medicine for women: Aligning your body's energies to boost your health and vitality*. New York: Jeremy P. Tarcher/Penguin.

Edinger, E. (1972). *Ego and archetype*. New York: Putnam.

Edinger, E. F. (1985). *Anatomy of the psyche: Alchemical symbolism in psychotherapy*. La Salle, IL: Open Court.

Eisenberg, D. (1995). *Encounters with Qi: Exploring Chinese medicine.* New York: W.W. Norton.

Eisenberg, D. M., Davis, R. B., Ettner, S. L., et al. (1998, November 11). Trends in alternative medicine use in the United States, 1990–1997. *Journal of the American Medical Association, 280*(18), 1569–1575.

Eisenberg, D. M., Kessler, R. C., Foster, C., Norlock, F. E., Calkins, D. R., & Delbanco, T. L. (1993). Unconventional medicine in the United States: Prevalence, costs, and patterns of use. *New England Journal of Medicine, 328*, 246–252.

Eliade, M. (1956). *The forge and the crucible: The origins and structures of alchemy.* Chicago: University of Chicago Press.

Eliade, M. (1958). *Rites and symbols of initiation.* New York: Harper Torchbooks

Eliade, M. (1959). *The sacred and the profane.* New York: Harcourt, Brace, & World.

Eliade, M. (1964). *Shamanism: Archaic techniques of ecstacy* (Bollingen Series). Princeton, NJ: Princeton University Press.

Eliade, M. (1965). *The two and the one.* New York: Harper & Row.

Eliade, M., & Trask, W. (1954). *The myth of the eternal return.* Princeton, NJ: Princeton University Press, Bollingen Foundation.

Engel, G. I. (1977). The need for a new medical model: A challenge for biomedicine. *Science, 196*, 129–136.

Engler, J. (1986). Therapeutic aims in psychotherapy and meditation. In K. Wilber, Engler, J., & D. Brown D. (Eds.). (1976). *Transformations of consciousness.* Boston: Shambhala.

Epstein, M., & Lieff, J. (1986). Psychiatric complications of meditation practice. In K. Wilber, J., Engler, J. & Brown, D. P. (Eds.). *Transformations of consciousness.* Boston, Shambhala.

Epstein, S. S. (1998). *The politics of cancer: Revisited.* Fremont Center, NY: East Ridge Press.

Erickson, M. (1948/1980). *The collected papers of Milton Erickson on hypnosis (IV).* New York: Irvington.

Feinstein, D. (2004a). *Energy psychology interactive* (Book and CD). Ashland, OR: Innersource.

Feinstein, D. (2004b). *State of the art,* from module in CD of *Energy psychology interactive.* ibid. Ashland, OR: Innersource.

Feinstein, D. (2006a, March-May). Energy psychology in disaster relief. *Shift: At the Frontiers of Consciousness.* The Institute of Noetic Sciences.

Feinstein D., & Eden, D. (2006b). *Six pillars of energy medicine: Clinical strengths of a complementary paradigm,* from www.energymedicineprinciples.com. Earlier article accepted and published: Feinstein, D., & Eden, D., (2008). Six pillars of energy medicine: Clinical strengths of a complementary paradigm, *Alternative Therapies in Health and Medicine, 14*(1), 44–54, January/ February.

Feinstein, D. (2006c). *Energy psychology in disaster relief: New applications for an age-old paradigm*, Draft version submitted for journal publication. Final published version is Feinstein, D. (2008). Energy psychology in disaster relief. *Traumatology.* 14(1), 124–137.

Feinstein, D., Eden, D., & Craig, G. (2005). *The promise of energy psychology.* New York: Jeremy P. Tarcher.

Feinstein, D. (2008). Energy psychology: A review of the preliminary evidence. *Psychotherapy: Theory, Research, Practice, Training.* 45(2), 199–213.

Feng, A. (2003). *The five animals play Qigong.* Oakland, CA: The Taoist Center.

Fingarette, H. (1963). *The self in transformation.* New York: Harper & Row.

Fitzgerald, P. B., et al. (2003). Low field magnetic stimulation in the treatment of depression: A double blind, placebo controlled trial. *Archives of General Psychiatry, 60,* 1002–1008.

Fleming, T. (1996). *Reduce traumatic stress in minutes: The tapas acupressure technique (TAT) workbook.* Torrance, CA: Author.

Fleming, T. (1999). *You can heal now: The tapas acupressure technique (TAT).* Redondo Beach, CA: TAT International.

Fox, R. E. (2006). Economics, politics, and psychological practice. *The National Psychologist. January/February,* 13.

Francis, B. K. (1993). *Opening the energy gates of your body.* Berkeley, CA: North Atlantic Books.

Francis, B. K. (1998). *The power of internal martial arts.* Berkeley, CA: North Atlantic.

Frankl, V. (1967). *Psychotherapy and existentialism: Selected papers in logotherapy.* New York: Simon and Schuster.

Frenier, C., & Hogan, L. S. (n.d.). *Engaging the imaginal realm: Doorway to collective wisdom.* Retrieved July 5, 2006, from www. collectivewisdominitiative.org papers/frenier_imaginal.htm#imaginal

Frese, E., Brown, M., & Norton, B. J. (1987). Clinical reliability of manual muscle testing. *Physical Therapy, 67,* 1072–1076.

Freud, S. (1899, 1965). *The interpretation of dreams.* New York: Avon Books.

Freud, S. (1923). *The ego and the id.* London: Hopgarthe Press.

Freud, S. (1933; 1990). *New introductory lectures on psychoanalysis.* New York: Norton.

Frost, R. (2002). *Applied kinesiology: A training manual and reference book of basic principles and practices.* Berkeley, CA: North Atlantic Books.

Gach, M. (1990). *Acupressure potent points.* New York: Bantam.

Gach, M. (2004). *Emotional healing with acupressure.* New York: Bantam.

Gach, M., & Marco, C. (1981). *Acu-yoga: Self help techniques to relieve tension.* New York: Japan Publications, Inc.

Gagne, D., & Toye, R. (1994). The effects of therapetuic touch and relaxation techniques in reducing anxiety. *Archives of Psychiatric Nursing, 8(3),* 183–189.

Gallo, F. P. (2000). *Energy diagnostic and treatment methods.* New York: Norton.

Gallo, F. P. (2002). *Energy psychology in psychotherapy: A comprehensive source book.* New York: W. W. Norton.

Gallo, F. P. (2004). Research in energy psychology. Retrieved from www.energypsych .com/Content/readings-num7.htm

Garber, J., & Seligman, M. E. (1980). *Human helplessness: Theory and applications.* New York: Academic Press.

Garlinkle, M. S., et al. (1998, November 11). Yoga-based interventional for carpal tunnel syndrome. *Journal of the American Medical Association, 280*(18), 1601–1603.

Gatchel, R. J., & Blanchard, E. B. (1993, 1998). *Psychophysiological disorders: Research and clinical applications.* Washington, DC: American Psychiatric Association.

Gendlin, E. (1962). *Experiencing and the creation of meaning.* Toronto, Ontario: Free Press of Glencoe.

Gendlin, E. (1978). *Focusing.* New York: Bantam Books.

Gendlin, E. (1986). *Let your body interpret your dreams.* Wilmette, IL: Chiron Publications.

Gerber, R. (1996). *Vibrational medicine.* Santa Fe, NM: Bear & Co.

Goleman, D. (1988). *The meditative mind.* New York: Jeremy P. Tarcher.

Goleman, D. (2003). *Destructive emotions.* New York: Bantam Books.

Goodheart, G. (1964). *Applied kinesiology.* Detroit, MI: Author.

Goodman, F. D. (1990). *Where spirits ride the wind: Trance journeys and other ecstatic experiences.* Indianapolis: IN: University Press.

Goodman, M. (1988, Winter). To touch or not to touch. *Psychotherapy, 25*(4), 492–500.

Gordon, D. (1978). *Therapeutic metaphors.* Cupertino, CA: Meta Publications.

Gore, B. (1995). *Ecstatic body postures.* Santa Fe, NM: Bear & Co.

Gorman, D. (2002, August 5). Why Tai Chi is the perfect exercise. *Time.*

Gorton, B. (1957). The physiology of hypnosis. *Journal of the American Society of Psychosomatic Dentistry, 4*(3), 86–103.

Grauds, C., & Childers, D. (2005). *The energy prescription: Giving yourself abundant vitality.* New York: Bantam Books.

Grauds, D. (1994). *Jungle Medicine.* San Rafael, CA: Center for Spirited Medicine.

Graves, R. (1955). *The Greek myths, I and II.* New York: Penguin.

Green, M. M. (2002). Energy applications in medical settings. In F. Gallo (Ed.), op. cit., 2002.

Gross, L., & Ratner, H. (2002). The use of hypnosis and EMDR combined with energy therapies in the treatment of phobias and dissociative, post-traumatic stress, and eating disorders. In F. Gallo (Ed.), op. cit., 2002.

Grosskurth, P. (1986). *Melanie Klein: Her world and her work.* New York: Alfred A. Knopf, Inc.

Grotstein, J. (1984). Forgery of the soul. In C. Nelson & M. Eigen (Eds.), *Evil, self, and culture*. New York: Human Sciences Press.

Gruen, W. (1972). A successful application of systematic self-relaxation and self-suggestions about postoperative reactions in a case of cardiac surgery. *International Journal of Clinical and Experimental Hypnosis, 20,* 141–151.

Guo, X., Zhou, B., Nishimura, T., Teramukai, M., & Fukushima, M. (2008). Clinical effect of Qigong practice on essential hypertension: A meta-analysis of randomized clinical trials, *Journal of Alternative and Complementary Medicine*, Vol. 14, No 1, pp. 27–37.

Guthrie, E. (1998). Somatization is essentially a normal process. *Advances in Mind-Body Medicine, 14,* 103–105.

Ha, F. (1995). *Stillness in movement; the practice of Tai Chi Chuan* (Video/DVD). San Francisco, CA: Vision Arts.

Ha, F., & Olsen, E. (1996). *Yiquan and the nature of energy*. Berkeley, CA: Summerhouse Publications.

Haas, M., Cooperstein, R., & Peterson, D. (2007). Disentangling manual muscle testing and applied kinesiology: Critique and reinterpretation of a literature review. *Chiropractic & Osteopathy*, 15:11.

Haddock, C. K., Rowan, A. B., Andrasik, R., Wilson, P. G., Talcotte, G. W., & Stein, R. J. (1997). Home-based behavioral treatments for chronic benign headache: a meta-analysis of controlled trials, *Cephalalgia, 17*(2), 113–118.

Hadhazy, V. A., Ezzo, J., Creanerm, C., & Berman, B. M. (in press). Mind-body therapies for the treatment of fibromyalgia: A systematic review. *Journal of Rheumatology.*

Hahn, R. A., Teutsch, S. M., Rothenberg R. B., & Marks, J. S. (1990). Excess deaths for nine chronic diseases in the United States. 1986. *Journal of the American Medical Association, 264*(20), 2654–2659.

Hall, M. (1988). *The secret teachings of all ages*. Los Angeles: The Philosophical Research Society.

Hamer, R. (1997). *Scientific chart of the new medicine*. Ontario, Canada: Quintessanz.

Hammer, L. (1990). *Dragon rises, red bird flies: Psychology and Chinese medicine*. New York: Station Hill Press.

Harner, M. (1990). *The way of the shaman*. New York: Harper & Row.

Harris, R., Porges, S., Clemenson-Carpenter, M., & Vincenz, L. (1993). Hypnotic susceptibility, mood state, and cardiovascular reactivity. *American Journal of Clinical Hypnosis, 36,* 15–25.

Hartman, C. A., Manos, T. M., Winter, C., Hartman, D. M., Li, B., & Smith, J. C. (2000, December). Effects of T'ai Chi training on function and quality of life indicators in older adults with osteoarthritis. *Journal of the American Geriatrics Society, 48*(12), 1553–1559.

Hartung, J. G., & Galvin, M. D. (2002). Combining eye movement desensitization and reprocessing (EMDR) and energy therapies. In F. Gallo (Ed.), *Energy psychology in psychotherapy,* op. cit., 2002.

Heinerman J. (1988). *Encyclopedia of Fruits, Vegetables and Herbs.* West Nyack, NY: Parker Publishing Company.

Hernandez-Reif, M., Field, T., & Thimas, E. (2001, April). Attention deficit hyperactivity Disorder: Benefits from Tai Chi, *Journal of Bodywork and Movement Therapies,* Vol. 5 Issue 2, pp. 120–123.

Heuscher, J. (1974). *Myths and fairy tales: Their origin, meaning and usefulness. A psychiatric study of fairy tales.* Springfield, IL: Charles C. Thomas.

Hilgard, E. (1965). *Hypnotic susceptibility.* New York: Harcourt.

Hilgard, E., & Hilgard, J. (1983). *Hypnosis in the relief of pain.* Los Altos, CA: William Kaufman, Inc.

Hillman, J. (1972). *The myth of analysis.* Evanston, IL: Northwestern.

Hillman, J. (1975). *Re-visioning psychology.* New York: Harper and Row.

Hillman, J. (1976, 1979a). Peaks and vales. In J. Needleman (Ed.), (1976). *On the way to self knowledge.* New York: A. A. Knopf. Also in J. Hillman, (Ed.), (1979). *Puer papers* (pp. 54–72). Irving, TX: Spring Publications.

Hillman, J. (1979b). *The dream and the underworld.* New York: Harper & Row.

Hilts, P. (1995, Winter). Spiritual side finds favor in medical field. *Qi: Journal of Traditional. Eastern Health & Fitness, 5*(4), 45. Reprinted from the *New York Times.*

Hinds, M. W., et al. (1985, March 15). Neonatal outcome in planned vs. unplanned out of hospital births in Kentucky. *Journal of the American Medical Association, 253*(11).

Hoffman, E. (1981). *The way of splendor: Jewish mysticism and modern psychology.* Boulder, CO: Shambhala.

Horner, A. (1990). *The primacy of structure: Psychotherapy of underlying character pathology.* Northvale, NJ: Jason Aronson, Inc.

Houston, J. (1992). *The hero and the goddess: The odyssey as mystery and initiation.* New York: Ballentine Books.

Hover-Kramer, D. (1996). *Healing touch: A resource for healthcare professionals.* Albany, NY: Delmar.

Hover-Kramer, D., & Murphy M. (2006). *Creating right relationships.* Albany, NY: Delmar.

Hover-Kramer, D., & Shames, K. H. (1997). *Energetic approaches to emotional healing.* Albany, NY: Delmar.

Huang, W. S. (1974). *Fundamentals of Tai Chi Chuan.* Hong Kong, China: South Sky Book Co.

Hui K. K. S., et al. (2000). Acupuncture modulates the limbic system and subcortical gray structures of the human brain. Evidence from MRI studies in normal subjects. *Human Brain Mapping, 9*(1), 13–25.

Huxley, A. (1969). *Brave new world.* New York: Perennial Library.

Huxley, A. (1970). *The perennial philosophy.* New York: Harper Colophon.

Idel, M. (1988). *The mystical experience in Abraham Abulafia.* Albany, NY: State University of New York Press.

Ingerman, S. (1991). *Soul retrieval: Mending the fragmented self.* New York: Harper Collins.

Irwin M., Pike, J., Cole, J., & Oxman, M. (2003). Effects of a behavioral intervention, Tai Chi Chih, on varicella-zoster virus specific immunity and health functioning in older adults. *Psychosomatic Medicine,* 65: 824–30. <http://ecam.oxfordjournals.org/cgi/ijlink?linkType=ABST&journalCode=psychmed&resid=65/5/824>

Irwin, M., Olmstead, R., and Motivala, S., (2008). Improving sleep quality in older adults with moderate sleep complains: A randomized controlled trial of Tai Chi Chih. *Sleep,* Vol. 31, No 7.

Irwin, M., Olmstead, R., and Oxman M., (2007). Augmenting immune responses to Varicella Zorster Virus in older adults: A randomized, controlled trial of Tai Chi, *Journal of the American Geriatrics Society.*

Irwin, M., Pike, J., & Oxman, M. (2004). Shingles immunity and health functioning in the elderly: Tai Chih as a behavioral treatment, *eCAM,* 1:223–32.

Iwao, M., Kajiyama, S., Mori, H., & Oogakio, K. K. (1999). Effects of Qigong walking on diabetic patients. *Journal of Alternative and Complementary Medicine, 5*(40), 353–358.

Jacob, R. G., Chesney, M. A., Williams, D. M., Ding, Y., & Shapiro, A. P. (1991). Relaxation therapy for hypertension. Design effects and treatment effects. *Annals of Behavioral Medicine, 13,* 9–17.

Jacobson, A., Hackett, T., Surman, O., & Silverberg, E. (1973). Raynaud's phenomenon: Treatment with hypnotic and operant technique. *Journal of the American Medical Association, 225,* 739–740.

Jacobson, E. (1964). *The self and object world.* New York: International University Press.

Jahnke, R. (2002a). *The healing promise of Qi.* New York: McGraw Hill.

Jahnke, R. OMD (2002b). Getting your immune system in shape. In *Boosting immunity: Creating wellness naturally.* Novato, CA: New World Library.

Janov, A. (1970). The primal scream. Delta Books.

Jansen, N., & Barron, J. (1988, Winter). Introduction and overview: Psychologist use of physical interventions. *Psychotherapy, 25.*

Jerosch, J., & Wustner, P. (2002). *Effect of a sensorimotor training program on patients with subacromial pain syndrome.* In German *Unfallchirurg* JID–8502736, *105*(1), 36–43. Also see *Time,* 2002. August 5, *160*(6), 68.

Jetter, A. (1996, September). The end of pain. *Hippocrates Magazine.*

Jin, P. (1944). Theoretical perspectives on a form of physical and cognitive exercise:

Tai Chi. In G. Davidson, (Ed.). (1994). Lessons-Oceania. Also see E. Sandlund, & N. Torsten, (2000). The effects of Tai Chi Chuan relaxation and exercise on stress responses and well-being: An overview of research. *International Journal of Stress Management, 7*(2).

Jing, G. (1988). Observations on the curative effects of Qigong self-adjustment therapy in hypertension. *Proceedings of the First World Conference for Academic Exchange of Medical Qigong,* Beijing, China. 115–117.

Johnson, C., Mustafe, S., Sejdijaj, X., Odell, R., & Dabishevci, J. (2001). Thought field therapy—soothing the bad moments of Kosovo. *Journal of clinical psychology, 57,* 1237–1240.

Johnson, J. (2000). *Chinese medical Qigong therapy: A comprehensive clinical text.* Pacific Grove, CA: The International Institute of Medical Qigong.

Johnston, M., & Vogele, D. (1993). Benefits of psychological preparation for surgery: A meta-analysis. *Annals of Behavioral Medicine, 15,* 245–256.

Joint National Committee on Detection, Evaluation, and Treatment of High BP (5th Report). (1993). *Archives of Internal Medicine, 153,* 154–183.

Jonas, W. B., & Levin, J. S. (2000). *Essentials of complementary and alternative medicine.* New York: Lippencott, Williams, & Wilkins.

Jonte-Pace, D. (1998). The swami and the Rorschach. In R. Forman (Ed.), *The innate capacity: Mysticism, psychology and philosophy.* New York: Oxford University Press.

Judith, A. (1990). *Wheels of life: A user's guide to the chakra system.* St. Paul, MN: Llewelyn.

Jung, C. G. (1936). *Yoga and the West* (Collected Works, Vol. 11). Princeton, NJ: Princeton University Press.

Jung, C. G. (1953). *Two essays on analytical psychology.* New York: World Publishing Company.

Jung, C. G. (1955). *Mysterium coniunctionis* (Collected Works, Vol. 14). Princeton, NJ: Princeton University Press.

Jung, C. G. (1957–1970). *The collected works of C. G. Jung* (Vols. 1–19, Bollingen Series). Princeton, NJ: Princeton University Press.

Jung, C. G. (1960). *The structure and dynamics of the psyche* (Bollingen Series XX). Princeton, NJ: Princeton University Press.

Jung, C. G. (1974). *Dreams* (Bollingen Series). Princeton, NJ: Princeton University Press.

Jung, E. (1974). *Animus and anima.* Zurich, Switerland: Spring Publications.

Kabat-Zinn, J. (1990). *Full catastrophe living: Using the wisdom of your body and mind to face stress, pain, and illness.* New York: Dell.

Kabat-Zinn, J. (2003). Mindfulness-based interventions in context: Past, present and further. *Clinical Psychology: Science and Practice, 10,* 144–156.

Kalsched, D. (1996). *The inner world of trauma: Archetypal defenses of the personal spirit.* London: Routledge.

Kaptchuk, T. (1983). *The web that has no weaver: Understanding Chinese medicine.* New York: Congdon & Weed.

Karasek, R., Baker, D., Marxer, F., Ahibom, A., & Theorell, T. (1981). Job decision latitude, job demands, and cardiovascular disease: A prospective study of Swedish men. *American Journal of Public Health, 71,* 694–705.

Kasamatsu, A., & Hirai, T. (1969). An electroencephalographic study on the Zen Meditation (Zazen). *Psychologia, 12,* 205–225.

Katie, B. (2002). *Loving what is.* New York: Harmony Books.

Keen, S., & Fox, A. (1989). Your mythic journey: Finding meaning in your life through writing and storytelling. New York: Jeremy P. Tarcher

Kelleman, S. (1985). *Emotional anatomy.* Berkeley, CA: Center Press.

Kerenyi, C. (1951/1979). *The gods of the Greeks.* London: Thames and Hudson.

Kerenyi, C. (1976). *Dionysos: Archetypal image of indestructible life* (Bollingen Series LXV-2). Princeton, NJ: Princeton University Press.

Kilburg, R. (1988, Winter). Psychologists and physical interventions: Ethics, standard, and legal implications. *Psychotherapy, 25*(4), 487–491.

Kingsley, P. (1999). *In the dark places of wisdom.* Inverness, CA: Golden Sufi Center.

Kirsteins, A. E., Dietz, F., & Hwang, S. M. (1991). Evaluating the safety and potential use of a weight-bearing exercise, Tai-Chi Chuan, for rheumatoid arthritis patients. *American Journal of Physical Medicine & Rehabilitation, 70*(3), 136–141.

Kober, A., Scheck, T., Greher, M., Lieba, F., Fleischhackl, R., Fleischhackl, S., Randunsky, F., & Hoerauf, K. (2002). Pre-hospital analgesia with acupressure in victims of minor trauma: A prospective, randomized, double-blinded trial. *Anesthesia & Analgesia, 95*(3), 723–727.

Kohn, L. (1989). *Taoist meditation and longevity techniques.* Ann Arbor, MI: Michigan University.

Kohn, L. (2001). *Daoism and Chinese culture.* Cambridge, MA: Three Pines Press.

Kohut, H. (1971). *The analysis of the self.* New York: International Press.

Kohut, H. (1977). *The restoration of the self.* New York: International Universities Press.

Kohut, H. (1971). *The analysis of the self.* New York: International Press.

Kornfield, J. (1993). Even the best meditators have old wounds to heal: Combining meditation and psychotherapy. In R. Walsh & G. Vaughn (Eds.), *Paths beyond ego* (pp. 67–68). New York: Jeremy P. Tarcher/Putnam.

Korte, D., & Scaer, R. (1992). *A good birth: A safe birth: Choosing and having the childbirth experience you want.* Cambridge, MA: Harvard Common Press.

Kostis, J., Rosen, R., Holzer, B., Randolph, C., Taska, L., & Miller, M. (1990). CNS side effects of centrally active anti-hypertensive agents: A prospective placebo-controlled study of sleep, mood state, and cognitive and sexual function in hypertensive males. *Psychopharmacology, 102,* 163–170.

Kramer, P. D. (1997). *Listening to Prozac.* New York: Penguin.

Krippner, S., & Conti, B. A. (2006). The furrows of reality: Scientific and spiritual implications of the reenchanted cosmos. In E. Laszlo (Ed.), *Science and the reenactment of the cosmos: The rise of the integral vision of reality,* (pp. 95–100). Rochester, VT: Inner Traditions.

Krippner, S., & Powers, S. M. (1997). *Broken images, broken selves: Dissociative narratives in clinical practice.* Washington, DC: Brunner/Mazel.

Kristof, N. (1991, April 14). China sets example in healthcare. *New York Times, Ann Arbor News,* A-6.

Krysal, H. (1978). Trauma and affects. *Psychoanalytic Study of the Child, 22,* 81–116.

Kuang, A., Wang, C., Xu, D., & Qian, Y. (1991). Research on the anti-aging effect of Qigong. *Journal of Traditional Chinese Medicine, 11*(2), 153–158; and *11*(3), 224–227.

Kuhn, T. (1996). *The structure of scientific revolutions.* Chicago, IL: University of Chicago Press.

Lam, K. C. (1999). *Chi Kung: The way of healing, Chinese exercises for quieting the mind and strengthening the body.* New York: Broadway Books.

Lammers, W. (2002). Inner child, inner parent resolution: Meridian-based treatment focused on archaic states and introjects. In F. Gallo (Ed.), op. cit., 2002.

Larson, S. (1990). *The mythic imagination: your quest for meaning through personal mythology.* New York: Bantam Books.

Lascow, L. (1998). *Healing with love.* San Francisco: Harper and Row.

Laszarus, D. (2005, March 1). Sleep: Can't get enough of it. *San Francisco Chronicle,* C4–5.

Laszlo E. (2004). *Science and the Akashic field: An integral theory of everything.* Rochester, Vermont, Inner traditions.

Laszlo, E. (2006). (Ed.). *Science and the reenchantment of the cosmos: The rise of the integral vision of reality.* Rochester, VT: Inner Traditions.

Lean, M., & Hankey, C. (2004). Aspartame and its effects on health. *British Medical Journal, 329,* 755–756.

LeDoux, J. (1986). *Mind and Brain: Dialogues in cognitive neuroscience.* New York: Cambridge University Press.

LeDoux, J. (1992). Emotion and memory: Anatomical systems underlying indelible neural traces. In S. A. Christianson (Ed.), *Handbook of emotion and memory* (pp. 269–288). Hillsdale, NJ: Eribaum.

Lee, M. S., et al. (2007). Qigong for hypertension: a systematic review of randomized clinical trials." *Journal Hypertension.* 2007 Aug; 25(8):1525–32.

Lee, M. S., Hwa, J., Jeong, H., Kim, B. G., Ryu, H., Lee, H., Kim, J., Taeg, H., & Chung, H. (2002). Effects of Qi-training on heart rate variability *The American Journal of Chinese Medicine, 30*(4), 463–470.

Lehrer, P. M., & Woolfolk, R. L. (Eds.). (1993). *Principles and practice of stress management* (2nd ed.). New York: Guilford.

Lerner, M. (1994). *Choices in healing.* Cambridge, MA: MIT Press.

LeShan, L. (1974). *How to meditate.* New York: Bantam Books.

Leveno, K. J., Cunningham, F. G., Nelson, S., Roark, M., Williams, M. L., Guzick, D., et al. (1986). A prospective comparison of selective and universal electronic fetal monitoring in 34,995 pregnancies. *New England Journal of Medicine, 315*(10). In J. Robbins, 1986, op. cit., p. 48.

Levine, P. A. (1997). *Waking the tiger: Healing trauma.* Berkeley, CA: North Atlantic.

Levy, B., et al. (1971, January). Reducing neonatal mortality rates with nurse-midwives. *American Journal of Obstetrics and Gynecology, 109.*

Li, F., et al. (2007). Tai Chi-based exercise for older adults with Parkinson's disease: A pilot-program evaluation. *Journal of Aging and Physical Activity,* April 15, 2:139–151.

Li, F., Fisher K., Harmer, P., Irbe, D., Tearse, R. & Weimer, C. (2001). Tai Chi and self-rated quality of sleep and daytime sleepiness in older adults: A randomized controlled trial. *Journal American Geriatric Society,* 52: 892–900.

Li, W., Pi, D. R., Zing, Z. H., et al. (1994). Clinical study of Qigong on hypertension (In Chinese), *TCM Res, 7,* 23–24. (As reported in X. Guo, 2008).

Liboff, A. R. (2004). Toward an electromagnetic paradigm for biology and medicine. *Journal of Alternative and Complimentary Medicine,* 10(1) 41–47.

Linden, W., & Chambers, L. (1994). Clinical effectiveness of non-drug treatment for hypertension: A meta-analysis. *Annals of Behavioral Medicine, 16,* 35–45.

Linden, W., Stossel, C., & Maurice, J. (1996). Psychosocial interventions for patients with coronary artery disease. *Archives of Internal Medicine, 156,* 745–752.

Lipton, B. (2005). *The biology of belief.* Santa Rosa, CA: Elite Books.

Lipton, B. (2006, May 4). *From keynote address at Association for Comprehensive Energy Psychology Conference.* Santa Clara, CA.

Little, P., Girling, G., Hasler, A., & Trafford, A. (1991). A controlled trial of low sodium, low fat, high fiber diet in treated hypertensive patients: Effect on anti-hypertensive drug requirement in clinical practice. *Journal of Human Hypertension, 5,* 175–181.

Lorig, K., Chastain, R., et al. (1989). Development and evaluation of a scale to measure perceived self-efficacy in people with arthritis. *Arthritis and Rheumatism, 32,* 37–44.

Lorig, K., et al. (1993). Evidence suggesting that health education for self-management in patents with chronic arthritis has sustained health benefits while reducing health care costs. *Arthritis and Rheumatism, 36*(4), 430–53.

Lorig, K., Laurin, J., Gines, G. E. (1984). Arthritis self-management. A five year history of a patient education program. *Nursing Clinics of North America, 19*(4), 637–645.

Lorish, C. D., Abraham, N., et al. (1991). Disease and psychosocial factors related to physical functioning in rheumatoid arthritis. *Journal of Rheumatology, 18,* 1150–1157.

Lowen, A. (1971). *The language of the body.* New York: Macmillan Books.

Lowen, A. (1975). *Bioenergetics.* New York: Penguin Books.

Luk, C. (1972). *The secrets of Chinese meditation.* New York: Samuel Weiser.

Luk, C. (1977). *Taoist yoga: Alchemy and immortality.* New York: Samuel Weiser.

Lv, Z. C., Yu, H. P., Liu, J. W., et al. (1987). Comparative analysis of Qigong, jogging and drug therapy on hypertension (In chinese). *Zgongguo Zgong Xi Yi Jie He Za Zhi,* 7 pp 462–464.

Lynch, J. (1977). *The broken heart: Medical consequences of loneliness.* New York: Basic.

Lynn, S., & Rhue, J. (Eds.). (1991). *Theories of hypnosis: Current models and perspectives.* New York: Guilford.

Mahler, M. (1952). On child psychosis and schizophrenia. *Psychoanalytic study of the child, 7,* 286–305.

Mahler, M., Pine, F., & Bergman, S. (1975). *The psychological birth of the human infant.* New York: Basic Books.

Manga report: Executive summary. (1994, July). *Townsend letter for doctors* (p. 814).

Mann, S. J. (2000). The mind/body link in essential hypertension: A time for new paradigm, *Alternative Therapies in Health and Medicine,* Vol 6, pp. 29–45.

Mannerkorpi, K. (2005, March). Exercise in fibromyalgia. *Current Opinions in Rheumatology, 17*(2), 190–194. Related articles, links.

Mannerkorpi, K., Arndorw, M. (2004, November). Efficacy and feasibility of a combination of body awareness therapy and Qigong in patients with fibromyalgia: A pilot study. *Journal Rehabilitation Medicine, 36*(6), 279–81.

Matthews, J., & Matthews, C. (1986). *The western way: A practical guide to the western mystery tradition. Volume II: The hermetic tradition.* London: Arkana Paperbacks.

Mayer, M. H. (1977). *A holistic language of meaning and identity: Astrological metaphor as a language of personality in psychotherapy.* Doctoral dissertation. San Francisco: Saybrook Institute.

Mayer, M. H. (1982). The mythic journey process. *The Focusing Folio, 2*(2).

Mayer, M. H. (1984). *The mystery of personal identity.* San Diego, CA: ACS Publications.

Mayer, M. H. (1993). *Trials of the heart: Healing the wounds of intimacy.* Berkeley, CA: Celestial Arts.

Mayer, M. H. (1996). Qigong and behavioral medicine: An integrated approach to chronic pain. *Qi: The Journal of Eastern Health and Fitness, 6*(4), 20–31.

Mayer, M. H. (1997a). *Psychotherapy and Qigong: Partners in healing anxiety.* Berkeley, CA: The Psychotherapy & Healing Center.

Mayer, M. H. (1997b). Combining behavioral healthcare and Qigong with one chronic hypertensive adult. *Mt. Diablo Hospital-Health Medicine Forum.* Unpublished study. (Video available from Health Medicine Forum, Walnut Creek, CA, www.alternativehealth.com).

Mayer, M. H. (1999). Qigong and hypertension: A critique of research. *Journal of Alternative and Complementary Medicine, 5*(4), 371–382. (Peer-reviewed).

Mayer, M. H. (2000). *Bodymind healing Qigong* (DVD). Orinda, CA: Bodymind Healing Center.

Mayer, M. H. (2001a). *Find your hidden reservoir of healing energy: A guided meditation for cancer* (Audio cassette). Orinda, CA: Bodymind Healing Publications.

Mayer, M. H. (2001b). *Find your hidden reservoir of healing energy: A guided meditation for chronic disease* (Audio cassette). Orinda, CA: Bodymind Healing Publications.

Mayer, M. H. (2003). Qigong clinical studies. In W. B. Jonas (Ed.), *Healing, intention, and energy medicine* (pp. 121–137). England: Churchill Livingston. (Peer-reviewed).

Mayer, M. H. (2004a). *Qigong: Ancient path to modern health* (DVD of keynote address to National Qigong Association). Orinda, CA: Bodymind Healing Publications.

Mayer, M. H. (2004b). *Secrets to living younger longer: The self-healing path of Qigong, standing meditation and Tai Chi.* Orinda, CA: Bodymind Healing Publications.

Mayer, M. H. (2004c). What do you stand for? *The Journal of Qigong in America,* Vol. 1, Summer.

Mayer, M. H. (2004d). Walking meditation: Yi Chuan Qigong. *The Empty Vessel: A Journal of Comtemporary Taoism,* Summer.

Mayer, M. H. (2005). Qigong: An age-old foundation of energy psychology. *The Energy Field, Association for Comprehensive Energy Psychology,* Vol. 6, (4), Winter.

Mayer, M. H. (2007). *Bodymind healing psychotherapy: Ancient pathways to modern health.* Orinda, CA: Bodymind Healing Publications.

Mayer, M. H. (2008). Mind-body treatment for anxiety and panic disorders. *California State Journal of Oriental Medicine,* Summer.

Mayer, M. H. (2009, Winter). Bodymind healing in psychotherapy: Towards an integral, comprehensive energy psychotherapy, *The Energy Field: International Energy Psychology News and Articles,* p. 13 (or online, www.bodymindhealing.com <http://www.bodymindhealing.com>).

McClare, C. W. F. (1974). Resonance in bioenergetics. *Annals of the New York Academy of Sciences, 227,* 74–97.

McDougall, W. (1911). *Body and Mind.* New York: Beacon Press.

McGee, C. & Chow, E. (1994). *Qigong: Miracle healing in China*. Coeur d'Alene, ID: Medipress.

McGinnis, J. M., & Foege, W. H. (1993). Actual causes of death in the United States. *Journal of the American Medical Association, 287*(20), 2711–2712.

McTaggart, L. (2003). *The field*. New York: Harper.

Medical Research Council Working party (1985). MRC trial of treatment of mild hypertension: Principal results. *British Medical Journal, 291*, 97–104.

Meier, C. A. (1967). *Ancient incubation and modern psychotherapy*. Evanston, IL: Northwestern University Press.

Merck manual of medical information (Home ed.). (1997). Whitehouse Station, NJ: Merck Research Laboratories.

Meyer, T. J., & Mark, M. M. (1995). Effects of psychosocial interventions with adult cancer patients: A meta-analysis of randomized experiments. *Health Psychology, 14*, 101–108.

Michaud, G., McGlowan, J. L., van der Jagt, R., Wells, G., & Tugwell, P. (1998). Are therapeutic decisions supported by evidence from health care research? *Archives of Internal Medicine, 158*(15), 1665–1668.

Miller, J., Fletcher, K., & Kabbat-Zinn, J. (1995). Three year follow-up and clinical implications of a mindfulness-base intervention in the treatment of anxiety disorders. *General Hospital Psychiatry, 17*, 192–200.

Mindell, A. (1985). *Working with the dreaming body*. Boston: Routledge.

Mindell, A. (2000). *Quantum mind*. Portland, OR: Lao Tse.

Ming, Y. J. (1986). *Advanced yang style Tai Chi Chuan*. Jamaica Plains, NY: Yang's Martial Arts Association.

Minor, M. A. (1991). Physical activity and management of arthritis. *Annals of Behavioral Medicine, 13*, 117–124.

Mollon, P. (2001). *Releasing the self: The healing legacy of Heinz Kohut*. London: Whurr Publishers.

Moncrieff, J., & Kirsch, I. (2005, Jul 16). Efficacy of antidepressants in adults. *British Medical Journal, 331*, 155–157.

Monte, D. A., Sinnott, J., Marchese, M., Kunkel, E. J., & Greenson, J. (1999). Muscle test comparisons of congruent and incongruent self-referential statements. *Perceptual & Motor Skills, 88*, 1019–1028.

Moore, T. (1992). Care of the soul: A guide for cultivating depth and sacredness in everyday life. New York: Harper Collins.

Moreland, K. (1998, August). The lived experience of receiving healing touch therapy of women with breast cancer who are receiving chemotherapy: A phenomenological study. *Healing Touch Newsletter, 8*, 3–5.

Morin, C. M., Culbert, J. P., & Schwartz, S. M. (1999). Non-pharmacological interventions for insomnia. American Academy of Sleep Medicine Review. *Sleep, 22*(8), 1134–1156.

Morin, C. M., Mimeault, V., & Gagne, A. (1999). Non-pharmacological treatment of late-life insomnia. *Journal of Psychomatic Research, 46*(2), 103–116.

Morris, L. (2000, April). Tai Chi: Relieving a painful shoulder injury. *Positive Health, 51,* 21–23.

Morrison, A. L. (1999). *The anti-depression sourcebook.* New York: Doubleday.

Murphy, M. (1992). *The future of the body.* Los Angeles: Jeremy P. Tarcher.

Murphy, M., & Donovan S. (1997). *The physical and psychological affects of meditation* (2nd Ed.). Petaluma, CA: Institute of Noetic Sciences.

National Institute of Health Technology Panel (1996). Integration of behavioral and relaxation approaches into the treatment of chronic pain and insomnia. In *Journal of the American Medical Association, 276*(4), 313–318.

Needham, J. (1956). Science and civilization in China (Vol. 2). England: Cambridge University Press.

Nemiah, J. C. (1991). Dissociation, conversion and somatization. In A. Tasman & A. Goldfinger (Eds.), *American Psychiatric Press Review of Psychiatry* (Vol. 10, pp. 248–260). Washington, DC: American Psychiatric Press.

Nerem, R., Levesqu, M. J., & Cornhill, J. F. (1980, June 27). Social environment as a factor in diet-induced artherioschlerosis. *Science, 208,* 1475–1476.

Neumann, E. (1954). *The origins and history of consciousness* (Bollingen Series). Princeton, NJ: Princeton University Press.

Neumann, E. (1956). *Amor and psyche.* Princeton, NJ: Princeton University Press.

Nims, L. P. (2002). *Be set free fast. Training manual.* Orange, CA: Author.

Noble, K. D. (1987). Psychological health and the experience of transcendence. *The Counseling Psychologist, 15,* 601–14.

Nordenstrom, B. E. (1983). *Biologically closed circuits: Experimental and theoretical evidence for an additional circulatory system.* Stockholm, Sweden: Nordic Medical Publications.

Nurse Healers-Professional Associates, Inc. (2000). *Compendium of therapeutic touch research to date.* Reson, VA. Retrieved from www.therapteutic touch.org (see here the Moreland, 1997 study).

O'Brien, J. (2004). *Nei Jia Quan: Internal martial arts.* Berkeley, CA: North Atlantic Books.

O'Connell, P. J., Wang, X., Leon-Ponte, M., Griffiths, C., Pingle, S. C., Gerard, P., & Ahern, G. P. (2006, February). A novel form of immune signaling revealed by transmission of the inflammatory mediator serotonin between dendritic cells and T cells. *Blood, 107*(3), 1010–1017.

Odanjnyk, W. V. (1988). Gathering the light: A Jungian exploration of meditation. *Quadrant, 21,* 35–51.

O'Meara K. P., Antidepressants may trigger violent behavior, www.mercola.com/2002/sep/18/luvox.htm.

Ornish, D., et al. (1993). Can lifestyle changes reverse coronary disease? *Lancet, 336,* 129–133.

Oschman, J. (2000). *Energy medicine: The scientific basis.* New York: Churchill Livingston.

Oxford English dictionary (Compact ed.). (1979). London: Oxford University Press.

Palmer, D. (2007). *Qigong fever: Body, science and utopia in China.* New York: Columbia University Press.

Papadakis, T. (1988). *Epidauros: The sanctuary of Asclepius.* Zurich & Athens: Verlag Schnell and Steiner Munchen.

Paske, B. (1982). *Rape and ritual.* Toronto, CA: Inner City Books.

Peat, F. D. (1997). *Infinite potential: The life and times of David Bohm.* New York: Addison-Wesley.

Pedraza, R. (1977). *Hermes and his children.* Zurich, Switzerland: Spring Publications.

Pelletier, K. R. (2000). *The best alternative medicine: What works? What does not?* New York: Simon & Schuster.

Pelletier, K. R. (2003, March 3). Conventional and integrative medicine—evidence based? Sorting fact from fiction. *Focus on Alternative and Complementary Therapies, 8*(1).

Pelletier, K. R. (2004). Mind-body medicine in ambulatory care: An evidence-based assessment. *Journal of Ambulatory Care Management, 27*(1), 25–42.

Pennebaker, J. W. (1993). Putting stress into words. Health, linguistic and therapeutic implications. *Behavior Research and Therapy, 31*(6), 539–548.

Pearlman, O. L., & McCann, L. O. (1992). Constructivist self-development theory. In D. K. Sakheim & S. K. Devine (Eds.), *Out of darkness.* New York: Lexington.

Perot, C., Meldener, R., & Gouble, F. (1991). Objective measurement of proprioceptive technique consequences on muscular maximal voluntary contraction during manual muscle testing. *Agressologie, 32*(10), 471–474.

Pert, C. B. (1997). *Molecules of emotion: The science behind mind-body medicine.* New York: Touchstone.

Pert, C. B. (2004). *Forward to energy psychology interactive.* Ashland, OR: Inner Source.

Pollare, T., Lithell, H., Selinus, I., & Berne, C. (1989). A comparison of the effects of hydrochlorothiazide and captopril on glucose and lipid metabolism in patients with hypertension. *British Medical Journal, 321,* 868–873.

Pollare, T., Lithell, H., Selinus, I., and Berne, C. (1989). Sensitivity to insulin during treatment with atenolol and metoprolol: A randomised, double blind study of effects on carbohydrate and lipoprotein metabolism in hypertensive patients, *British Medical Journal, 298* (6681) April 29.

Pomeranz, H., & Bhavsar, A., (2005). Nonarteritic ischemic optic neuropathy developing soon after use of Sildenafil (Viagra): A report of seven new cases, *Journal of Neuro-Ophthalmology,* Vol 25, No. 1.

Popp, F. A., Li, K., & Gu, Q. (Eds.). (1992). *Recent Advances in Biophoton Research.* Singapore: World Scientific.

Propst, L. R. (1988). *Psychotherapy in a religious framework: Spirituality in the emotional healing process.* New York: Human Sciences Press.

Province, M., Hadley, E., Hornbrook, M., Lipsitz, A., Miller, P., Mulrow, C., Ory, M., Sattin, R., Tinetti, M, & Wolf, S. (1995, May 3). The effects of exercise on falls in elderly patients: A pre-planned meta-analysis of the FICSIT trails. *Journal of the American Medical Association (JAMA), 272*(17), 1341–1347.

Pulos, L. (2002). Integrating energy psychology and hypnosis. In F. Gallo (Ed.), *Energy psychology in psychotherapy,* op. cit., pp. 167–178.

Quinn, J., & Stelkaudal, A. J. (1993). Psychoimmunologic effects of therapeutic touch on practitioners and recently bereaved recipients. *Advances in Nursing Science, 12*(4), 13–26.

Rael, L., & Rudhyar, D. (1980). *Astrological aspects.* New York: ASI Publishers.

Rama, S., Ballentine, T., & Weinstock, A. (1976). *Yoga and psychotherapy: the evolution of consciousness.* Honesdale, PA: Himalayan Institute.

Rampton, S., & Stauber, J. (2001). *Trust us we're experts: How industry manipulates science and gambles with your future.* New York: Tarcher.

Rauch, S. L., van der Kolk, B. A., Fisler, R. E., et. al. (1996). A symptom provocation study of post-traumatic stress disorder using positron emission tomography and script-driven imagery. *Archives of General Psychiatry, 53,* 380–387.

Reich, W. (1970). *Character analysis.* New York: Farrar, Straus, & Giroux.

Rein, G. (1992). *Quantum biology.* Northpoint, NY: Quantum Biology Research Labs.

Reinhardt, E. (2004). *Journal of the American Medical Association, 202*(10), 1227–1230. From handout at professional seminar by Dr. Ken Pelletier, "Stress-Free for Good," slide on International Medical Expenditures.

Requena, Y. (1989). *Character and health: The relationship of acupuncture and psychology.* Brookline, MA: Paradigm Pub.

Reuther, I., & Laderidge, D. (1998). Qigong Yangsheng as a complementary therapy in the management of asthma. *The Journal of Alternative and Complementary Medicine, 4*(2), 173–183.

Rinpoche, S. (1993). *The Tibetan book of living and dying.* San Francisco: Harper Collins.

Ritter, C. & Aldridge, D. (2001). Qigong Yangsheng as a therapeutic approach for the treatment of essential hypertension in comparison with a western muscle relaxation therapy: A randomized controlled pilot (In German). *Chinesische Medizin,* 16: 48–63.

Robbins, J. (1996). *Reclaiming our health: Exploding the medical myth and embracing the source of true healing.* Tiburon, CA: H. J. Kramer.

Roberts, S. J. (1994). Somatization in primary care: the common presentation of psychosocial problems through physical complaints. *Nurse-Practitioner, 19*(47), 50–56.

Rohan, M., et al. (2004). Low field magnetic stimulation in bipolar depression using an MRI based stimulator. *American Journal of Psychiatry, 161,* 93–98.

Rosch, E. (1999). Is wisdom in the brain? *Psychological Science. 10,* 222–224.

Rosen, M. (1989). *The cesarean myth.* New York: Viking.

Rosen, S. (1982). *My voice will go with you: The teaching tales of Milton H. Erickson.* New York: W. W. Norton.

Rossi, E. (1986). *The psychobiology of mind-body healing: New concepts of therapeutic hypnosis.* New York: Norton.

Rossi, E. (1990). Mind-molecular communication: Can we really talk to our genes? *Hypnosis, 17*(1), 3–14.

Rossi, E. (2002). *The psychobiology of gene expression: Neuroscience and neurogenesis in hypnosis and the healing arts.* New York: W. W. Norton & Co.

Rossi, E., & Cheek, D. (1988). *Mind-body therapy: Methods of ideodynamic healing in hypnosis.* New York: Norton.

Rowe, J. (2005, July). The effects of EFT on long term psychological symptoms. *Counseling and Psychology Journal, 2*(3), 104–111.

Rubik, B. (2002). The biofield hypothesis: It's biophysical basis and its role in medicine. *Journal of Alternative and Complementary Medicine, 8,* 703–717.

Ruden, R. A. (2005, Summer). Why tapping works: Speculations from the observable brain. *The Energy Field, 6*(2), 1–4.

Rudhyar D. (1970). *The astrology of personality.* New York: Doubleday.

Rudhyar D. (1975). *From humanistic to transpersonal astrology.* Palo Alto, CA: The Seed Center.

Salt, W. B., & Neimark, N. F. (2002). *Irritable bowel syndrome and the mind-body-spirit connection.* Columbus, OH: Parkview.

Sancier, K. (1996a). Anti-aging benefits of Qigong. *Journal of the International Society of Life Information Science, 14*(1), 12–21.

Sancier, K. (1996b). Medical applications of Qigong. *Alternative Therapies, 2*(1), 40–46.

Sancier, K. M., & Holman, D. (2004). Multifaceted health benefits of medical Qigong. *Journal of Alternative and Complementary Medicine, 10*(1), 163–166.

Sapolsky, R. M. (1998). *Why zebras don't get ulcers: An updated guide to stress, stress-related diseases, and coping.* New York: W. H. Freeman & Company.

Schafer, E. (1977). *Pacing the void: T'ang approaches to the stars.* Berkeley, CA: University of California Press.

Schmitz-Hubsch, T., et al. (2005, October 14). Qigong exercise helps reduce the motor and non-motor symptoms of Parkinson's disease: A randomized controlled pilot study. *Movement Disorders.*

Schneider, M. S. (1994). A beginners guide to constructing the universe. New York: HarperCollins.

Schneider, R. H., Alexander, C. N., et al. (2005). A randomized controlled trial of stress reduction in African Americans treated for hypertension for over one year. *American Journal of Hypertension, 18,* 8–98.

Schneider, R. H., Staggers, F., Alexander, C. N., Sheppard, W., Rainforth, M., Kondwani, D., Smith, S., & King, C. G. (1995). A randomized controlled trial of stress reduction for hypertension in older African Americans. *American Heart Association, Hypertension, 226,* 820–827.

Scholem, G. (1969). *Jewish mysticism.* Jerusalem: Schocken Publishing House.

Schoninger, B. (2001). *Thought field therapy in the treatment of speaking anxiety.* Unpublished doctoral dissertation. Cincinnati, OH: Union Institute.

Schore, A. N. (2003). *Affect regulation and the repair of the self.* New York: W. W. Norton & Company.

Schram, S. (2002, October). Tefillin: An ancient acupuncture point prescription for mental clarity. *Journal of Chinese Medicine, 70,* 5–8.

Schure, E. (1977). *The great initiates.* New York: Steiner Books.

Seem, M. (1989). *Bodymind energetics: Toward a dynamic model of health.* Rochester, VT: Healing Arts Press.

Segall, S. G. (2003). *Encountering Buddhism: Western psychology and Buddhist teachings.* New York: SUNY Press.

Selfridge, N., & Peterson, F. (2001). *Freedom from fibromyalgia: The five week program proven to conquer pain.* New York: Three Rivers Press.

Selye, H. (1975). Confusion and controversy in the stress field. *Journal of Human Stress, 1,* 37.

Sha, Z. G. (2003). *Power Healing: Four keys to energizing your body, mind, and spirit.* San Francisco: Harper Collins.

Shapiro, D., & Astin, J. (1998). *Control therapy.* New York: Wiley.

Shapiro, D. H., & Giber, D. (1978). Meditation and psychotherapeutic effects: Self-regulation strategy and altered states of consciousness. *Archives General Psychiatry, 35,* 294–302.

Shapiro, F. (1995). *Eye movement desensitization and reprocessing.* New York: Guilford Press.

Shapiro, R. (1997). *Minyan: Ten principles for living a life of integrity.* New York: Random House.

Shearer, A. (1982). *The yoga sutras of patanjali.* New York: Random House.

Sheldrake, R. (1988). *The presence of the past: Morphic resonance and the habits of nature.* Park Street Press.

Shepard, A. (2005). *Monkey: A superhero tale from China.* Skyhook Press.

Silver, L., & Wolfe, S. (1992). Unnecessary sections: How to cure a national epidemic. *Public Citizen Health Research Group,* Washington, DC. Quoted in D. Koret, *A good birth, a safe birth: Choosing and having the childbirth experience you want* (p. 135). Cambridge, MA: Harvard Common Press.

Smith, R. (1991). Where is the wisdom? The poverty of medical evidence. *British Medical Journal, 303,* 798–799.

Smith, R. W. (1972). *Pa-kua: Chinese boxing for fitness and self-defense.* New York: Harper & Row.

Smith, R. W. (2003). *Hsing-I: Chinese mind-body boxing.* Berkeley, CA: North Atlantic Books.

Smith, T. W., Peck, J. R., et al. (1988). Cognitive distortion in rheumatoid arthritis: Relationship to depression and disability. *Journal of Consulting and Clinical Psychology, 56,* 412–516.

Snell, B. (1969). *The discovery of mind.* New York: Harper & Row.

Song, R., Lee, E., Lam, P., & Bae, S. (2003). Effects of Tai Chi exercise on pain, balance, muscle strength, and perceived difficulties in physical functioning in older women with osteoarthritis: A randomized clinical trial, *Journal of Rheumatology,* Vol. 30:2039–44.

Sparks, T. (1993). *The wide open door: The twelve steps, spiritual tradition and the new psychology.* Center City, MI: Hazeldon.

Sperry, L. (2001). *Spirituality in clinical practice: Incorporating the spiritual dimension in psychotherapy.* Philidelphia, PA: Brunner-Routledge.

Starfield, B. (2000). Is U.S. health really the best in the world? *Journal of the American Medical Association, 209*(20), 2651–2662.

Stein, M. (1982). *Jungian analysis.* London: Open Court.

Stein, M., Wallston, K. A., et al. (1986). Correlates of a clinical classification schema for the arthritis helpless subscale. *Arthritis and Rheumatism, 31,* 876–881.

Steiner, R. (1973). *Mystery knowledge and mystery centres.* London: Rudolf Steiner Press.

Sternbach, R. (1986). Survey of pain in the United States: The Nuprim pain report. *The Clinical Journal of Pain, 1,* 49–53.

Stolorow, R. D., Brandchaft, F., & Atwood, G. E. (1987). *Psychoanalytic treatment: An intersubjective approach.* Hillsdale, NJ: The Analytic Press.

Stone, M. (1976). *When God was a woman.* New York: Harcourt, Brace, Jovanovich.

Storm, H. (1972). *Seven arrows*. New York: Harper& Row.

Sturgis, L., & Coe, W. (1990). Psychological responsiveness during hypnosis. *International Journal of Clinical Hypnosis, 38*(3), 196–207.

Suares, C. (1973). *The cipher of genesis*. Berkeley, CA: Shambhala.

Suares, C. (1976). *The sepher yetsira*. Boulder, CO: Shambhala.

Suzuki, M., et al. (1993). Clinical effectiveness of the AST Chiro method on chronic renal failure and hypertension. Japanese Mind Body Science 2(1): 15–22.{0918–2489, from San Francisco Qigong Database: http://www.qigonginstitute.org/html/database.php.}

Swingel, P. (2000a, May). *Effects of Emotional Freedom Techniques (EFT) method on seizure frequency in children diagnosed with epilepsy*. Paper presented at the annual meeting of the Association for Comprehensive Energy Psychology, Las Vegas, NV.

Swingle, P., Pulos, L., & Swingle, M. (2000b). Neurophysiological correlates of successful EFT treatment of post-traumatic stress disorder. Manuscript submitted for publication. In F. Gallo (Ed.), 2002, op. cit., p. 172.

Taggart, H. M., Arslanian, C. L., Bae, S., & Singh, K. (2003, September-October). Effects of Tai Chi exercise on fibromyalgia symptoms and health-related quality of life. *Orthopedic Nursing, 22*(5), 353–60.

Tart, C. (1968). *Altered states of consciousness*. New York: John Wiley & Sons.

Taylor, R. (1988). *The Confucian way of contemplation*. University of South Carolina Press.

Taylor, S. (1991). *Health psychology* (2nd ed.). New York: McGraw Hill.

Teeguarden, I. M. (1978). *Acupressure way of health: Jin Shin Do*. Tokyo: Japan Publications.

Teeguarden, I. M. (1988). *The joy of feeling: Bodymind acupressure*. Tokyo: Japan Publications.

Tiller, W. A. (1997). *Science and human transformation: Subtle energies, intentionality, and consciousness*. Walnut Creek, CA: Pavior.

Tloczynski, J., & Tantriells, M. (1998). A comparison of the effects of Zen breath meditation on college adjustment. *Psychologia, 41*, 32–43.

Tomio, N. (1994). *The Bodhisattva warriors*. New York: Samuel Weiser.

Travis, F., Arenander, A., & Dubios, D. (2002). Psychological and physiological characteristics of a proposed object-referral/self-referral continuum of self-awareness. *Consciousness and Cognition. 13*, 401–420.

Trieschmann, R. B. (1999). Energy medicine for long-term disabilities. *Disability and Rehabilitation, 21*(5), 269–276.

Tsang, H. W., Cheung, L., & Lak D. C. (2002). Qigong as a psychosocial intervention for depressed elderly with chronic physical illnesses. *International Journal of Geriatric Psychiatry. 17* (12), December, 1146–1154.

Tsang, H. W., Mok, Y. T., Yeung A., & Chan S. Y. (2003). The effect of Qigong on general and psychosocial health of elderly with chronic physical illnesses: A randomized clinical trial. *International Journal of Geriatric Psychiatry.* 18, (5), May, 441–449.

Ulansey, D. (1989). *The origins of the Mithraic mysteries.* Oxford: Oxford University Press.

van der Kolk, B. A. (1987). *Psychological trauma.* Washington, DC: American Psychiatric Press.

van der Kolk, B. A. (1994). The body keeps the score: Memory and the evolving psychobiology of post-traumatic stress. *Harvard Review of Psychiatry, I, 253–265.*

van der Kolk, B. A. (2002). Beyond the talking cure: Somatic experience and subcortical imprints in the treatment of trauma. In F. Shapiro (Ed.), *EMDR, Promises for a paradigm shift,* APA Press.

van der Kolk, B. A., et. al. (1996). *Traumatic stress: The effects of overwhelming experience on mind, body, and society.* New York: Guilford Press.

van der Kolk, B. A., & Fisler, R. E. (1995). Dissociation and the fragmentary nature of traumatic memories: Overview and exploratory study. *Journal of Traumatic Stress,* 8, 505–525.

van Deusen, J., & Harlowe, D. (1987). The efficacy of the ROM dance program for adults with rheumatoid arthritis. *American Journal of Occupational Therapy, 41(2), 90–95.*

van Tulder, M. J. W., Ostelo, R., Vlaeyen, J. W., Linton, S. J., Morley, S. J., & Assendelft, W. J. (2000). Behavioral treatment for chronic low back pain: A systematic review with the framework of the Cochrane back review group. *Spine, 25(20),* 2688–2699.

Wade, J. F. (1990). *The effects of the Callahan phobia treatment techniques on self concept.* Unpublished doctoral dissertation. San Diego, CA: The Professional School of Psychological Studies.

Wagner, M. (1993, Fall). An epidemic of unnecessary cesareans, *Mothering, Fall,* 72.

Wain, H., Amen, D., & Oetgen, W. (1984). Hypnotic intervention in cardiac arrhythmias. *The American Journal of Clinical Hypnosis, 27(1),* 70–75.

Waite, W. L., & Holder, M. D. (2003, Spring/Summer). Assessment of the Emotional Freedom Technique: An alternative treatment for fear. *The Scientific Review of Mental Health Practice, 2(1),* 20–26.

Wallas, L. W. (1985). *Stories for the third ear.* New York: W. W. Norton.

Walsh, R. (1999). *Essential spirituality: The seven central practices.* New York: Wiley.

Walsh, R., & Shapiro, S. (2006, April). The meeting of meditative disciplines and Western psychology. *American Psychologist, 61(3),* 227–239.

Walsh, R., & Vaughn, F. (1993). *Paths beyond ego.* Los Angeles: Jeremy Tarcher.

Wang, C., Xu, D., Qian, Y., Shi, W., Bao, Y., & Kuang, A. (1995). The beneficial effects of Qigong on the ventricular function and microcirculation of deficiency in heart energy hypertensive patients. *Chinese Journal of Internal Medicine, 1,* 21–23.

Ware, J. E., & Sherbourne, C. D. (1992). The medical outcomes study 36-item short-form health survey (SF-36). *Medical Care, 30(6),* 473–483.

Warnke, G. (1987). *Gadamer: Hermeneutics, tradition and reason (key contemporary thinkers).* Stanford, CA: Stanford University Press.

Watkins, M. (1984). *Waking dreams.* New York: Gordon & Breach.

Watts, A. W. (1961). *Psychotherapy east and west.* New York: Ballentine.

Wayne, P. M. & Kaptchuk, T. J. (2008). Challenges inherent to Tai Chi research: Part I–Tai chi as a complex multicomponent intervention, *Journal of Alternative and Complementary Medicine,* Vol. 14, No 1, pp. 95–102.

Weil, A. (1995). *Spontaneous healing.* New York: Alfred Knopf.

Weil, A. (2004, September). *Self-healing newsletter.*

Weinstein, E., & Au, P. (1991). Use of hypnosis before and after angioplasty. *American Journal of Clinical Hypnosis, 34,* 29–37.

Weintraub, M. I. (2001). Qigong and neurologic illness. *Alternative and Complementary Treatments in Neurologic Illness, 15,* 197–220. As reported on www.Qigonginstitute.org

Weizel, M. S. et al. (1998). Courses involving complementary and alternative medicine at U.S. medical schools. *Journal of the American Medical Association, 280,* 784–787.

Wells, S., Polglase, K., Andrews, H., Carrington, P., & Baker, A. H. (2003). Evaluation of a meridian-based intervention, Emotional Freedom Techniques (EFT) for reducing specific phobias of small animals. *Journal of Clinical Psychology, 59(9),* 943–966.

Wheeler, M. S. (2002). Integrating past and present: The early recollection techniques. In F. Gallo (Ed.), 2002, op. cit.

Wickramasekera, I. (1998). Secrets kept for the mind but not the body of behavior: The unsolved problems of identifying and treating somatization and psychophysiological disease. *Advances, 14,* 81–132.

Wilbur, K. (1980). *The atman project.* Wheaton, IL: Quest Books.Wilbur, K. (2000). *The eye of the spirit: An integral vision for a world gong slightly mad* (Vol. 7). *The collected works of Ken Wilber.* Boston: Shambhala.

Wilbur, K., Engler, J., & Brown, D. P. (Eds.). (1986). *Transformations of consciousness. Conventional and contemplative perspectives on development.* Boston: Shambhala/New Science Library.

Wilhelm, R. (1931, 1963). *The secret of the golden flower.* New York: Harcourt, Brace, & Jovanovich.

Wirth, D. (1991). The effect of non–contact therapeutic touch on the healing rate of full thickness dermal wound. *Journal of Subtle Energies, I(1),* 1–20.

Wiseman, R., & Schliz, N. (1997). Experimenter effects and remote detection of staring. *The Journal of Parapsychology, 61,* 201–207.

Wolf, E. S. (1988). *Treating the self.* New York: Guilford Press.

References

Wolf, S. L., Coogler, C., & Xu, T. (1997). Exploring the basis for Tai Chi Chuan as a therapeutic exercise approach. *Archives Physical Medical Rehabilitation, 78*, 886–890.

Wollam, G., & Hall, W. (Eds.). (1988). *Hypertension management: Clinical practice and therapeutic dilemmas.* Chicago: Yearbook Publishers. Quoted by R. Rosen, E. Brondolo, & J. Kostis (1998). Non-pharmacological treatment of essential hypertension: Research and clinical applications. In R. Gatchel, & E. Blanchard (Eds.), *Psychophysiological disorders: Research and clinical applications* (pp. 63–100). Washington, DC: American Psychological Association.

Wolpe, J. (1958). *Psychotherapy by reciprocal inhibition.* Stanford, CA: Stanford University Press.

Wu, R., & Liu, Z. (1993). Study of Qigong on hypertension and reduction of hypotension. *Proceedings of Second World Conference for Academic Exchange of Medical Qigong,* Beijing, China, *125.* From Sancier, Qigong Computerized Database, op. cit., record #7970, full article provided by author translated into English.

Wu, W. H., Bandilla, E., Ciccone, D. S., Yang, J., Cheng, S., Carner, N., Wu, Y., & Shen, R. (1999, January). Effects of Qigong on late-stage complex regional pain syndrome. *Alternative Therapies, 5*(1). Peer reviewed.

Wuthnow, R. (1978). Peak experiences: Some empirical tests. *Journal of Humanistic Psychology, 18*(3), 59–75.

Yanovski, A. (1962). The feasibility of alteration of cardiovascular manifestations in hypnosis.

Yapko, M. (1997). Breaking the patterns of depression. New York: Doubleday.

Young, L. D. (1993). Rheumatoid arthritis. In R. J. Gatchel & E. B. Blanchard (Eds.). *Psychophysiological disorders.* Washington, DC: American Psychological Association.

Zamara, J. W., Schneider, R. H., et al. (1996). Usefulness of the transcendental meditation program in the treatment of patients with coronary artery disease. *American Journal of Cardiology, 78*, 77–80.

Zautra, A. J., & Manne, S. E. (1992). Coping with rheumatoid arthritis: A review of a decade of research. *Annals of Behavioral Medicine, 14*, 31–39.

Zeig, J. K. (1985). *Ericksonian psychotherapy: Clinical Applications* (Vols. I and II). New York: Brunner Mazel.

Zur, O. (2005, January/February). Boundaries and dual relationships in psychotherapy. *The National Psychologist, 14* (1), 12.

NOTES

Preface

1. I have used Chinese spellings from the two Chinese-to-English translation systems (Pin Yin and Wade-Giles) throughout this book, according to the way they are used colloquially, feel appropriate to Western sensibilities, and convey appropriate symbolic meaning or fit with ease of usage. For example, the Pin Yin term *Qigong* is used in this book instead of the Wade-Giles term *Chi Kung* or *Chi Gung*. But the Wade-Giles term *Tai Chi Chuan* is used instead of the Pin Yin term *Taiji Quan*. (Please note that the academically correct usage of the Wade-Giles term is spelled *T'ai Chi Ch'uan,* but for ease of the Western readership I have used the term *Tai Chi Chuan,* without the apostrophes.) I made these choices because most Westerners are more familiar with the terms *Qigong* and *Tai Chi Chuan*; and furthermore, in the main text of my book *Secrets to Living Younger Longer* (Mayer, 2004b), I discussed how the letter *Q* conveys a symbolic meaning better fitting with the deep meaning of *Qigong* and *Qi* than does the *C* in *Chi* or *Chi Kung*. It is important that you realize that the term *chi* (in Wade-Giles and *Qi* in Pin Yin) is not the Chinese character in the Wade-Giles spelling of *Tai Chi*. Many people assume that the *chi* in *Tai Chi* refers to life energy; but rather the Chinese character *T'ai Chi* (*Taiji* in Pin Yin spelling) refers to the meeting place of opposites where the shady and sunny side of a mountain meet and the *axis mundi,* which connects heaven and earth (Mayer, 2004b). The term *Chuan* from the Wade-Giles is used because the term *Quan* is not common in Western usage and it does not fit with Western sensibilities. In some instances in this book, in a single phrase Pin Yin and Wade-Giles are combined as can be seen in the choice of spelling of term *Yi Chuan*—the *Yi* comes from Pin Yin and *Chuan* comes from Wade-Giles. The spelling *I Chuan* (Wade-Giles) or *Yi Quan* (Pin Yin) does not fit Western sensibilities, either. (Again, the Wade-Giles term is actually spelled *Ch'uan,* but for ease of reading, I am using the term *Chuan,* without the apostrophe in all references to *Chuan* throughout this book.) In addition, there could easily be confusion about the pronunciation of the *I* in *I Chuan*—the pronunciation of the term *I* or *Yi* is *yee*. Therefore, I chose to use the hybrid term *Yi Chuan*.

2. This integrated medical clinic has recently changed its name and location. It is now called The Health Medicine Center, located in Walnut Creek, California. If interested, visit the Web site at www.alternativehealth.com.

Introduction

1. Some of these age-old traditions touched upon in this book are ancient sacred wisdom traditions, such as symbolic process traditions of alchemy, astrology, and mythology. Also incorporated into the definition of *primordial Self* in Bodymind Healing Psychotherapy (BMHP) are the teachings contained in the books *The Mystery of Personal Identity* (1984) and *Trials of the Heart* (1993), regarding the use of symbolic process traditions to activate the elements of the primordial Self for ourselves and our relationships. It should be noted that this concept of the primordial Self incorporates the concept of "progressions" in our natal birth chart, and so it is not a regressive moving back to an idealized past self, but instead it represents a progressing, learning, evolving life force. Similar, therefore, to Carl Jung's ideas about the axis that connects the ego and collective unconscious to form the Self, my concept of the primordial Self contains an axis (axis mundi) that connects the "face before you were born," the instinctual and archetypal aspects of the Self, and the absorbed learning of that Self as it progresses through time. Also underlying BMHP's definition are the teachings from the book *Secrets to Living Younger Longer* (Mayer, 2004b), which shows the importance of Bodymind Healing Qigong practices to help cultivate the primordial Self—particularly animal movements stemming from static and dynamic postural initiation traditions. In the book *Bodymind Healing Psychotherapy* (Mayer, 2007) and in this book, my viewpoint is presented on the psychological/emotional/affective dimensions of what it means to connect with our primordial Selves. It should be noted that there are many pathways to the primordial Self, in addition to the ones mentioned above. Teilhard de Chardin perhaps best captures my meaning of the primordial Self when he wrote, "What is the work of works for man if not to establish in and by each one of our selves an absolutely original centre in which the universe reflects itself in a unique and inimitable way, and those centres are our very selves and personalities."

2. To see the illustration of this commonly known first Tai Chi movement called Commencement, or Raising and Lowering the Chi, see any Tai Chi Chuan manual or *Secrets to Living Younger Longer* (Mayer, 2004b, p.158).

3. It is not my aim to review the many forms of energy psychology. There are those who focus on the chakra systems of Hinduism, applied kinesiology, and so on. My focus in this book is to stick to the particular system of energy psychology that I have developed. For one fairly comprehensive overview of the arena of energy psychology in psychotherapy, see Gallo, F.P. (2000), op. cit.

Chapter 1

1. The most often heard about solution to our bodily complaints are pharmaceutical drugs. Fueled by the patented pharmaceuticals industry, which is by far the most

profitable business in the world, our culture is mass hypnotized through advertisements to see the solution to our maladies in pharmaceutical medications. In 2002 alone the American patent drug industry raked in $35.9 billion in profit—not total sales and revenue (that number's closer to $200 billion)—but *pure profit*. This followed 2001's banner year of $37.2 billion. Since the late 1990s, the top ten U.S. drug makers raked in many times the average annual profit margins of all other Fortune 500 companies combined. In 2001 and 2002, the top ten U.S. drug companies have averaged around 17.5 percent raw profit—more than *five times as much* as the 3.3 percent median return of the Fortune 500. This data comes from Jonathan Wright, MD, the recipient of the prestigious Linus Pauling Award for lifetime achievement in medicine, who calls the effects of pharmaceutical companies a "Pharma-geggon." He says that the government's getting a big chunk of the action through corporate and sales taxes and approval and application fees which amount to about $250 million per drug. http://www.isecureonline.com/Reports/NAH/E6EAHCCG/Default.cfm?o=1407910&u=15786079&l=836690&g=1362&PAGE=2&PCODE=E6EAHCCG&ALIAS=all.

2. The International Society for the Study of Subtle Energies and Energy Medicine (ISSSEEM) has compiled hundreds of very well researched studies, as has the scholarly research compendium of Daniel Benor (1992). For an easier read, Dr. Richard Gerber (1996) presents a good overview of the field in his book *Vibrational Medicine*, as does Andy Baggott (1999) in *The Encyclopedia of Energy Healing*.

3. Paraphrased from Gerber, R. (1966). *Vibrational medicine.* (Bear & Co.) p. 43.

4. For a description of Dr. Mehmet Oz and Julie Motz's work, see Benor, D. (1992). *Spiritual healing: Scientific validations of a healing revolution*, pp. 95–96.

5. Burr, H.S. (1957), *Yale Journal of Biology and Medicine*, 30, p. 161. As reported by Church, D., *The genie in your genes*, Elite Books, 2007, p. 124.

6. Nordenstrom, B.E. (1983). *Biologically closed circuits: Experimental and theoretical evidence for an additional circulatory system.* (Stockholm, Sweeden: Nordic Medical Publications). See Heilberg, E. (1983, Winter.) ISSEEM, 4 (4), 5. One must be cautious about interpreting this research because electricity has been shown to increase as well as decrease tumors.

7. Hu, F., & Tanasescu, M., Specific types of exercise level can significantly reduce risk of heart disease among men. *Journal of the American Medical Association,* October 23, 2002. Gibala, Short bursts of very intense exercise as good as traditional endurance training, "No time to exercise is no excuse," Gibala, *Journal of Physiology,* Changes in human skeletal muscle ultrastructure and force production after acute resistance exercise, *J Appl Physiol* 78: 702–708, 1995. The Pace program is one training program that builds on the Harvard Health Professionals study. Dr. Sears, author of *The Doc-*

tor's Heart Cure, is the founder of PACE, which stands for Progressively Accelerating Cardiopulmonary Exertion. See http://www.alsearsmd.com/pace/.

8. At the First World Conference for Academic Exchange of Medical Qigong, which was held in Beijing in October 1988, many scientific papers were presented giving data to support claims of the effectiveness of Qigong in healing. Of 137 papers presented, only three were from the United States, one was from Canada, almost all of the others were from China. The research described in the abstracts does not always meet strict scientific standards; but taken as a whole, the favorable results suggest that there should be more rigorously executed follow-up studies to determine how Qigong can improve Western health care. A Qigong database of 1,000 abstracts of the papers presented from these proceedings, including articles from 160 scientific journals, has been prepared by the Qigong Institute of San Francisco, 450 Sutter Street #2104, San Francisco, CA 94108.

9. Lu, G. (1993). Second World Conference for Academic Exchange of Medical Qigong. Record 8010, Database from Qigong Institute of San Francisco.

10. Shen, F., Hubei College, Wuhan China, 1993. Second World Conference. See record 8090 Qigong Institute Database.

11. Wang, S., Annual Conference, Henan Tumor Hospital, Zhengzhou, China. Since 1985, cancer patients have been prescribed long-term Qigong exercises side-by-side combined with routine treatments, such as chemotherapy, radiotherapy, and surgery. Results seem to show that this combination of Qigong-chemotherapy in the management of cancer has the advantage of raising the curative rate, extending the tumor-free survival time of the patients, lessening nausea, increasing strength, improving appetite, and bettering the quality of patients' survival. See McGee, C., & Chow, E. (1994). *Miracle healing from China.* (Coeur d'Alene, ID: Medipress), p. 173.

12. See McGee, C., & Chow, E. (1994). *Miracle healing from China.* (Coeur d'Alene, ID: Medipress), pp. 203–210.

13. For copies of their materials and conference proceedings, contact ISSSEEM, 356 Goldco Circle, Golden, CO 80403.

14. Many psychophysiological measures are affected by practicing Qigong. There are psychophysiological correlates to the relaxation response, including change in brain-wave patterns and neurochemical release. One research study from Japan indicates Qigong's ability to affect the immune system and endorphin levels. In this study a sitting control group experienced a thirty-five percent decrease in endorphins after one hour sitting, whereas the Qigong group showed an increase in endorphins after practicing Qigong. Higucchi, Y. (September 1996). Endocrine and immune response during Qigong meditation. *Journal of International Society of Life Information Science (ISLIS)*, 14(2). Many questions remain as to whether studies on Qi have proved the

existence of Qi, or whether some epiphenomenon is being measured. One researcher, Voll, measured the electrical conductance of the skin above individual acupuncture points of Qigong practitioners and found significant differences. It should be kept in mind that this does not necessarily measure Qi; it measures its effects. See Sancier, K. (1996a and b). The effect of Qigong on therapeutic balancing measured by electro-acupuncture according to Voll. *Acupuncture and Electro-Therapy Research International Journal, 19*, 119–127. See reports of Feng Li Da's ability to increase or decrease bacteria cell growth with Qigong, in McGee, C., & Chow, E. (1994). *Qigong: Miracle healing in China.* (Coeur d'Alene, ID: Medipress). Likewise, this study points to the effects of a Qigong master's hands over a medium and does not necessarily show whether Qi exists. In the past, Western scientists have viewed with skepticism the actuality of energy existing in the meridians of the human body, but recent research is exploring the ancient notion that meridian lines of energy in the body in fact exist. On the side of Qi being objectively real, see Kaptchuk, T. (1983). *The web that has no weaver.* (New York: Congdon & Weed). Thermally sensitive film shows Qigong masters' emission of energy down lines similar to classical acupuncture meridians in Lerner, M. (1994). *Choices in healing.* (Cambridge, MA: MIT Press), p. 389. Credit should be given to the early research of Becker, R. (1985) who has shown the healing effects of electrical energy in a Western context (pp. 234–237). Also see Serizawa, K., et al. (1964). *Individual pattern changes in the distribution of skin temperature and electrical resistance.* (University of Tokyo School of Medicine); and *The distribution of skin temperature and point meridian phenomena.* (1976), as cited in Teeguarden, I. M. (1988) *The joy of feeling.* (Tokyo: Japan Publications), p. 23. In general, see the vast literature on acupuncture. A hypothesis for this stage of our knowledge is that Qigong practice simultaneously induces effects in many areas of human anatomy: energetic dimensions, brain-wave functioning, and biochemical measures, such as endorphin levels and so forth.

15. Schmitz-Hubsh, T., et al. (2005, October 14). Qigong exercise helps to reduce the motor and non-motor symptoms of Parkinson's disease: A randomized controlled pilot study *Movement Disorders*. The abstract reads as follows: "Irrespective of limited evidence, not only traditional physiotherapy, but also a wide array of complementary methods are applied by patients with Parkinson's disease (PD). We evaluated the immediate and sustained effects of Qigong on motor and non-motor symptoms of PD, using an add-on design. Fifty-six patients with different levels of disease severity (mean age/standard deviation, 63.8/7.5 years; disease duration 5.8/4.2 years; 43 men {76%} were recruited from the outpatient movement disorder clinic of the Department of Neurology, University of Bonn, Germany. We compared the progression of motor symptoms assessed by Unified Parkinson's Disease

Rating Scale motor part (UPDRS-III) in the Qigong treatment group (n = 32) and a control group receiving no additional intervention (n = 24). Qigong exercises were applied as 90-minute weekly group instructions for 2 months, followed by a 2 months pause and a second 2 month treatment period. Assessments were carried out at baseline, 3, 6, and 12 months. More patients improved in the Qigong group than in the control group at 3 and 6 months (P = 0.0080 at 3 months, and P = 0.0503 at 6 months; Fisher's exact test). At 12 months, there was a sustained difference between groups only when changes in UPDRS-III were related to baseline. Depression scores decreased in both groups, whereas the incidence of several non-motor symptoms decreased in the treatment group only."

16. At the UCLA Neuropsychiatric Institute in Los Angeles, doctor and psychiatrist Michael Irwin's 2004 study reports that three Tai Chi classes a week for fifteen weeks boosts shingles immunity by about fifty percent. Irwin wrote, "There's nothing currently available to boost shingles immunity to match what we did.... We found significant improvements in the older adults who practiced Tai Chi and their ability to carry out day-to-day tasks." This research was reported by www.ivanhoe.com who offers medical alerts by email.

17. An overview of Tai Chi and Qigong research can be found at www.Qigong-institute.org, where you can also find the Computerized Qigong Database, referenced in the 2001 *Journal of Alternative and Complementary Medicine*, 7(1), 93–95. You can search a wide variety of medical applications of Qigong on this database. Also see www.worldtaichday.org, for a good overview.

18. In volume I, Appendix I of my book *Secrets to Living Younger* (Mayer, 2004b), I outlined how the Bodymind Healing Qigong system can be applied to various health issues including hypertension, chronic pain, joint problems, and so on.

19. There are Qigong traditions, such as Taoist Alchemy, that are oriented to transcendence. However for the most part, Qigong and Tai Chi foster greater bodily awareness and being in the present. It is true that psychotherapy is oriented more to being present in one's "emotional body;" and for that reason, the blending of traditions is beneficial to incorporate presence of both greater body awareness (which can develop from Qigong) and emotional self-awareness (which comes from Western psychotherapy).

Chapter 2

1. See, for example, The Energy Field, *Journal and Newsletter for the Association for Comprehensive Energy Psychology*, P. O. Box 910244, San Diego, CA 92121 or www.energypsych.org. Other sources for the voluminous publications in the field of energy psychology are listed in one of the classic overviews in the field: Gallo, F. (2002).

Energy psychology in psychotherapy. (New York: W. W. Norton). Also see Feinstein, D. (2004a). *Energy psychology interactive.* (Ashland, OR: Innersource).

2. For an more extensive examination of research on the field of energy psychology see Dr. David Feinstein's article, *An overview of research in energy psychology,* at: http://www.innersource.net/energy_psych/epi_research.htm. For a broader view of references to Qigong research, see index of this book, and Volume I (Mayer, 2004b, op. cit.).

3. Updated reports can be found at www.eftupdate.com/ResearchonEFT.html.

4. Some references that relate to this material on brain research are Schore, A. N. (2003), op. cit. and Ruden, R. A. (2005), op. cit.

5. I gleaned this information from a workshop by Dr. Jim Lane at a conference sponsored by the Association for Comprehensive Energy Psychology in May 2006. Dr. Lane's Web site is www.weheal4u@cs.com.

6. In *Secrets to Living Younger Longer,* I showed how touch and tapping is incorporated in various parts of the Bodymind Healing Qigong system—for example, in Wild Goose Taps Its Chest, Tapping the Belly Clock, and Beating the Heavenly Drum (Mayer, 2004b).

7. I completed the 150-hour certification program at the Acupressure Institute of Berkeley, California, and I recommend it as one source of training for psychotherapists or anyone who wants further training in these methods.

8. Energy psychologists might take umbrage at saying there is a one-size-fits-all approach. And there is some truth to this in that there are different treatment protocols in some energy psychology approaches for phobias, trauma, hypertension, and so forth. However, the sophistication of Chinese medicine involves much more ideographic, patient-specific, time-tested diagnostic and treatment methods for any single disorder. In favor of the energy psychology tradition is that the power of point touching is enhanced by the power of the mind, and the life issue behind the disorder, as it is focused upon in energy psychotherapy. In later chapters I will show why in Bodymind Healing Psychotherapy (BMHP) there is a focus on the unique meaning of a patient's healing solutions that are expressed in symbols, movements, and stances that derive from the depths of that person's unconscious (see Chapter Five). BMHP does not preclude, at appropriate times, the suggestion of holding or tapping places on the body that seem fitting with the patient's sensibilities. In this way BMHP in general is more aligned with phenomenological and inner-directed, rather than prescriptive, solutions. Though from the more metasystematic, medicine wheel perspective outlined in Chapter Two, whatever works is used.

9. For a more complete review of the literature on muscle testing and applied kinesiology, see Feinstein, D. (2002). *Energy psychology interactive: Studies pertaining to energy*

checking (muscle testing). Compiled by the International College of Applied Kinesiology, www.icakusa.com. For an excellent article on the subject of muscle testing involving a trialogue between three experienced clinicians examining the values and problems with muscle testing, see Durlacher, J., & Scott, W. (2002). For an updated review of the literature in support of the reliability and validity of muscle testing, see Cuthbert, S. C., & Goodheart, G. J. (2007). On the other side of the debate, Hass, M., et al. (2007, p. 11) gives a critical review of methodological deficiencies of many studies, including the aforementioned Cuthbert (2007) review, and Hass concludes that "the use of manual muscle testing for the diagnosis of organic disease or putative pre/subclinical conditions is insupportable." (http://www.chiroandosteo.com/content/15/1/11). Also see "Applied Kinesiology" in Wikipedia.

10. See Chapter Twenty-two of *Bodymind Healing Psychotherapy* for a discussion of ethical issues regarding combining methods from other traditions with psychotherapy. This chapter addresses specifically combining Qigong and psychotherapy (Mayer, 2007, pp. 259–266).

11. One of these scales is the Stanford Hypnotic Susceptibility Scale (see Wickramasekera, I., 1998).

Chapter 3

1. Gold, S. (2006, March 3). From the Shabbat service Torah reading at temple Chochmat Halev in Berkeley, California. Written commentary on the *parsha* (part) of the Torah, called Terumah of the Old Testament for the week of March 3, from Rabbi Shefa Gold.

2. Temple Chochmat Halev in Berkeley, California, has a training program in Jewish Spirituality and Meditation. In this program and during their Friday night Shabbat services, such songs are introduced, see www.chochmat.org.

3. The Taoist tradition actually contains both transcendent and immanent dimensions and practices. For example, the human being is seen as being comprised of a *hun* (heavenly) soul and a *po* (earthly) soul; it is believed that the *hun* soul rises up to the heavens after death, and the *po* soul descends back to the earth. There are practices, such as Wuji Standing Meditation and various Taoist Alchemy practices, that are oriented to activate a path to the transcendent state of *wuji* (the mother of Qi, the void); and there are immanent practices, including the meditative focus on the belly (Tan Tien) and the practice of the animal forms of Qigong.

4. Erickson, M. (1948/1980). *The collected papers of Milton Erickson on hypnosis IV.* (New York: Irvington), p. 38. See Rossi, E. (1986). *The psychobiology of mind-body healing,* op. cit, p. 67.

5. Such esoteric traditions as alchemy, which uses metals and chemical processes as

metaphors (Edinger, 1985), and astrological symbols, which use the celestial bodies as metaphors (Mayer, 1984), are examples, as are the everyday metaphors of life, to make a link to the wider whole of which we are a part (Gordon, 1978; Wallas, 1985).

6. For example, Wilhelm Reich advocated a bioenergetic psychology, and he was put in jail for advocating the use of orgone energy. It is true that nowadays forefront psychological educational institutions have somatic psychology training programs, and leading-edge thinkers are advocating the incorporation of the body in psychotherapeutic training. However, this is not mainstream psychotherapy quite yet.

7. Papadakis, T. (1988). *Epidauros: The sanctuary of Asclepius.* (Zurich, Switzerland: Verlag Schnell), p. 6. Stories also say he "raised from the dead" the heroes Lycurgos and Tyndareos.

8. See, for example, the teaching tale of the gnostics called "The Hymn of the Pearl" discussed in Mayer, M. H. (1994). *Trials of the heart,* Berkeley, CA: Celestial Arts.

Chapter 4

1. See Bandler, R., & Grindler, J. (1975). *The structure of magic, II.* (Palo Alto, CA: Science and Behavior Books). Hypnotherapists have shown that different people have strengths and weaknesses in accessing a "trance" state through a given representational system—visual, kinesthetic, auditory, and olfactory. The art of hypnotherapy is in how to blend and cross over from one to the other to facilitate activating an individual's healing resources.

2. In addition to the best-known sources of Microcosmic Orbit Breathing (Wilhelm, 1931; Cleary, 1991), there are numerous descriptions, such as Huang, W. S. (1974). *Fundamentals of Tai Chi Chuan.* (Hong Kong, China: South Sky Book Co.); Chia, M. (1986). *Iron shirt Chi Kung healing.* (Huntington, NY: Healing Tao Books). The Microcosmic Orbit Breathing method that is outlined throughout this book combines classical Microcosmic Orbit Breathing with the River of Life method that I developed. The river merges into the Sea of Elixir.

3. Chan, L. (1995, October). A visit to a unique Qigong hospital. *T'ai Chi Magazine, 19*(5), 34–35.

4. In a personal communication from Dr. Larry Stoler—psychologist, past president of the Association for Comprehensive Energy Psychology, and one of Luke Chan's students—he said Luke reported that on the day he videotaped this healing, five out of seven people's tumors disappeared. Professor Feng Li Da of Beijing reports that the ability of Qigong masters to increase or decrease bacteria cell growth in multiple laboratory settings by placing their hands over a cell culture of bacteria or cancer cells. See Eisenberg, D. (1995). *Encounters with Qi.* (New York: W. W. Norton).

Thermally sensitive film shows Qigong masters emitting energy down lines similar to classical acupuncture meridians. According to Eisenberg, D. (1990, Spring). *Energy medicine in China.* (Noetic Science Review). As cited in Lerner, M. (1994). *Choices in healing.* (Cambridge, MA: MIT Press), p. 389. There is a need for replicating the scientific validity of these studies in order to investigate the reality of these reported effects. See also Sancier, K. (1996b, January). Medical applications of Qigong. *Alternative Therapies, 2*(1). For more current research on this topic, Dr. Garret Yount, of the California Pacific Medical Center, and Beverly Rubik, of The Institute of Frontier Science (brubik@earthlink.net), are two of the top researchers in this field. Right now, on the growing edge of research, it seems that such results do occur but not consistently; therefore, scientific research questions whether such results are merely due to chance. The Qigong master's mental set needs to be considered as a confounding variable.

5. See Achterberg, J. (1985, p. 198). *Imagery and healing.* Basmajian, J. V. (1963, August) Control and training of individual motor units, *Science Magazine, 2,* 440–441.

Chapter 5

1. The term *Self* is deliberately spelled with a capital *S* in many places in this book, following Dr. Carl Jung's indication that as a key element of his analytic psychology, a depth psychological perspective on healing necessitates a Self wider than the ego. Dr. Jung felt that this Self, which he spelled with a capital *S*, was defined by an axis between the collective unconscious, the home to the energy potentials (archetypes of the collective unconscious), and the ego. Throughout this book I will build on this foundation to show that the *psychoid* (body-oriented, rather than just mentally psychic) nature of the archetypes includes body, mental, and energy components; and when these elements combine, verbal therapy is best able to reach the goal of healing the primordial Self.

2. In one of its earliest usages, the term *transpersonal* implied "beyond and through the person," thereby including both transcending and transmuting aspects in its definition. Dane Rudhyar (1975) said that the "transpersonal attitude may be one involving a reaching beyond the personal—an ascent of consciousness, to seek to attain greater heights and peak experience.... But *transpersonal* also implies a descent of spiritual power focusing itself through a person, as diffused solar light is focused through a clear lens" (p. 38). Rudhyar used *transpersonal* this way in a small magazine called *The Glass Hive,* in 1930, then wrote about it in his 1948 book, *Modern man's conflict: The creative challenge of a global society.* (New York: Philosophical Library). See Rudhyar's chapter entitled "The Transpersonal Way and the New Manhood." I was honored to have been able to study, and meet privately, with Dane

Rudhyar during my doctoral dissertation years. I still appreciate the deep influence he had on the development of my way of seeing the world.

3. Hillman, J. (1979b). *The dream and the underworld*; Gendlin, E. (1986). *Let your body interpret your dreams.*

4. The idea of a "true self" is not a fixed concept in the Western mystery tradition. For example, the astrological metasystem includes the notion of a natal chart, which is a mandala for meditation through which a person reflects upon his or her beginning essential nature. Additionally, there is a progressed chart whereby one reflects upon the self that has developed and progressed to a given moment in time. The symbols of the astrological mandala enable one to reflect upon his or her life's meaning and identity. For more information on this phenomenological meaning reorganization point of view (Fingarette, 1963)—which transcends the issue regarding the objective correspondence between the celestial sphere and one's personality—see *The mystery of personal identity* (Mayer, 1984). It was the first book to show how astrological symbols could function as a metaphorical tool in depth psychotherapy to help a patient come to terms with his or her life's meaning and identity.

5. It would be an interesting subject of research to examine the biochemical differences between just imagining versus imagining with the use of Microcosmic Orbit Breathing. For more on how this research has already begun, see Lascow, L. (1998).

6. See *Secrets to living younger longer: The self-healing path of Qigong, standing meditation and Tai Chi* (Mayer, 2004b). Orinda, CA: Bodymind Healing Publications. Also see *Bodymind healing Qigong DVD* (Mayer, 2000) available at www.bodymindhealing.com.

7. See Gendlin's early research that showed from listening to psychotherapy tapes of many different types of therapy that this type of focusing is what made psychotherapy work regardless of which tradition was being used. Gendlin, E. (1962). *Experiencing and the creation of meaning.* (Toronto, Ontario: Free Press of Glencoe); and Gendlin, E. (1978). *Focusing.* (New York: Bantam Books).

8. Actually the state-specific state of consciousness of White Crane Spreads Wings is not just a transcendent state. One hand is up by the third eye, which can represent the crane's transcendent, rising above ability; however, a grounded dimension is also experienced in this posture as the practitioner places the other hand down by the belly, pressing down toward the earth, while the practitioner stands grounded on one leg. (For an illustration, see *Secrets to Living Younger Longer* (Mayer, 2004b).

9. On the topic of scientific measurement of psychotherapy practice, psychoanalyst and author Adam Phillips says: "Since at least the middle of the nineteenth century, Western societies have been divided between religious truth and scientific truth, but none of the new psychotherapies are trying to prove they are genuine religions. Nor is there much talk, outside of university literature departments, of psy-

chotherapy trying to inhabit the middle ground of arts, in which truth and usefulness have traditionally been allowed a certain latitude (nobody measures Shakespeare or tries to prove his value).... It would clearly be naïve for psychotherapists to turn a blind eye to science, or to be 'against' scientific methodology. But the attempt to present psychotherapy as a hard science is merely an attempt to make it a convincing competitor in the marketplace. It is a sign, in other words, of a misguided wish to make psychotherapy both respectable and servile to the very consumerism it is supposed to help people deal with. In the so-called arts it has always been acknowledged that many of the things we value most—the gods and God, love and sexuality, mourning and amusement, character and inspiration, the past and the future—are neither measurable or predictable. Indeed, this may be one of the reasons they are so abidingly important to us. The things we value most, just like the things we most fear, tend to be those we have least control over. If psychotherapy has anything to offer, and this should always be in question, it should be something aside from the dominant trends in the culture. And this means now that its practitioners should not be committed either to making money, or to trivializing the past, or to finding a science of the soul...." Phillips, A. (2006, February 26). A mind is a terrible thing to measure. *New York Times.*

10. This is spoken of in terms of "from Qi (energy) to Yi (intention)," which refers to the ability to "first cultivate, then utilize, then manifest," as Master Fong Ha says. Or, as the founding grandmaster of the Yi Chuan tradition says, "Big circles are very good, small circles are even better, and no circles are best."

11. Parallels between the ancient concept of underworld journeys and modern psychotherapy are discussed in Meier, C.A. 1967, op. cit., pp. 93–112; and Hillman, J. 1979b, op. cit., p. 21.

Chapter 6

1. Los Angeles Times, (1995, April 24). *Billions spent on new hypertension drugs*, p. A-17. Prescriptions for just one class of antianxiety drugs, the benzodiazapines, are estimated at costing between $100–800 million a year. A variety of questions have been raised regarding whether the new drugs that are coming on to the market are really superior to the old ones. New drugs, including calcium antagonists and ACE inhibitors, add $10 billion to consumer costs over old diuretics and beta-blockers, with scanty evidence to prove that they are superior.

2. Altrocchi, J. (1994). Nondrug treatment of anxiety. *American Family Physician, 10,* 161–6. Altrocchi reports that ten percent of adults have an anxiety disorder, yet only one-fourth of them receive treatment. Treatment is usually given in a general medical setting rather than through the mental-health system. Most patients with

anxiety disorders are treated by nonpsychiatrist physicians who are generally more familiar with pharmacological management of anxiety. However, nondrug treatment can be more effective and may be both more time-efficient and less risky.

3. National Institute of Health Technology Assessment Panel. (1996, July 24). Integration of behavioral and relaxation approaches into the treatment of chronic pain and insomnia. *Journal of the American Medical Association, 276*(4). See also Hilts, P. (1995, Winter). Spiritual side finds favor in medical field. *Qi: Journal of Trad. Eastern Health & Fitness, 5*(4), 45. Reprinted from the *New York Times*.

4. For example, Elmer Green, in the Copper Wall Project at the Menninger Clinic, at Topeka, Kansas, scientifically documented the energy activated by healers from a variety of traditions entering into a meditative altered state. See Green, E., et al. (1991). Anomalous electrostatic phenomena in exceptional subjects. *Subtle Energies, 2*(3), 69–94.

5. See *Secrets to living younger longer: The self-healing path of Qigong, standing meditation and Tai Chi* (Mayer, 2004b). Orinda, CA: Bodymind Healing Publications. Also see *Bodymind healing Qigong DVD* (Mayer, 2000) available at www.bodymindhealing.com.

6. The use of a holographic/energetic model to healing in Bodymind Healing Psychotherapy seemingly goes in a different direction from the managed care approach that wants brief, solution-oriented approaches. The conservative, Newtonian, economically based viewpoint of managed care moves away from holistic approaches and seeks to legislate a narrower range of approaches to fix specific psychological issues, that is, cognitive-behavioral therapy, drug therapy, and so forth. Further research needs to be done to compare the two approaches to explore whether—paradoxically—deeper, more integrative models are better in their ability to achieve long-lasting results, and more cost-effective over a long time span, than "brief therapies" are.

7. Elevator Breathing is a simple variation I developed to simplify the commonly used Taoist breathing practice of Microcosmic Orbit Breathing, which emphasizes circulating the breath up the Governing Vessel *(Du,* or the *Tu Mei,* channel) on the back on the inhalation, and down the front Conception Vessel *(Ren,* or the *Jen Mei,* channel) of the body on the exhalation. Whereas Elevator Breathing emphasizes the up and down of raising the spirit and sinking the Qi. The Taoists believe that by cultivating the breath in such a way, through focus on the center of the body at the Tan Tien, one can become more centered and revitalized and can enter into an experience of discovering the reservoir of universal Qi, which aids in healing and activates transcendental awareness. My preliminary clinical research with Elevator Breathing shows promising results as an adjunct to treatment with a wide variety of psychological issues, such as over intellectualization, anxiety and panic disor-

ders, borderline issues, obsessive traits, substance abuse issues, general stress reduction, and as part of hypnotherapy for trance induction. Further research is needed to validate these preliminary results. Two audiocassettes are available from the following conferences where I presented: Mayer, M. H. (1987). *An integrated approach to anxiety and phobias.* From the Eighth Annual Conference and Training Institute on Phobias and Related Anxiety Disorders, sponsored by Langley Porter Neuropsychiatric Institute. San Francisco; and Mayer, M. H. (1997). *Psychotherapy & Qigong: Partners in healing anxiety.* From the Second World Congress on Qigong. San Francisco: Conference Recording Services.

8. There are some patient populations that have more difficulty feeling the sinking of Qi than others, such as those who suffer from severe dissociative conditions and some schizophrenic patients. The use and adaptation of this method to different clinical populations is refined through experience.

9. Before doing this exercise and others like it, have yourself checked by a Western medical doctor to be sure you do not have any medical problems that could be exacerbated by pressing in on your stomach. In particular, please check with a doctor first if you have high blood pressure, a heart condition, an aneurysm; or if you have had a stroke or suffer from circulation problems, detached retinas, diabetes, varicose veins, and/or clotting or inflammation of a blood vessel. And, for comfort, it is best to practice this massage when your bladder is not full. For a more complete exposition of this technique, and contraindications and cautions, see Chia, M., & Chia, M. (1990). *Chi Nei Tsang: Internal organ massage.* (Huntington, NY: Healing Tao Books).

10. See Gendlin, E. (1978). *Focusing.* (New York: Bantam Books). It is best to learn this method from a trained Focusing teacher or guide, because there are many subtle intricacies to its steps. See www.focusing.org. This way of inner accessing won an award from the American Psychological Association. It is an invaluable technique to help find felt meaning; and it has been used in a wide variety of settings, such as the Simonton Cancer Center). I use this method as a center post of Bodymind Healing Psychotherapy (BMHP).

11. The Macrocosmic Orbit Breathing comes down the front of the body down the *Ren* channel and out the feet through the Bubbling Well points (Kidney-1). See Huang, W. S. (1974). *Fundamentals of Tai Chi Chuan.* (Hong Kong, China: South Sky Book Co.), p. 472.

12. I suggested this idea about "clearing a space" to Dr. Gendlin when I was his Focusing Training Coordinator of the East Bay-San Francisco area, and he enthusiastically supported my idea to combine Focusing and Taoist breathing methods. Then

in the early 1980s, I wrote about this integration in the Transpersonal Psychology Association's newsletter.

13. Archetypes, as Carl Jung said, are "energy potentials." When internal representations of the people in our own lives are insufficient as healing images, our wider psyches can activate archetypally energized images from the wider whole of which we are a part to promote healing. I discuss this idea of moving from the personal to archetypal level as a therapeutic strategy in Chapter Twenty-three of *Bodymind Healing Psychotherapy* (Mayer, 2007) using Tai Chi Push Hands movements as an initiatory analogy.

14. An alternative is to place the whole hand over this area, which gives a more expansive, but less focused, feeling.

15. For example, I presented this concept in my presentation, *An Integrated Approach to Anxiety and Phobias,* at the Eighth Annual Conference and Training Institute on Phobias and Related Anxiety Disorders, sponsored by Langley Porter Neuropsychiatric Institute, in San Francisco, in 1987.

16. I learned two traditions of Standing Meditation in my three decades of Qigong practice. From Sifu Fong Ha's kind introduction to three masters, I learned Wuji Qigong from Master Cai Songfang of Canton, China; and Yi Chuan Standing, also called Zhan Zhuang, from Master Han Xiyuan and Master Sam Tam. I continued these practices with Master Fong Ha. *Wuji* means the void or stillness from which movement and Tai Chi derives. Ken Cohen, author of *The Way of Qigong* (Ballantine Books, 1997), whom I taught these methods to, says that they are the million-dollar secret of Qigong. For more information, see Mayer, M. H. (2004b). *Secrets to living younger longer,* op. cit. Also see Diepersloot, J. (1995). *Warriors of stillness.* (Walnut Creek, CA: Center for the Healing Arts).

17. See Note 3 in Chapter Twenty-one for some research on Standing Meditation regarding increasing coherence between left and right hemispheres of the brain and other positive health effects.

Chapter 7

1. Ortho McNeil Pharmaceutical and Louis Harris and Associates, Inc. *The pain and absenteeism report: A study of full-time employees and employee benefit managers.* (1996, June). For a copy of this report, fax 212–885–0570.

2. The cost of $90 billion includes compensation claims, time off from work, medication, disability allowance, and direct treatment. See Taylor, S. (1991). *Health psychology* (2nd Ed.). (New York: McGraw Hill). Quoted by Groth-Maarnat, G. (1996). Professional psychologists in general health-care settings: A review of the financial

efficacy of direct treatment interventions. *Professional Psychology: Research and Practice, 27*(2), 166. The statistic of $100 billion for pain remedies, includes temporary pain relief from colds, headaches, chronic pain, and the like. Taylor, S. (1991). *Health psychology,* (2nd Ed.), New York: McGraw Hill. Quoted by Groth-Maarnat, G. (1996). Professional psychologists in general healthcare settings: A review of the financial efficacy of direct treatment interventions. *Professional Psychology: Research and Practice, 27*(2), 161–174.

3. For a review of the literature on various relaxation and behavioral techniques for relieving chronic pain, see (National Institute of Health (NIH) Technology Assessment Panel. (1996, July 24). Integration of behavioral and relaxation approaches into the treatment of chronic pain and insomnia. *Journal of the American Medical Association, 276*(4). The NIH panel reviewed numerous well-designed studies of pain relief that used a variety of behavioral medicine approaches, including such relaxation methods as progressive relaxation (tightening and loosening various muscles of the body), meditation, hypnosis, autogenic training, biofeedback, and cognitive-behavioral therapy.

4. One source for a wide review and discussion of the medical literature on pain medication is the Roxane Pain Institute, www.Roxane.com. In terms of medical devices, there are a wide variety, such as electrical transcutaneous electrical nerve stimulation (T.E.N.S. units). These electrical stimulation devices give relief to many who suffer from sports-related and other kinds of pain. Some of the modern drugs that are used for pain relief are coumarin (a chemical compound found in many plants) that has collagen-reducing effects; corticosteroids; percodan; elavil; and heparin. The most recent advertised "panacea" for severe pain are the long-acting opiates, such as morphine—now given in graduated doses to provide steady relief, but no euphoria. The idea behind this pharmacological advance is that graduated doses will lessen addiction to these drugs; and there is some evidence to prove this. Addiction is composed of two factors: tolerance—the compulsive craving for increasing amounts of a drug over time—and dependence, the withdrawal symptoms that come from stopping a drug abruptly. The evidence is still inconclusive, but research at this time seems to show that when taken properly, long-acting opiates do not produce tolerance in most people; however, they can produce dependency. See Jetter, A. (1996, September). The end of pain. *Hippocrates*, p. 45.

5. Side effects of various drugs need to be carefully weighed in the decision as to whether and when to use various medications. Speak with your physician about this and check for yourself such books as the *Physicians Desk Reference, (PDR); Worst pills, best pills II,* Public Citizens Health Research Group, 1993; Breggin, P., *Toxic psychiatry.* (New York: St. Martin's Press).

6. Different points of view about taking medication are presented in Jetter, A. (1996, September). The end of pain. *Hippocrates*, p. 45. On the critical-of-opiates side of the debate is John Loeser, a neurosurgeon from the University of Washington School of Medicine in Seattle. On the pro-opiate side is Dr. James Campbell, who runs the pain clinic at John Hopkins Hospital in Baltimore. Also, Dr. Russell Portnoy, a neurologist at New York's Sloan Kettering Hospital, reports that his cancer patients who took opiates did not develop tolerance (the compulsive craving for increased amounts of the drug).

7. Chopra, D. (1990). *Quantum healing.* (New York: Bantam Books), pp. 62–63. Rossi (1986) says the placebo effect is responsible for about fifty-five percent of cure rates as determined by meta-analytic studies (p.16).

8. Another very well-designed, double-blinded study by Wirth (1991) showed the effect of noncontact therapeutic touch (a form of external emission Qigong) on wound healing. Due to its focus on external emission rather than self-healing practices, it is outside the scope of this book.

9. Two sources for research on the beneficial results of using imagery in healing are Achterberg, J. (1985). *Imagery in healing: Shamanism and modern medicine.* (Boston: New Science Library) and Rossi, E. & Cheek, D. (1988). *Mind-body therapy: Methods of ideodynamic healing in hypnosis.* (New York: W. W. Norton).

10. Look at an acupuncture chart to see the exact location of K-I, which is slightly forward of the bottom center of the foot. One good source of point location is Gach, M. (1990). Acupressure potent points. (New York: Bantam Books).

11. There is voluminous research demonstrating that by imagining something to be real in the body, physiological changes take place. For example, see Achterberg, J. (1985), Chopra, D. (1990), and Rossi, E. (1986).

12. In China there are a wide variety of reports that Qigong masters can emit energy from their hands and affect cell cultures, increasing or decreasing bacteria, and even killing cancer cells. See Sancier, K. (1991). Medical application of Qigong and emitted Qi on humans, animals, cell cultures, and plants: Review of selected scientific research. *American Journal of Acupuncture, 19*(4). Also see McGee, C. & Chow, E. (1994). *Qigong: Miracle healing in China,* pp. 164–165, op. cit., for reports of Feng Li Da's controlled study whereby killing and inactivation of thirty-one percent of cancer cells occurred in the experimental group with emitted Qi. All cancer cells survived in the control group. Reported at the First Medical Conference for Medical Exchange of Medical Qigong, 1988. The line is difficult to draw between whether studies on Qi emission prove emission of Qi or prove it is a function of hypnosis, some psychokinetic phenomenon, biochemical release of endorphins, or other neurotransmitters, and so on. Also, there are often replicability issues with these studies—one

problem seems to be the condition of the Qigong master on the day of the experiment. This emerging field needs to be subjected to further research and analysis. In private correspondence Dr. Sancier reported that low frequency sound in the 3–12 hertz range has been measured from the Lao Gong points on the palms. There are those who have developed "Qi Machines," such as Richard Lee (China Healthways 1-800-743-5608), that attempt to replicate the vibratory rate of Qi. Further research needs to be done to learn how these machines compare to Qigong practice and what the positive and negative side effects of the machines may be.

13. See Hilgard, E., & Hilgard, J. (1983) *Hypnosis in the relief of pain.* (Los Altos, CA: William Kaufman Inc.), pp. 241–250. Arlene Morgan and Josephine Hilgard standardized the scale.

14. For example, one energy gate in the center of the palms is called the Lao Gong point or Pericardium-8. It can be found by making the fingers curl inward into a fist, where the middle finger presses into the inner palm between the extensions of the bones of the two inner middle fingers. These points are useful on a cold day to generate heat in the hands. Massage practitioners and healers who practice Qigong use these points for emitting Qi to heal others.

15. *Yi Chuan Qigong,* also called Zhan Zhuang (Standing like a Tree), has been one of my main practices for thirty years. One person I taught it to was Taoist scholar Ken Cohen. He describes this method as the million-dollar secret of Qigong in his *Way of Chi Gung Tapes* (Boulder, CO: Sounds True Catalogue). One written source for learning how to work with the ball of magnetic force between the hands in the Zhan Zhuang tradition is Chuen, L. (1991). *The way of energy.* (London: Gaia Books), p. 127. Also see Diepersloot, J. (1995, 1999). *Warriors of stillness.* (Walnut Creek, CA: Center for Healing and the Arts). Paul Dong (1990) in *Chi Gong: The ancient Chinese way to health.* (New York: Marlowe & Co.), p. 127, reports that the Zhan Zhuang standing meditation practice began two thousand years ago with Taoist philosopher Wang Chong-Yang. Yi Chuan Qigong is also used to embark upon the path toward developing the much talked about "empty force," *(kung jing),* whereby the practitioner supposedly discharges a fellow practitioner without touching them. For a realistic appraisal of this issue, see Ha, F. (1991, August). Is empty force real? *Tai Chi Magazine, 15*(4); Dong, P. (1990). *Chi Gong.* (New York: Marlowe and Co.); and Dong, P., & Raffill, T. (2006). *Empty force: The power of Chi for self-defense and energy healing.* (New York: Random House).

16. For more specific instructions, see Ha, F., & Olsen, E. (1996), Diepersloot, J. (1995), Mayer, M. H. (2004b). The best way to learn these methods and assure proper posture and training is to study with a teacher of the Yi Chuan. For example, when standing, we can imagine four points in a straight line to activate our center-line.

(The four points are the point between the two feet, the Huiyin point between the anus and genitals, the center point between the Tan Tien and Ming Men right below the navel, and the Baihui point at the top of the head.) Without postural corrections from a teacher, limitations or pitfalls in practice can arise.

17. Taoists use this energy center, two or three fingers' width beneath the navel, as a key point for meditation.

18. Some evidence to support the idea that Qi is emitted from the Lao Gong points, also called Pericardium-8, can be found in McGee, C., & Chow, E. (1994). *Qigong: Miracle healing from China*. (Coeur d'Alene, ID: Medipress), pp. 37–38. Measures include Raman spectra, ultraviolet spectra, and infrasonic emission at low frequencies in the 1–12 hertz range, microwave emissions, magnetic field generation, and electrostatic field generation. Reports in this book say that Qigong Master Yan Xin could affect the decay rate of a radioactive compound. The studies reported in this book often were not footnoted or subjected to Western scientific methodology standards, and they need to be further documented and replicated. Scientists who I have privately corresponded with have many doubts about some of the data, in particular on Raman spectra and the effects on radioactive compounds. These sources say reports on infrasonic emissions from the hands may be more likely to have validity. (See Qigong Database from the Qigong Institute of San Francisco, Lascow, L. [1998] *Healing with love*. San Francisco: Harper & Row). Dr. Leonard Lascow, another clinician and researcher, reports an eighteen percent reduction in tumor cells in a controlled study of measuring the ability of magnetic field emission from his hands while practicing Microcosmic Orbit Breathing. See Lascow, L. (1998). *Healing with love*. (New York: Harper and Row), p. 306.

19. Stone, J. (1996). *Tai Chi Chih*. (Beverly Hills, CA: Interarts Productions). Tai Chi Ruler can also be practiced without the technological devices of the ruler or balls by doing circular movements with the hands held apart like a ball. This is a key practice of the Bodymind Healing Qigong tradition used for chronic diseases as seen on the *Bodymind Healing Qigong* DVD (Mayer, 2000).

20. Jou, T. (1980). *The Tao of Tai Chi Chuan*. (Rutland: Vermont: Charles Tuttle), pp. 77–78. He discusses the classic notion of how Tai Chi—the yin and yang of creation—derives from *wuji*, or nothingness. One of the feelings associated with wuji and Qi is of heaviness and lightness at the same time. For more about the Wuji Qigong tradition that I have studied with Masters Cai Songfang and Fong Ha, see Diepersloot, J. (1995) and Mayer, M. H. (2004b).

21. It would be interesting to have further research to determine if the methods used in the case of Terry would enhance healing in other cases of chronic pain compared to a nontreated control group.

22. Quizhi, S., & Zhao, L. (1993). Clinical observation of Qigong as a therapeutic aid for advanced cancer patients. *Proceedings of the Second World Conference for Academic Exchange of Medical Qigong*, Beijing, China. See Sancier, K. (1996b, January). Medical Applications of Qigong. *Alternative Therapies, 2*(1), 43.

23. Quizhi, S., & Zhao, L. (1993). Clinical observation of Qigong as a therapeutic aid for advanced cancer patients. *Proceedings of the Second World Conference for Academic Exchange of Medical Qigong*, Beijing, China. See Sancier, K. (1996b, January). Medical Applications of Qigong. *Alternative Therapies, 2*(1), 43.

24. There is well-documented evidence of the use of Mindfulness Meditation in reducing pain at the Stress Reduction Clinic at the University of Massachusetts Medical Center. In one study there, meditators showed a thirty-six percent improvement in pain on the McGill-Melzack Pain Rating Index (PRI), while nonmeditators showed no improvement; meditators showed a eighty-seven percent improvement in mood, while the nonmeditators showed only a twenty-two percent improvement; meditators showed a seventy-seven percent improvement in psychological distress, nonmeditators had an eleven percent improvement. Kabat-Zinn (1990) also reports that several laboratory experiments with acute pain have shown that "tuning into sensations is a more effective way of reducing the level of pain experienced when the pain is intense and prolonged than is distracting yourself" (p. 291).

Chapter 8

1. Cognitive Restructuring Therapy was developed by Dr. Aaron Beck (1967), a psychologist who used cognitive restructuring therapy with his depressive patients. The method has now been adapted to treat a wider variety of psychological issues, including anxiety and self-esteem issues.

2. Such scientists as David Bohm and F. David Peat (1997) subscribe to the theory that mind creates physical reality. *Bottom-up* theories posit that consciousness is a by-product of molecules that create mind, while *top-down* theories propose just the opposite—that consciousness is the creative force of the universe. This is a matter of ongoing debate (Tiller, 1997), but many mind-body clinicians use the term *bottom-up* loosely to speak about the need in certain psychological syndromes to emphasize the role of the body in creating new, more healthy cognitive and affective abilities. See also van der Kolk, B. A. (2002, p. 68). From a Taoist perspective, why dichotomize between the creative powers of above and below? From a cross-cultural mythological perspective, there are creation myths of gods of the earth and the heavens; for example, see Von Franz, M. L. (1982). *Creation myths*. (Zurich, Switzerland: Spring Publications).

3. See Volume I (Mayer, 2004b) to read about my experience of how the practice of Tai Chi helped in healing my early trauma experience.

Chapter 10

1. Cooper, A. (2006, March 9). Asleep at the wheel. *CNN*. This information came from CNN anchor Anderson Cooper who reported cases of some people who "woke up" after driving in an erratic manner, and they didn't remember getting into the car to drive to the store in the middle of the night.

2. See Volume I for specific complementary movements for repetitive stress syndrome, such as Commencement in Tai Chi, and Moving a Snake through Your Joints. First, the Qi needs to be built up with practices, such as Wuji Standing or Sitting Meditation.

Chapter 11

1. See Chapter Twenty-one, note 3, about the study by Yang Sihuan (1993) Second World Conference for Academic Exchange on Medical Qigong, reported in the Qigong Database: Qigong Institute of San Francisco. This study analyzed the EEG patterns of young students and reported that Qigong training had affected coherence of EEGs between the two frontal regions, between the two occipital regions, and between the two temporal regions of the brains of the Qigong group students while they meditated.

Chapter 12

1. Visit: http://www.mercola.com/2004/dec/18/vioxx.htm; additionally, I discuss the corporatization of health care in Chapter 1 of *Bodymind Healing Psychotherapy* (Mayer, 2007, pp. 3–22).

2. Reuters. Retrieved May 16, 2005, from http://msnbc.msn.com/id/7876902.

Chapter 13

1. *Chronic Diseases:* Adding to the research discussed throughout this book and in Chapter One, I created an audiotape for my patients that takes the listener through a healing meditation. Called *Find Your Hidden Reservoir of Healing Energy: A Guided Meditation for Chronic Diseases*, this tape was reformatted into a CD called the River of Life practice. This audiotape and CD is used by some therapists and hospitals to supplement the healing methods of other health professionals and can be helpful at-home aids to enhance relaxation and healing (Mayer, 2001b).

   Cancer: In Chapter One of *Bodymind Healing Psychotherapy* (2007), I reviewed some of the literature about the successful use of adjunctive mind-body approaches to cancer treatment (Devine & Westlake, 1995; Meyer & Mark, 1995; Hamer, 1997). In addition, I discussed some of the research on the use of Qigong as a complementary treatment helpful in raising the curative rate, extending the tumor-free survival time of patients (McGee & Chow, 1994, p. 173), lessening nausea, increasing strength, improving appetite, and bettering the quality of their survival (Sancier, 1996b; Chen & Yeung, 2002).

From my work with a cancer patient, I created a guided meditation audiotape, which I discussed in the preface of this book. Called *Find Your Hidden Reservoir of Healing Energy: A Guided Meditation for Cancer*, it is a duplicate of the aforementioned tape on chronic disease; but marketed for use by cancer patients (Mayer, 2001a). Some references for the use of Qigong with cancer can also be found in the appendixes of *Secrets to Living Younger Longer,* Volume I. My publications are available at www.bodymindhealing.com.

Death and Dying: A DVD of a presentation I gave on the Bodymind Healing Psychotherapy approach to death and dying was filmed by one of my students, a retired internist, and is in the production process.

2. Reuter's Health. (2005). *Tai Chi may lessen arthritis pain*. New York: Reuters. Retrieved January 6, 2005, from energeticsart@yahoogroups.com.

3. One respected source of knowledge on natural herbal remedies is herbologist Karen Sanders, who does the *Herbal Highway* show on KPFA radio, 94.1 FM, Berkeley, CA or go to http://www.kpfa.org/archives/index.

4. This study is reported by Pelletier, K. R. (2000), op. cit., p. 144.

5. You might also try Horse Whipping Tail, which increases circulation to the shoulders and arms. This practice is done by swinging the waist from side to side, allowing the arms to whip around naturally over the shoulders (Mayer, 2004, p. 102).

6. Pelletier, K.R. (2000) reports this 1991 study by Hanerdos on the efficacious treatment of fibromyalgia with hypnosis (p. 70).

7. For pictures and a discussion of the Tiger Qigong Animal Frolic movements, see *Secrets to Living Younger Longer* (Mayer, 2004b, p. 135–137).

Chapter 14

1. An exception to confidentiality laws, the Tarasoff law requires psychotherapists to report someone who is "dangerous to self or others" to the appropriate authorities. Additionally, it requires the therapist to let the intended victim know of the potential danger.

2. In Tai Chi Push Hands, one learns to be with their center-line and find their central equilibrium. In "emotional push hands," one practices not being overreactive. In Tai Chi Push Hands, a person learns to deal with the oncoming force of another

by yielding, taking in the other's force and then returning that to another unde-fensively and without attack. In relationships influenced by Tai Chi Push Hands, the practitioner takes in his or her partner's viewpoint and from their center responds appropriately. Another basic principle of pushing hands, and the train-ing of Master Ha, is "don't collide and don't separate." Instead of the dysfunc-tional human tendency to collide with and separate from others, the Tai Chi practitioner substitutes a practice involving "sticking with" the other person, and when "pushing back" doing that with sensitivity and a dot of yin in our yang (like the Tai Chi symbol). That is why oftentimes "pushing hands practice" is called "joining hands" or "sticking hands." For example, in a relationship when our part-ner says something critical of us, we may have the inclination to attack them back verbally (colliding) or break off the relationship (separating) saying, "I'm not going to be with someone like this." When embodying the Tai chi Push Hands metaphor, at a time like this, the practice is to learn to stick with the feeling behind our part-ner's criticism; and as we respond to that criticism, we empathize with his or her feeling and what is wanted; but we keep our center and respond appropriately to any judgmental language. "Modulating affects" in psychology is parallel to the Tai Chi Joining Hands practices of "using the least amount of force."

Chapter 15

1. For more on dual relationship issues, see Chapter Twenty-two of *Bodymind Healing Psychotherapy* (Mayer, 2007) and check the most recent American Psychological Association Guidelines for Ethical Practice at www.apa.org.

Chapter 16

1. Mayer, M. H. (1993). In *Trials of the heart*. Berkeley, CA: Celestial Arts., I suggested a method for constructive clearing of negative feelings for interpersonal relationships, which partially involves (1) positive intention, (2) expressing one's feelings as *I feel* versus expressing them as *you are* statements, and (3) *I want* statements. For an illus-tration of this method see Chapter Nineteen of this energy psychology book.

Chapter 17

1. For an illustration of this Tai Chi posture, see any illustrated Tai Chi Chuan book or *Secrets to Living Younger Longer,* (Mayer, 2004b, p.159).

Chapter 18

1. Castelman, S. (1995, September). Beginners mind. *Spirit Rock Meditation Newslet-ter*, p. 14. (Fairfax, California).

2. For more on dual relationship issues, see Chapter Twenty-two of *Bodymind Healing Psychotherapy* (Mayer, 2007) and check the most recent American Psychological Association Guidelines for Ethical Practice, www.apa.org.

3. One victim of rape was working with another therapist and was a Tai Chi student of mine for a year. One day a man approached her at a laundromat and put his hand on hers, coming on to her sexually. She adeptly and instinctively warded off his touch in such a way that fear came over his face. She told me that this was an important step in her re-empowerment and recovery.

Chapter 19

1. For a good introduction to transpersonal psychology, see the many publications of Ken Wilber; or for a current overview of the field, go to the Association for Transpersonal Psychology Web site at www.atpweb.org.

2. It should be noted that energy psychology does not just use single energy psychology interventions. From the perspective of energy psychology, this patient would be looked at as involved in a case of "psychological reversal"; and energy psychology has its methods for dealing with such imbedded patterns that stand in the way of patients finding a sense of love for themselves. See, for example, Feinstein, D. (2004a, pp. 75–91).

3. In *Secrets to Living Younger Longer* (Mayer, 2004b, pp.104–110), I outline and illustrate a "healing the internal organs medical Qigong" set, which corresponds to the five elements of fire, earth, metal, water, and wood. They are also illustrated on the *Bodymind Healing Qigong* DVD. (Bodymind Healing Publications, 2000, available at www.bodymindhealing.com).

4. In *Trials of the Heart: Healing the Wounds of Intimacy* (Mayer, 1993), I provide many examples of how this process has helped to improve couples' relationships and marriages.

Chapter 20

1. From the front of the brochure of the Association for Transpersonal Psychology's Second East Coast Conference, Asilomar: California, November 1984.

2. See Hillman, J. (1975), op. cit., and Bly, R. (1975), op. cit. Also see Gimbutas, M. (1982). *The goddesses and gods of old Europe.* (University of California Press); Von Franz, M. L. (1982). *Individuation in fairy tales.* (Zurich, Switzerland: Spring Publications); Salant, N. S. (1989). *The borderline personality: Vision and healing.* (Chiron Publications); and Krippner, S., & Feinstein, D. (1988). *Personal mythology.* (Los Angeles: Tarcher Publications).

3. For an excellent discussion of the use of "story" to enhance self-awareness, see Keen, S. (1973). *Telling your story.* (New York: New American Library).

4. Edinger, E. (1972). *Ego and archetype.* (New York: Putnam).

5. Gendlin, E. (1968). Focusing ability in psychotherapy, personality, and creativity. *Research in Psychotherapy, 3.*

6. For a more complete discussion of the Focusing process, see Gendlin, E. (1978). *Focusing.* (New York: Bantam Books).

7. Several references to the journey to the underworld are in Harner, M. (1980). *The way of the shaman.* (New York: Harper and Row); Eliade, M. (1972). *Shamanism.* (Princeton, NJ: Princeton University Press); Halifax, J. (1982). *Shaman: The wounded healer.* (Crossroad Pub.); Meier, C. A. (1967). *Ancient incubation and modern psychotherapy.* (Evanston, IL: Northwestern University Press); and Campbell, J. (1978). *The mysteries.* (Princeton, NJ: Princeton University Press).

8. For a more complete understanding of this type of breathing meditation, see Huang, W. S. (1974). *Fundamentals of Tai Chi Chuan.* (Hong Kong, China: South Sky Book Co.); Luk, C. (1972). *The secrets of Chinese meditation.* (New York: Samuel Weiser); and Jou, T. H. (1980). *The Tao of Tai Chi Chuan.* (Rutland, Vermont: Charles Tuttle). I also discuss this method in Chapter Four.

9. See Gendlin's *Focusing* for a discussion of the distinction between a feeling and a *felt sense.* A feeling is clear and well defined, whereas the felt sense is an unclear "edge" around the feeling that contains its wider *felt meaning,* that is, what the feeling is "all about." Gendlin's method is a way of getting to an "ah-ha" experience. Gendlin gives an example of a woman whose husband spilled some milk after a job promotion. The feeling she had was anger; when she tuned into the felt sense, she discovered that she was afraid of being left behind in life.

10. I learned this particular way of getting in touch with the felt sense from shared Focusing sessions with Ann Weiser, when we were both district coordinators of Focusing in the San Francisco area.

11. The person here was referring to the Maiden of the Lake (in the story of King Arthur), who helped repair the sword that Arthur broke when he angrily struck Lancelot. The Maiden of the Lake appeared after Arthur repented and lamented that he did not deserve the sword for his violent use of it against such a pure knight.

12. Participants in my workshops usually choose from the complete set of movements illustrated in *Secrets to Living Younger Longer* (Mayer, 2004b), which has an accompanying *Bodymind Healing Qigong* DVD.

13. The Mythic Journey Process brings together my past books and this one into an energy psychology circle—like three uroboric dragons biting each other's tails and

feeding each other. The Qigong emphasis in *Secrets to Living Younger Longer* (Mayer, 2004b) gives us practices that feed the psychologically oriented bodymind healing practices emphasized in my *BMHP* book and in this energy psychology book, and vice versa.

14. For more on the healing power of "the name," see Mayer, M. H. (1984). *The mystery of personal identity.* (San Diego, CA: ACS Publications).

Chapter 21

1. Jahnke, R. OMD, (2002b). Getting your immune system in shape. In *Boosting Immunity: Creating Wellness Naturally*, (Novato, CA: New World Library). From the old Web site of the Health Medicine Institute, now relocated as The Health Medicine Center, www/alternativehealth.com.

2. I want to express my profound gratitude to my respected teachers and sources from whom and from which I have synthesized my Bodymind Healing Qigong system over three decades of training, practice, and teaching. I am not making a representation that this system is a direct representation of my honored teachers' transmissions; rather, I have adapted each of their teachings to fit with my own understanding, healing imagery methods, and experience with Western bodymind healing traditions. I have trained in Standing Meditation Qigong for thirty years with Master Fong Ha with additional training from Masters Han Xingyuan, Cai Songfang, and Sam Tam. I learned the Dispersing Stagnant Qi exercises from my friend and colleague Ken Cohen as part of our sharing our traditions; I learned Tai Chi Ruler from Master Ha, and to make an East/West self-healing ritual, I added a guided visualization practice to it (available in video on the front page of www.bodymindhealing.com). I first learned Ocean Wave Breathing in a workshop by Arnold Tayam and Shoshanna Katzman, at a National Qigong Association conference; I adapted and added to Moving a Snake through the Joints from trainings with various Qigong Masters; I learned Crane Walking and Flying from training with Sifu Dr. Alex Feng; and I learned Yi Chuan Walking Meditation Qigong from training with Masters Ha, Xingyuan, Cai, and Tam.

3. Yang, S. (1993). *Second World Conference for Academic Exchange on Medical Qigong.* This study analyzed the EEG patterns of young students, seventeen to twenty years old, who had been practicing Zhan Zhuang Qigong (Standing like a Tree) for one year. Thirty-two persons in the Qigong group and thirty-five persons in the control group were involved in this experiment. During a one-year period of observation, the subjects of the Qigong group practiced Qigong for forty minutes every day. The EEGs of the Qigong group were analyzed every half-year in meditation, and the EEGs were also recorded before learning Qigong. The students in the con-

trol group did not take part in the Qigong training and their EEGs were investigated at rest twice within an interval of one year. In the test eight channels of EEGs were simultaneously processed by a computer online for twenty minutes. Yang summarized, "The results showed that Qigong training had affected coherence of EEGs between the two frontal regions, between two occipital regions and between two temporal regions of the Qigong group in meditation. The most significant is that, with the increase of training period, the total coherence value between the left and right temporal areas went up. It seems that there is certain dosage effect relationship." Another study on Zhan Zhuang is by Li, C. (1995). Preliminary exploration on the scientific proof of being sober-minded, sharp-eyed and energetic after practicing Zhan Zhuang. Reported at the *Fourth International Conference on Qigong, Vancouver, 200–24.* This study reports improvement in uric acid level after practice. See Qigong Database from the Qigong Institute of San Francisco.

4. For more information on Opening the Golden Ball of Your Heart, see *Secrets to Living Younger Longer* (Mayer, 2004b, p. 95). For more on Wild Goose Says Hello and Good-bye, see p. 103 of the same book.

5. For those of you who want to add other Dispersing Stagnant Qi exercises to your repertoire, see *Secrets to Living Younger Longer* (Mayer, 2004b, p. 101), where you will find the Three Methods for Electromagnetic Cleansing of the Skin, including self-massage, tapping methods, and Horse Tapping Feet.

Afterword

1. See previous discussion in Chapter Five about the "psyche," or "soul," which is defined as our own unique composition of the elements of nature and of the universe (Hillman, 1975; Rudhyar, 1970).

INDEX

Also by Michael Mayer

Bodymind Healing Psychotherapy: Ancient Pathways to Modern Health

*Secrets to Living Younger Longer: The Self-Healing Path of Qigong,
    Standing Meditation and Tai Chi*

Trials of the Heart: Healing the Wounds of Intimacy

Bodymind Healing Qigong (DVD)

Qigong: Ancient Path to Modern Health (DVD)

For more information or to purchase Dr. Mayer's publications, please see www.bodymindhealing.com. For information about Dr. Mayer's energy psychology workshops and private sessions (also available worldwide through video conferencing), please email: drmichael@bodymindhealing.com.

ABOUT THE AUTHOR

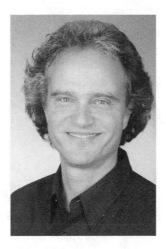

MICHAEL MAYER, PhD, is a licensed psychologist, hypnotherapist, and Qigong/Tai Chi teacher who specializes in giving his patients self-healing methods for health problems. Dr. Mayer presents his approach to bodymind healing at professional conferences, national/international workshops, hospitals, and universities, and he is a keynote speaker. He cofounded and is a practitioner at The Health Medicine Institute (now called the Health Medicine Center), a multidisciplinary medical clinic practicing integrative health care.

Pioneering the integration of Qigong and psychotherapy, Dr. Mayer was the first person in the United States to train doctoral psychology students in these methods. The World Institute for Self-Healing presented him with an award for outstanding research and contribution to the advancement of mind-body medicine. He is the author of twenty publications on bodymind healing, including five books, audiotapes on cancer and chronic disease, and articles on chronic pain and anxiety.

Dr. Mayer has trained for over thirty years with some of the most respected Tai Chi Chuan and Qigong masters. His guiding image of "two streams becoming one" inspires him as he blends East and West, mind and body, and ancient and modern in his life's work.